L. Handl-Zeller (ed.)

Interstitial Hyperthermia

Springer-Verlag Wien New York

Dr. Leonore Handl-Zeller
University Clinic of Radiotherapy
Vienna, Austria

Printed in Germany by Konrad Triltsch, D-W-8700 Würzburg

Printed on acid-free paper

With 84 Figures

Library of Congress Cataloging-in-Publication Data
Interstitial hyperthermia / L. Handl-Zeller (ed.).
p. cm.
ISBN 3-211-82280-1. – ISBN 0-387-82280-1
1. Cancer–Thermotherapy. 2. Radioisotope brachytherapy.
I. Handl-Zeller, L. (Leonore), 1952–
[DNLM: 1. Combined Modality Therapy. 2. Hyperthermia, Induced.
3. Neoplasms–therapy. QZ 266 I6192]
RC271.T5I579 1992 616.99′406832–dc20 91-5228

ISBN 3-211-82280-1 Springer-Verlag Wien New York
ISBN 0-387-82280-1 Springer-Verlag New York Wien

Foreword

Local hyperthermia of malignant tumours coupled with radiotherapy or chemotherapy is attracting increasing attention in both experimental and clinical applications. However, this involves a number of technical problems, not only in the generation of the heat, but above all in physically determining the distribution of this heat in the target area.
Radiological brachytherapy has enjoyed a massive revival thanks to the afterloading methods, which have made possible the safe application of radiation without affecting operating personnel. It was therefore a logical step to combine brachytherapy with hyperthermia. This led to a new and promising method of treatment in oncology, and it is highly praiseworthy that Dr. HANDL-ZELLER has undertaken the task of bringing together the leading scientists and clinicians on this specialised sector at the present time to publish their experimental and clinical findings and results in book form.
It is not possible to list and describe all the valuable contributions at this juncture. However, I should just like to mention HORSMAN's results in connection with matching up ionizing radiation and heat, HAHN's fundamental contributions on brachytherapy and hyperthermia, and URANO's work on hyperthermia in combination with chemotherapy. The book is perfectly rounded off by descriptions of technical procedures, such as STEA's use of interstitial hyperthermia with ferromagnetic seed implants, or the practice described by SEEGENSCHMIEDT of interstitial microwave hyperthermia iridium brachytherapy, and finally the results and technical specifications of animal experiments involving the use of interstitial hot-water hyperthermia by HANDL-ZELLER et al and BUDIHNA.
By way of conclusion, I should like to stress the fact that hot-water hyperthermia combined with interstitial brachytherapy – as introduced by HANDL-ZELLER, SCHREIER, BUDIHNA and LESNICAR – represents a simple, safe and clinically effective method that is also easily reproducible. This has been proved both in animal experiments and with phantoms, with the result that there will probably be growing clinical use of this method. It should then soon be possible to obtain comparable results on the effect of ionizing radiation in combination with hyperthermia as opposed to radiation alone.
For this reason, this book not only presents the current state-of-the-art, but above all provides an incentive to all those working and interested in this field to extend their clinical co operation It is to be hoped that it will be widely among cancer therapists.

March 1991 **K. H. Kärcher**

Contents

List of Contributors

Arian-Schad, K. S.
Bey, P.
Brady, L. W.
Budihna, M.
Cetas, T.
Hackl, A.
Hahn, G. M.
Hand, J. W.
Handl, O.
Handl-Zeller, L.
Hoffstetter, S.
Horsman, M. R.
Kahn, J.
Kapp, D. S.
Karlsson, U. L.
Kittelson, J.
Leitner, H.
Lesnicar, H.
Majima, H.
Marchal, C.
Overgaard, J.
Pernot, M.
Prionas, S. D.
Sauer, R.
Schreier, K.
Seegenschmiedt, M. H.
Shimm, D.
Stea, B.
Stücklschweiger, G.
Urano, M.

1

Brachytherapy and Hyperthermia: Biological Rationale

G. M. Hahn

Department of Radiation Oncology, Stanford University School of Medicine, Stanford, California, U.S.A.

Introduction

The purpose of this chapter is to survey the existing literature on effects of heat on cells and on animal tumors, specifically as these relate to clinical use of interstitial hyperthermia used in conjunction with brachytherapy. Biology remains biology, however, so that much of other research on hyperthermia and its interaction with ionizing irradiations remains applicable, even though the research was carried out for purposes not related to the topic of this book. If indeed this is the case (and it seems fairly obvious that it is), then why write a special review chapter? In part, the answer to this question is that there are aspects of hyperthermic biology that are of unique importance for the topic of this volume; in part also, because there is a body of literature that describes experiments that were performed for the specific purpose of exploring aspects of this combined modality. Finally, it seems that a book such as this has to make its formal bow to laboratory science.

Hyperthermia and X-irradiation

One of the first papers to appear on the subject of cell killing *in vitro* by x-rays as a function of environmental temperature was that of Ben-Hur and Elkind (1974). It involved low dose rate irradiation, and in that sense, it was the forerunner of investigations that have led to the combination of hyperthermia and brachytherapy. These workers irradiated Chinese hamster cells at 0.033 Gy/min (or rather 3.3 rads/min, since these authors preferred the older units) and varied the ambient temperature between 0 and 42°C. Survival was maximum when the temperature was between 34 and 37°C (Fig. 1). At higher temperatures, cytotoxicity was increased. Changes in the shapes of the survival curves were in an orderly progression: as the temperature increased, survival progressively dropped. Ben-Hur et al interpreted their findings as meaning that between 34 and 37°C there was maximum repair of sublethal damage. As the temperature increased, repair was inhibited, and hence, survival decreased. Survival curves ob-

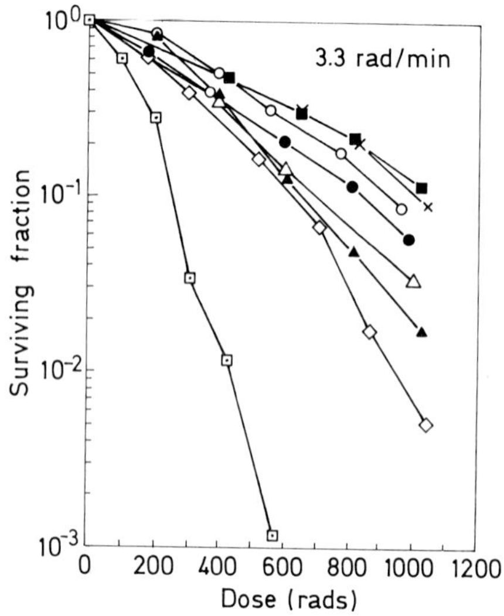

Fig. 1. Survival of cells exposed to 3.3 rad/min at various temperatures. Chinese hamster cells (V-79) were irradiated at specific temperatures for the dose indicated on the abscissa. Survival was maximum when the temperature was 34–37°C. Increasing the temperature reduced survival. This decrease was interpreted as showing that heat inhibited repair of sublethal damage. Consistent with this idea was the survival curve obtained at 0°C. At that temperature, repair of sublethal damage is completely inhibited. The additional cytotoxicity seen at 42°C then represents true sensitization. ■ 34°; × 37°; ○ 23°; ● 39°; △ 40°; ▲ 41°; ◊ 0°; ⊡ 42°. Data redrawn from Ben-Hur et al (1974)

tained at 41°C closely matched those seen at 0°C (Fig. 1). This result suggests that at 41°C repair from sublethal damage was completely inhibited, since presumably at 0°C such repair could not take place. The details of this explanation are somewhat open to question since there might have been a combination of low rate of repair coupled with some sensitization. If the temperature was raised further, then survival was even lower, suggesting that, at the temperatures exceeding 41°C, not only was repair maximally inhibited, but that the cells were actually sensitized to ionizing radiation. I should make it clear that in the experiments of Ben-Hur et al, the temperature was maintained constant during the entire time of irradiation. Cells were irradiated to a total dose of 11 Gy; they were therefore kept at the higher temperature for about 5 hr (since the dose rate was 3.3 cGy/min). This is far longer than is the case in most clinical applications where the maximum duration of hyperthermia is usually 2 hr; 1 hr at the beginning of treatment, the other at the completion of therapy. It is therefore not clear that the data of Ben-Hur et al are in any significant way applicable to the treatment of human cancers, at least as these treatments are now carried out. Further, in most clinical situations, the treatments are not simultaneous. In order not to expose the medical personnel to unnecessarily high levels of ionizing radiations, heating is done before and/or after brachy-therapy, not concurrently. Curiously, however, there are no data in the literature of studies that attempt, *in vitro*, to mimic the clinical situation. In fact, there are only a very few reports that describe results from experiments involving low dose rate irradiation and hyperthermia in tissue culture. Results that have been reported by others (Harisiadis et al, 1978; Gerner et al, 1983) are not greatly at variance with those of Ben-Hur and associates.

General consideration of the heat sensitivity of mammalian cells

Some laboratories have obtained data that do pertain to interstitial hyperthermia and radiotherapy. These relate primarily, though not only, to the role that

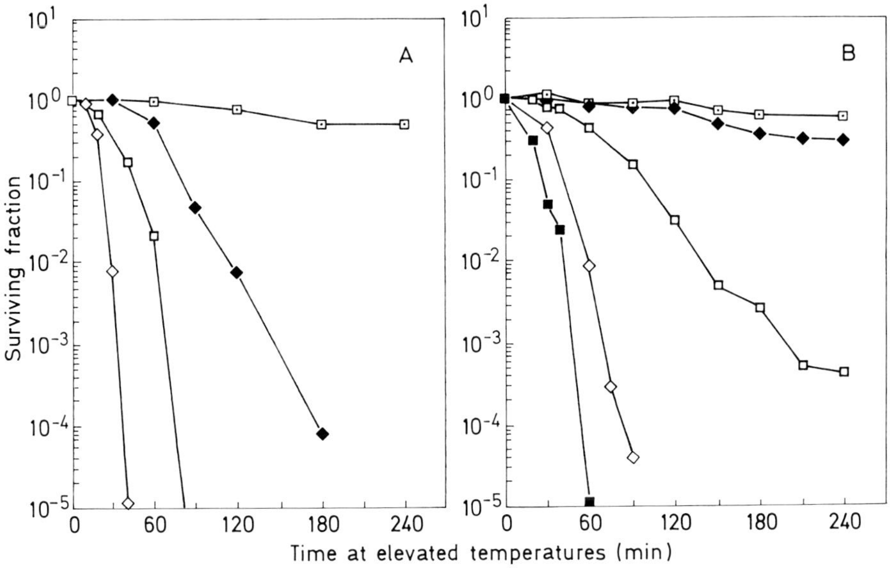

Fig. 2. Survival of mouse or human fibrosarcoma cells exposed to elevated temperatures. Cells were exposed to the indicated temperature for a time period as shown on the abscissa. Their survival was then assayed by colony formation. Note that the human cells (panel B) are more resistant to heat at all temperatures tested, with the biggest differences at 43 and 44°C. Panel A: murine fibrosarcoma cells (RIF-1). Panel B: human fibrosarcoma cells (HT1080). ⊡ 42°; ◆ 43°; □ 44°; ◊ 45°; ■ 46°. Data from HAHN et al (1989)

the tumor environment plays in affecting radiation sensitivity and hyperthermic sensitivity. While these are not uniquely applicable to interstitial hyperthermia, there are points that may have special relevance to that modality.

First, I should point out that almost all the data in the literature on cell survival at elevated temperatures have been obtained in experiments performed with rodent cells. Survival curves of mammalian cells exposed to elevated temperatures take on two different shapes depending upon the temperature and the species from which the line was obtained originally. In Fig. 2, I show a comparison of such curves obtained from cells derived either from a mouse or a human fibrosarcoma line in culture. While qualitatively the two sets of curves are similar, there are important quantitative differences. The human cells are not only more resistant at all the temperatures shown, but in addition, the temperature at which the shape of the curve changes is different. This "break" occurs between 42 and 43°C for the murine line, while the human line "breaks" between 44 and 45°C. While the survival data shown for the mouse line is more or less typical for rodent cells, not enough data are available to make that statement about the human cells. Nevertheless, these results have important implications for treatment. First, a dose concept based upon the shapes of the murine lines (SAPARETO and DEWEY, 1984) very likely is not applicable in the clinic. It could lead to serious undertreatment of tumors, particularly in the clinically very important 42–45°C range. Secondly, the human cells are more heat resistant at all the

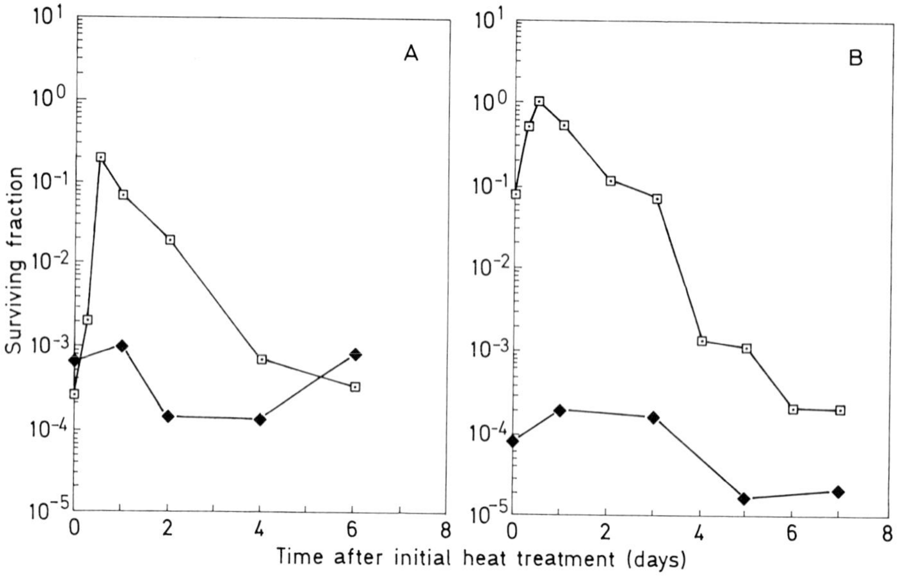

Fig. 3. Decay of thermotolerance in mouse and human fibrosarcoma cells. Cells were given an induction dose (open symbols) (45°, 10 min for murine RIF-1 cells; 46°, 10 min for human HT1080 cells) and then returned to the incubator at 37° for the time indicated on the abscissa. They were then given a test dose (45°, 45 min for murine cells; 46°, 45 min for human cells) and survival assayed by colony formation. Control cells (closed symbols) were exposed to the test dose without pretreatment. The murine cells (panel A) lose tolerance completely by day 4; in human cells (panel B), even at 6 days, survival has not returned to control values (8×10^{-5}). Data from HAHN et al (1989)

temperatures tested. As a result, treatment times and temperatures in human protocols must be based on results with human cells and not rodent cells. Failure to take into account the different responses of cells could lead to dangerous undertreatments of patients.

An interesting aspect of survival of cells to heat is the phenomenon of thermotolerance, i.e., the heat-induced temporary resistance of cells to heat. Comparable data for the mouse cells and human cells described earlier are shown in Fig. 3. Thermotolerance is shown by the rapid rise in cellular resistance as the interval between heat exposures is increased from 0 to 6 hr. Decay of tolerance (i.e., its disappearance with time) is slower in the human line. In the murine line, when the interval between the two treatments approaches 72 hr, tolerance has essentially disappeared. Not so in the human line. Here, tolerance is clearly measurable even 144 hr after the induction. The implication for clinical hyperthermia is that if treatments are not separated by more than a week, only the first treatment will have full efficacy, at least as far as direct cytotoxicity is concerned. For brachytherapy, this last finding may not be relevant, except that it does bring into question the current practice of treating twice, i.e., before and after irradiation.

The sensitivity of cells to killing by heat is modified by a variety of external factors.

Most important among these appears to be the triad of oxygenation, pH and nutritional status. These are not independent, a finding usually ignored in the literature. For example, it is generally accepted that cells are much more sensitive to heat if they are suddenly transferred from their normal pH to a low pH environment. But if these cells are overlaid with a balanced salt solution rather than the usual full growth medium, much of this pH sensitivity is lost. Perhaps the cell, in the absence of nutrients, devotes all its available energy to stabilizing intracellular pH. Hypoxia per se neither protects nor sensitizes cells to heat. But if cells are already deprived of nutrients, they become more sensitive if not given access to sufficient oxygen. Very likely, the unifying aspect is the cells' need to maintain a cross membrane proton gradient. This requires energy (approximately 60% of the cells' total ATP production is expended to maintain various membrane gradients). In addition, the cells attempt to maintain their internal pH at 7.4; at low pH, this requires additional expenditures of energy. Oxygen enters into this picture because in the absence of oxygen, the cells are forced to utilize anaerobic metabolism and ATP synthesis becomes inefficient. This places an additional burden on the metabolic system of the cells. How does all this relate to interstitial hyperthermia? Tumors frequently contain regions that are deficient in the availability of nutrients and, because of the accumulation of lactic acid, are also at low pH. Cells existing in this environment are frequently radiation resistant, because of hypoxia and, perhaps, because of their ability to repair potentially lethal damage. These cells are, however, readily killed by heat.

Physiology

There is another part to this equation. Blood flow is the major factor that determines the nutrient and oxygen environment of the cell. But blood flow also is the major factor involved in influencing the conversion of absorbed energy to elevated temperatures. In addition, it also modifies the pattern of heat diffusion. Blood is an efficient coolant, so that tumor volumes high in blood flow are difficult to heat. Conversely, regions that have low blood flow rates are readily heated if the elevation of temperature is achieved by techniques that depend upon local absorption of energy. Many investigators assume that the situation is different for interstitial heating; they suggest that blood flow plays less of a role in determining temperature distributions than is the case for externally induced hyperthermia. This very likely is a rosy view of the situation. While detailed temperature distributions during interstitial heating have only been reported by a very few investigators, one very carefully done study suggested that interstitial heating utilizing RF electrodes yielded temperature distributions that were only marginally superior to those obtained with external heating. When interstitial heating is combined with brachytherapy, the obvious and compelling advantage for the combination is that those tumor volumes likely to be resistant to one modality should be precisely the ones most readily treated successfully with the other. Well perfused tumor volumes should respond well to x-irradiation, poorly perfused volumes should respond to hyperthermia.

Response of mouse tumors to low dose rate radiations and hyperthermia

Does the literature on response of animal tumors that were treated with the combination of heat and brachytherapy confirm these educated speculations based on *in vitro* results? Unfortunately, there simply are not enough published data to give an unequivocal answer to this question. Curiously, although clinically the combination of brachytherapy and hyperthermia has found many practitioners, there are only a few published studies that analyze the effects of these modalities on tumors in experimental animals. Sapozink et al implanted intradermally inoculated RIF-1 tumors and also normal skin of C3H mice with Iodine 125 seeds of variable activities. Tumors and normal skin were then subjected to 0–3 radiofrequency treatments. Each of these lasted 30 min and raised the tumor temperature to 44°C. Neither radiofrequency treatments by themselves nor low dose rate irradiation (up to 180 Gy) cured any of these tumors. However, combined treatments at a total dose of 80 Gy or more were able to sterilize many of the lesions. Cure rate increased with total irradiation dose. One heat exposure was significantly better than no exposures; two were better than one, but three were no better than two. Radiation-induced normal tissue effects were also enhanced by hyperthermia, although one treatment appeared to cause the same enhancement as multiple treatments.

In conjunction with hyperthemia, is internal irradiation, i.e., brachytherapy more or less efficacious than external irradiation? Two studies have tried to answer this question. Moorthy et al (1983) compared external therapy with that generated by Iridium-192. These investigators concluded that irradiation given at a rate of 41.5 cGy/hr was essentially equivalent to fractionated radiotherapy given from an external source at much higher dose rates. They measured a very high thermal enhancement ratio (3.4–3.9), considerably higher than the 1.3–1.8 usually reported in the literature. This is proably related to the immunogenicity of the tumor used, a methylcolanthrene induced fibrosarcoma. When a less immunogenic tumor was used (the KHT sarcoma syngeneic in C3H mice) rather similar results were found with respect to dose rate, although the thermal enhancement found was only about 1.5 (Baker et al, 1987).

All the studies that I have described so far utilized external hyperthermia given either via waterbaths or utilizing external electromagnetic or ultrasound transducers. In the clinic, however, when heat is used in conjunction with brachytherapy, heating is also done interstitially, usually utilizing the same geometry for heating and for irradiation. Does this affect results? Only two groups of investigators has examined this possibility. Miller et al (1978) used implanted radium 226 needles; these served to provide irradiation at a dose rate of 0.67 cGy/min and also acted as electrodes for radiofrequency heating. The two arms of the study were irradiation alone, and irradiation plus hyperthermia. The latter was given immediately after the implant of the radium needles and temperature was maintained for 1 hr at about 43°C. Tumor volume was measured 4 days after heating. The average tumor volume was reduced by 60% in the combined group, but only by 29% in the radium only group. It is not clear if the combined treatment resulted in greater cell killing, or if hyperthermia only increased the rate at which tumor regression occurred. In a recent study, Papado-

POULOS and associates (1989) used the AC33 mammary carcinoma as their model. Irradiation was with Iridium-192, while heating was accomplished with an interstitial microwave antenna operating at 915 MHz. A quantitative comparison between the results obtained with the interstitial heating system and those obtained with external heating systems is not very meaningful. Temperature distributions are surely less homogeneous when one internal radiator is the only energy source; in any case, no data exist for the same tumor system. But my interpretation of the results obtained by PAPADOPOULOS et al is that internal heating did not produce any unexpected results. Heating was not as effective in terms of causing tumor regrowth delay as that reported by other investigators. But that is to be expected in view of the poorer temperature distributions. Heat modestly enhanced the irradiation effects; again the enhancement was less than that reported by others, and again the reason very likely is the heterogeneous temperature distribution. What about timing? What is the optimum sequence for heat and low dose rate irradiation? Or indeed does such an optimum even exist? I have already pointed out that for practical reasons most clinical treatments involve heating before and/or after irradiation. Can this be improved? Timing and sequencing was examined to some extent in the study of BAKER et al (1987). Unfortunately, the design of that study was such that it really did not test the clinically important options: heat before, in the middle, or after brachytherapy. Instead, what was examined was the timing of combined treatments. A more relevant study was the recent one of JONES et al (1989). The vehicle of study was another mammary carcinoma (MTG-B). Irradiation was accomplished by placing a noninvasive cap containing three iodine 125 seeds over the tumor. Dose rates ranged from 14–40 cGy/hr while the total dose varied between 830 and 2378 cGy over the treatment period (48–72 hr). Heating was from a waterbath, with tumor temperatures at 44 or 45°C for 15 min. Hyperthermia was given before, after or in the middle of the irradiation. Heating in the middle of the brachytherapy was most efficacious, heating after least. The differences were not inconsequential: Thermal enhancement was 1.07 if heating was before radiation, while it was 1.64 if the hyperthermia was applied in the middle of brachytherapy. These rather limited studies do suggest that while the present clinical schedules are probably acceptable, they are very likely not optimum. Heating that at least partially overlaps the irradiation appears to maximize antitumor effects. With the development of new equipment it should be possible to heat, at low temperatures (perhaps 39–40°C) for long periods of time, even as long as is required to match the entire radiation period. Experiments on the possible efficacy of such treatments are badly needed, since the early experiments of BEN-HUR et al strongly suggest that continuous heating could greatly enhance the radiation efficacy.

Heat and brachytherapy in other animal systems

Rabbits were inoculated in the suprachoroidal space with Greene melanomas (MIELER et al, 1989). The resulting tumors were treated with a plaque containing ferromagnetic seeds and/or iodine 125 seeds. Hyperthermia was generated by introducing an electromagnetic field that heated the ferromagnetic seeds. The study was primarily a feasibility study and no quantitative tumor responses were described. This, to my knowledge represents the only study on animals other than mice.

Summary

The current biological literature on the interaction of brachytherapy and hyperthermia is readily summarized. Tissue culture data show that if low dose irradiation is carried out at elevated temperatures, then the cytotoxicity is enhanced, even at temperatures that do not cause any independent cell killing. Partial inhibition by heat of the repair of x-ray induced damage is very likely the most reasonable explanation. It must be emphasized again that in these experiments the temperature was elevated during the entire time irradiation was carried out, a situation not matched in clinical protocols. These involve heating before and/or after brachytherapy. For such protocols, the current evidence strongly suggests that hyperthermia and heat act as independent modalities affecting different tumor cell populations.

Studies on animal models have also not provided any surprises. Except possibly for the case of extremely low dose rates (e.g. in the studies of Sapozink et al, 1984) the thermal enhancement provide by one or two heat exposure is very similar to that observed with high rate external beam therapy, i.e., on the order of 1.5. One group of scheduling experiments suggests that hyperthermia given during or in the middle of brachytherapy is optimum; heating after irradiation provides the least benefits. Two hyperthermic treatments may be a good as a larger number. No data exist on the combination of brachytherapy with continuous low temperature (38–41 deg). Such data would be of interest because current equipment development should make it possible to carry out simultaneous treatments in the clinic.

References

Baker DG, Sager HT, Constable WC (1987) The response of a solid tumor to X-radiation as modified by dose rate fractionation, and hyperthermia. Cancer Invest 5: 409–416

Ben-Hur E, Bronk VB, Elkind MM (1974) Thermally enhanced radioresponse of cultured Chinese hamster cells: Inhibition of repair of sublethal damage and enhancement of lethal damage. Radiat Res 58: 38–51

Gerner EW, Oval JH, Manning MR, Sim DA, Bowden GT, Hevezi JM (1983) Dose rate dependence of heat radiosensitization. Int J Radiat Oncol Biol Phys 9: 1401–1404

Hahn GM, Ning SC, Elizaga M, Kapp DS, Anderson RL (1989) A comparison of thermal responses of human and rodent cells. Int J Radiat Biol 56: 817–825

Harisiadis L, Sung D, Kessaris L, Hall E (1978) Hyperthermia and low dose rate irradiation. Radiology 12: 195–198

Jones EL, Lyons BE, Douple EB, Dain BJ (1989) Thermal enhancement of low dose rate irradiation in a murine tumour system. Int J Hyperthermia 5: 509–523

Levendag PC, Ruifrok AC, Marijnissen JP, van Putten WL, Visser AG (1989) Preliminary experience with interstitial radiation, interstitial hyperthermia and in-

terstitial photodynamic therapy in a simple animal model. Strahlenther Onkol 165: 56–60
Ling CC, Robinson E (1989) Moderate hyperthermia and low dose rate irradiation. Radiat Res 114: 379–384
Marmor JB, Pounds D, Hahn N, Hahn GM (1978) Treating spontaneous tumors in dogs and cats by ultrasound-induced hyperthermia. Int J Radiat Oncol Biol Phys 4: 967–973
Mieler WF, Jaffe GJ, Steeves RA (1989) Ferromagnetic hyperthermia and iodine 125 brachytherapy in the treatment of choroidal melanoma in a rabbit model. Arch Ophthalmol 107: 1524–1528
Miller RC, Leith JC, Veomett RC, Gerner EW (1978) Effects of interstitial radiation alone, or in combination with localized hyperthermia on the response of a mouse mammary carcinoma. Radiat Res 19: 175–180
Moorthy CR, Hahn EW, Kim JH, Feingold SM, Alfieri AA, Hilaris BS (1984) Improved response of a murine fibrosarcoma (Meth-A) to interstitial radiation when combined with hyperthermia. Int J Radiat Oncol Biol Phys 10: 2145–2148
Papadopoulos D, Kimler BF, Estes NC, Durham FJ (1989) Growth delay effect of combined interstitial hyperthermia and brachytherapy in a rat solid tumor model. Anticancer Res 9: 45–47
Sapareto SA, Dewey WC (1984) Thermal dose determination in cancer therapy. Int J Radiat Oncol Biol Phys 10: 787–803
Sapozink MD, Palos B, Goffinet DR, Hahn GM (1983) Combined continuous ultra low dose rate irradiation and radiofrequency hyperthermia in the C3H mouse. Int J Radiat Oncol Biol Phys 9: 1357–1365

2

Simultaneous and Sequential Treatment with Radiation and Hyperthermia: A Comparative Assessment

M. R. Horsman and *J. Overgaard*

Danish Cancer Society, Department of Experimental Clinical Oncology, Aarhus, Denmark

Acknowledgements: The authors would like to thank Ms. DORRIT RASMUSSEN for preparation of the manuscript.

Supported by grant no. 90-7598 from the Danish Cancer Society.

Introduction

Hyperthermia is a modality which on its own probably has no role to play in the curative treatment of tumours in humans (OVERGAARD, 1985). Its most likely clinical application is in combination with other cancer treatments, especially radiation. Numerous experimental studies have now established that moderate hyperthermia can enhance the response of animal tumours to ionizing radiation (for review, see HORSMAN and OVERGAARD, 1989). There is now also good evidence from clinical Phase I and II studies showing that heat can enhance the radiation effect to a significant degree in a variety of human tumours (OVERGAARD, 1989a). However, it is still not entirely clear as to how the radiation and heat should be combined clinically, in order to obtain the greatest therapeutic advantage. In the following chapter we would therefore like to discuss the basic mechanisms underlying the interaction between hyperthermia and radiation and then to consider how these modalities should be given to produce the maximal therapeutic benefit in a given clinical situation.

Mechanisms for the interaction

Hyperthermic cytotoxicity

Radioresistant hypoxic cells, found in many solid tumours *in vivo* (MOULDER and ROCKWELL, 1984), are now known to compromise the success of radiotherapy of human tumours (OVERGAARD, 1989c). These same cells have also been found to be sensitive to hyperthermia. *In vitro* studies have reported that cells under hypoxic conditions are more sensitive to heat than the same cells in a well oxygenated environment (OVERGAARD and BICHEL, 1977; GERWECK et al, 1979; SUIT and GERWECK, 1979). This is not a consequence of hypoxia *per se* because under well-defined nutrient conditions, acute hypoxia does not significantly alter cellular response to heat (GERWECK et al, 1974, 1979; POWER and HARRIS, 1977). However, prolonged oxygen deprivation or chronic hypoxia will increase cellular heat sensitivity (GERWECK et al, 1979; OVERGAARD and NIELSEN, 1980; NIELSEN, 1981). Prolonged hypoxia generally leads to metabolic changes, which in turn alter several other parameters such as acidity, and it is these changes which are responsible for the increased sensitization to hyperthermia (GERWECK et al, 1974; HAHN, 1974; OVERGAARD and BICHEL, 1977; OVERGAARD and NIELSEN, 1980). This effect can also be demonstrated *in vivo*. If the blood supply to a tumour is substantially reduced, the corresponding decrease in available oxygen will result in an increase in tumour hypoxia. Under such conditions a significant increase in tumour sensitivity to heat is observed. This is seen when tumour blood flow is reduced by clamping (SUIT, 1975; THRALL et al, 1975; DEWEY et al, 1977; HILL and DENEKAMP, 1978; WALLEN et al, 1986); by physiological agents like hydralazine (HORSMAN et al, 1988, 1989; KALMUS et al, 1990) or glucose (URANO et al, 1983; HIRAOKA and HAHN, 1990); and treatments which damage the tumour vascular supply such as flavone acetic acid (HORSMAN et al, 1991), tumour necrosis factor (KALLINOWSKI et al, 1988; WATANABE et al, 1988) or photodynamic therapy (WALDOW and DOUGHERTY, 1984; HENDERSON et al, 1985; LEVENDAG et al, 1988).

The mechanisms by which tumour cells are directly killed by heat are not clear although effects on membrane function, inhibition of metabolism and macromolecular synthesis, and changes in the cytoskeleton have been suggested (for reviews see DEWEY et al, 1980; LEEPER, 1985). *In vivo*, hyperthermia also causes severe vascular damage (SONG et al, 1980; RHEE et al, 1984; VAUPEL and KALLINOWSKY, 1987) which indirectly will result in tumour cell death.

It is unlikely that the cytotoxic action of heat will affect normal tissues to the same degree as it does tumours. In general, normal tissues have oxygen concentrations equivalent to a partial pressure of about 40 mm Hg and although some tissues in the body may have lower oxygen levels they do not contain the significant proportion of heat sensitive hypoxic cells normally found in tumours (HILL, 1987). Furthermore, the vasculature of normal tissues and tumours are different (FOLKMAN, 1976) and tumour blood vessels have been shown to be more susceptible to heat damage than vessels in certain normal tissues (REINHOLD et al, 1978; EDDY, 1980).

Hyperthermic radiosensitization

Radiation and hyperthermia are also known to interact to produce sensitization of the tumours. The mechanism of this interaction is not entirely clear. A heat treatment may simply increase the sensitivity of cells to radiation, which may be a general effect occurring in all cells or specifically only in those which are normally radioresistant. *In vitro* studies have shown a hyperthermia-induced increase in both radiation-induced DNA strand breaks (MILLS and MEYN, 1981) and DNA-protein cross-links (CLARK et al, 1981; BOWDEN et al, 1982). It has also been reported that the cell cycle dependent sensitivity of heat and radiation are complementary (WESTRA and DEWEY, 1971; RAAPHORST and AZZAM, 1984). Moreover, if heat and radiation are combined a flat cell cycle response is obtained (RAAPHORST and AZZAM, 1984). Increasing the sensitivity of only the radioresistant hypoxic cells might be a possibility, since although hyperthermia generally leads to vascular collapse in tumours, a small shortlived increase in blood flow is often seen during the heating period (SONG, 1984). Such an effect could conceivably result in an increase in oxygen delivery to tumours with a concomitant, albeit transient, decrease in the level of tumour hypoxia.

Alternatively, hyperthermia may affect the repair of sublethal or potentially lethal damage induced by the radiation itself. The ability of heat to inhibit the repair of radiation damage in mammalian cells has been well documented in several investigations (CORRY et al, 1971; CLARK et al, 1981; LUNEC et al, 1981; MILLS and MEYN, 1981, 1983; JORRITSMA and KONINGS, 1983; RADFORD, 1983; MITCHEL and BIRNBOIM, 1985; MITTLER, 1986), and this inhibition has been shown to affect both the rate and extent of the radiation-induced DNA strand break repair.

The lack of *in vivo* data makes it difficult to predict which mechanisms are actually responsible for the effects in tumours and normal tissues. Most of the *in vitro* data show that these hyperthermic radiosensitization mechanisms actually occur at low heat doses, which on their own are nonlethal. In addition, as we shall see later, giving heat and radiation together *in vivo* as a truly simultaneous treatment, in which the hyperthermic radiosensitization mechanism clearly predominates, generally does not lead to a therapeutic advantage. This suggests that for the radiosensitization effect, unlike with the hyperthermic cytotoxicity, the same mechanisms are probably operating to a similar degree in both tumours and normal tissues.

Single treatments

Treatment interval

In Fig. 1 is shown the effect of introducing an interval between the radiation and heat treatments to a C3H mouse mammary carcinoma and its surrounding skin. For the tumour, the thermal enhancement ratio (TER; ratio of the radiation doses for radiation alone and radiation with heat to produce the same effect) is greatest when the radiation and heat are given simultaneously. As the time interval between the two treatments increases the TER decreases, reaching a plateau with an interval of 4 hours and which appears to persist for at least 24 hours. These effects are independent of the sequence between the heat and radiation. Similar trends are seen in other tumour models (Fig. 2) although individual differences do occur. In both the fibrosarcoma of STEWART and DENEKAMP (1978) and the squamous carcinoma of HILL and DENEKAMP (1979) a rise in TER was actually seen when the treatments were separated by 3 and 2 hours, respectively, while for the NT carcinoma no significant change in response was found with any time interval between the heat and radiation. It is not clear why these different effects were obtained, but it should be born in mind that the results shown in Fig. 2 were generated using different assay procedures (regrowth delay and tumour control). Furthermore, only in the studies by GILLETTE and ENSLEY (1979) and OVERGAARD (1980) were truly simultaneous treatments given. The importance of this aspect is illustrated in Fig. 3A, in which even when tumours are irradiated immediately before or after

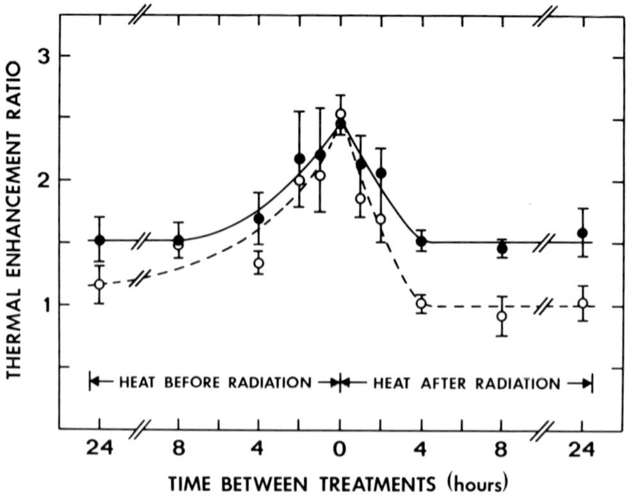

Fig. 1. Thermal enhancement ratios in a C3H mouse mammary carcinoma and its surrounding skin as a function of time interval and sequence between hyperthermia (42.5°C; 60 min) and radiation. Thermal enhancement ratios were determined from full dose response curves and represent the ratios of the radiation doses for radiation alone and radiation + heat to produce either local control in tumours (●) or moist desquamation in skin (○) in 50% of treated animals. Values are means ±95% confidence intervals. (Redrawn from OVERGAARD et al, 1987.)

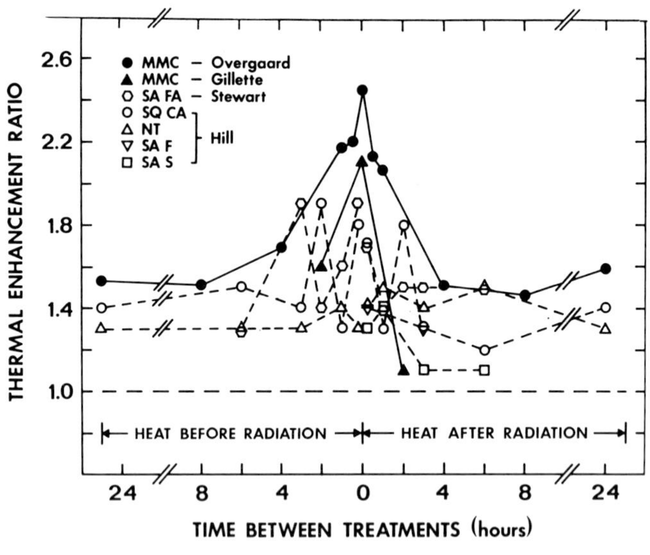

Fig. 2. Thermal enhancement ratios in different tumours as a function of time interval and sequence between hyperthermia (42.5°C; 60 min) and radiation. Thermal enhancement ratios were calculated using either a regrowth delay (STEWART and HILL) or a local tumour control (OVERGAARD and GILLETTE) assay and represent the ratio of the radiation doese for radiation alone and radiation + heat to produce the same effect. (Redrawn from OVERGAARD, 1982.)

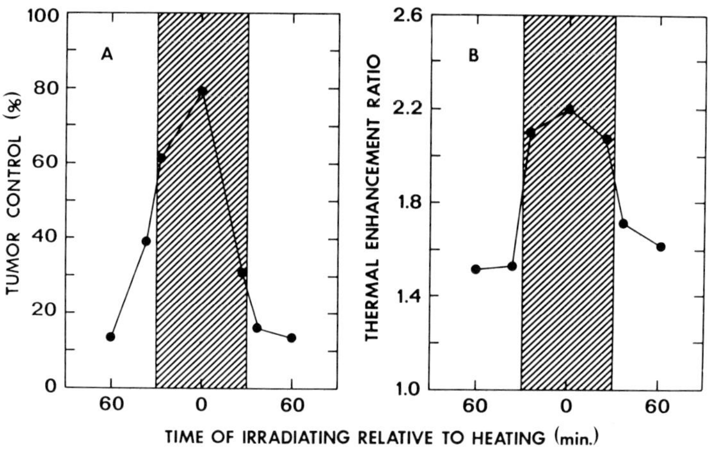

Fig. 3. The importance of interval between radiation and heat treatment in a C3H mouse mammary carcinoma and normal foot skin. Tissues were irradiated at various times before, during, or after heating with 42.5°C for 60 minutes. (A) Results represent the percentage of mice showing local tumour control 120 days after a combined heat and radiation (26 Gy) treatment. (B) Thermal enhancement ratios were determined from full does response curves and represent the ratios of the radiation doses for radiation alone and radiation + heat to produce moist desquamation in skin in 50% of treated animals. (Redrawn from OVERGAARD, 1985.)

hyperthermia there is a significant reduction in the TER compared to that observed when the radiation is administered in the middle of the heating period.

The TER obtained in normal skin with a truly simultaneous heat and radiation treatment is also significantly reduced when the radiation is given immediately before or after heat (Fig. 3B). From Fig. 1 it is also clear that this TER is further reduced with longer time intervals between the heat and radiation. However, when heat proceeds the radiation there is a persistent TER, but if the heat follows the radiation the TER is actually eliminated with a 4 hour interval. These trends are also seen in other normal tissues (Fig. 4).

The TER obtained with a simultaneous treatment is probably due primarily to hyperthermic sensitization, whereas the TER remaining in tumours after a 4 hour separation between the heat and radiation is most likely a consequence of heat killing the radioresistant hypoxic cells. This seems a likely explanation when one considers that most normal tissues are likely to be devoid of any significant hypoxia and the TER values in all the normal tissues shown in Fig. 4 are virtually eliminated when the heat follows radiation by at least a 4 hour interval. The presence of a TER in normal tissues when heat precedes radiation may be indicative of a persistent thermoradiosensitization mechanism.

It is obvious that the variations in TER for tumours and normal tissues will influence the therapeutic gain. This is shown in Fig. 5. No therapeutic advantage is to be expected from a simultaneous treatment, if the tumour and

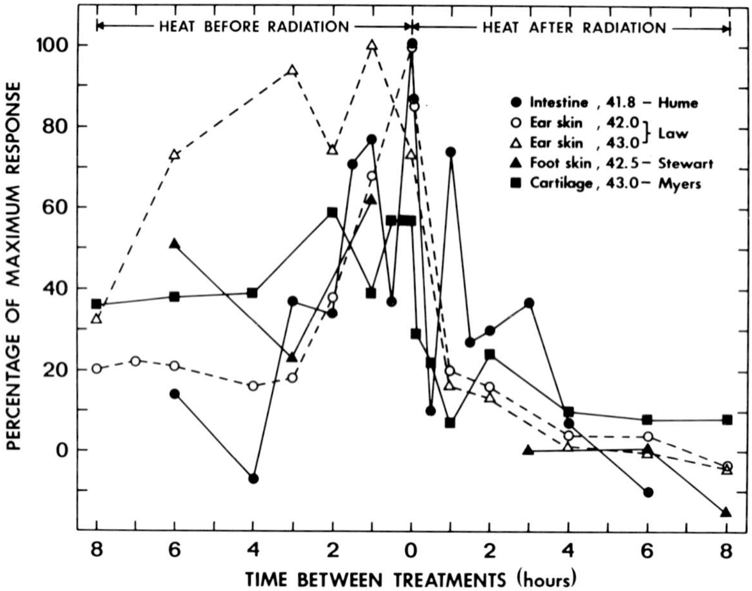

Fig. 4. The time course of decay of the heat potentiation of radiation damage in normal tissues. Several mouse tissues and rat cartilage were heated at various temperatures for 60 min either before or after irradiation. Thermal enhancement ratios are shown after normalization to the percentage of the maximum response for each curve. (Redrawn from FIELD and BLEEHEN, 1979.)

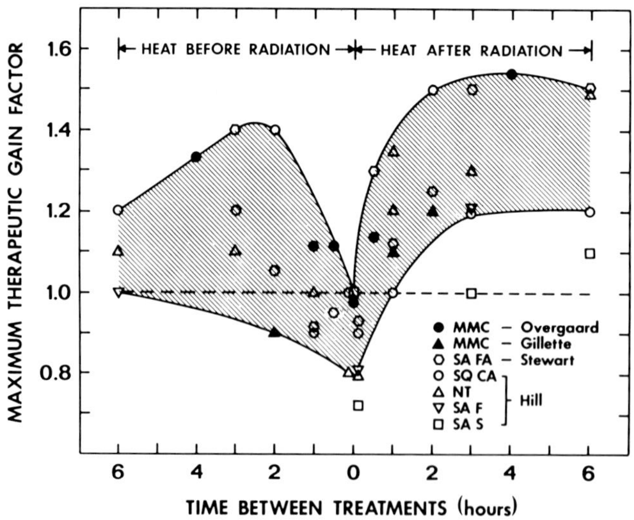

Fig. 5. Maximum therapeutic gain factor as a function of time interval between radiation and hyperthermia (42.5°C; 60 min). This figure is a survey of studies where tumour and normal tissues have been compared. The shaded area indicates the range of all the values obtained, with the exception of the slow-growing sarcoma. (Redrawn from OVERGAARD, 1982.)

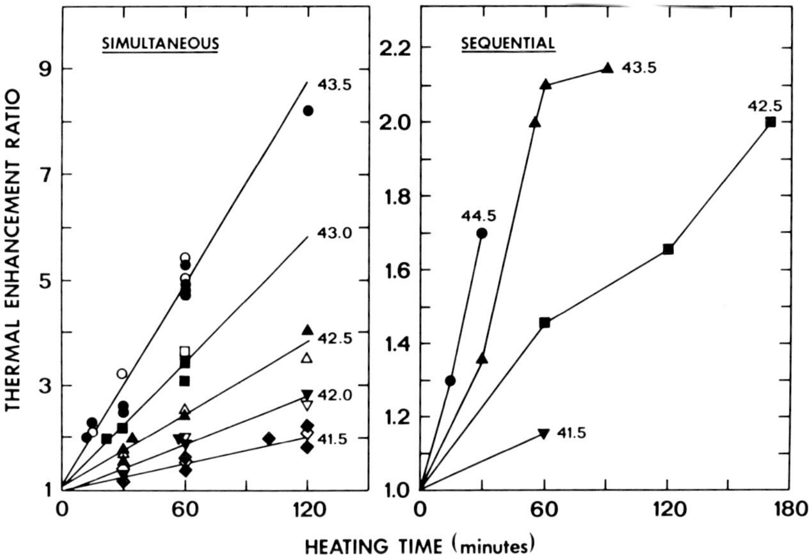

Fig. 6. The influence of heating time and temperature on the thermal enhancement ratio when heat and radiation are combined in either a simultaneous or sequential (heat 4 h after radiation) protocol. Thermal enhancement ratios were determined from the ratios of the radiation doses for radiation alone and radiation + heat to produce either local tumour control (closed symbols) or moist desquamation in skin (open symbols) in 50% of treated animals. Numbers on the figures indicate the treatment temperatures. (Redrawn from OVERGAARD, 1987.)

normal tissue are heated to the same degree. While perhaps at best only a small therapeutic gain will be seen when radiation follows hyperthermia, simply because the TER of the normal tissue is high. However, the rapid recovery from thermal radiosensitization in the normal tissues when heat is given after radiation contrasts to the prolonged TER observed in the tumours, thus a therapeutic gain is apparent with an interval of several hours.

Temperature and heating time

The TER values obtained in tumours and normal tissues are dependent on the treatment temperature and the time of heating. This is illustrated in Fig. 6 for both simultaneous and sequential treatments. A simultaneous treatment is not likely to give a therapeutic gain if the tumours and normal tissues are heated to the same extent, but a sequential treatment will be beneficial because of the lack of normal tissue damage. However, if a preferential tumour heating is achieved an improved therapeutic effect should be possible with the simultaneous protocol, with the magnitude of the effect depending on the temperature difference between the tumour and surrounding normal tissues. If we look at the treatment time required to produce the same thermal enhancement at each temperature, we find that the time-temperature relationship is different from a simultaneous and sequential treatment (Fig. 7).

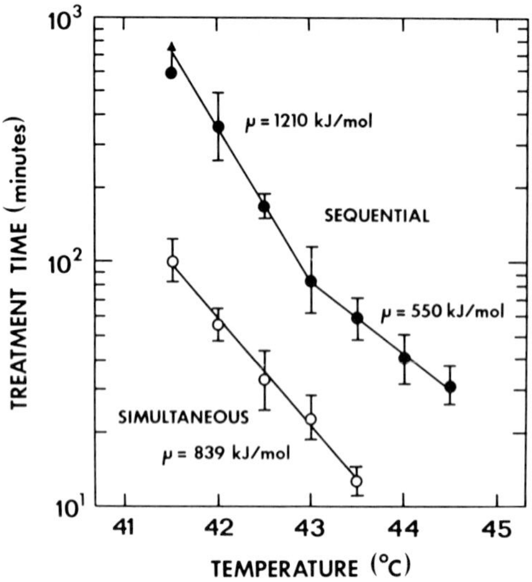

Fig. 7. The time-temperature relationship for heat and radiation combined as either a simultaneous or sequential (heat 4 h after radiation) treatment. Results show mean values (±95% confidence intervals) of the time required to produce a thermal enhancement ratio of 2, using a local tumour control assay in a C3H mouse mammary carcinoma. (Redrawn from Overgaard, 1984.)

Over a temperature range of 41.5–43.5°C the simultaneous treatment results in an activation energy equivalent to 839 kJ/mol. For the sequential treatment a steep time-temperature relationship is observed below 43.0°C resulting in an activation energy of 1210 kJ/mol, but at higher temperatures the relationship is less steep and a value of 550 kJ/mol is obtained. This biphasic pattern is similar to that observed with heat alone (Lindegaard and Overgaard, 1987) and supports the suggestion that the effect of sequential radiation and heat is due to an additive effect of the two modalities.

Blood flow and tumour size

The response of any tissue to hyperthermia will be strongly dependent on the tissue's vascular supply. Blood flow is one of the major vehicles by which heat is dissipated, thus the vascular supply will influence the ability to heat the tissue. It is also important in determining the type of environment that exists in tumours. Tumour blood flow is heterogeneous in nature and in general is of a lower flow rate than the normal tissue of origin (Peterson, 1979; Reinhold, 1988; Vaupel et al, 1989). It is this poor blood supply that results in large areas which are nutrient deprived, low in oxygen and high in acidity (Vaupel, 1979; Wike-Hooley et al, 1984) and as previously discussed, cells in these areas are heat sensitive. More importantly, as tumour size increases there is a relative decrease in blood flow (Peterson, 1979; Vaupel, 1979), thus tumour size can influence tumour response to hyperthermia. In fact, several studies have shown that the sensitivity of tumours to heat does increase with increasing tumour size (Urano et al, 1980, 1982). Since this is primarily the result of an increase in heat sensitive areas one would expect it to be reflected by an increase in the hyperthermic cytotoxic effect and not hyperthermic radiosensitization. This is demonstrated in Fig. 8 in which the TER for a sequential radiation and heat treatment changes with tumour size, whereas a simultaneous treatment is independent of tumour volume. The observation that large tumours tend to be

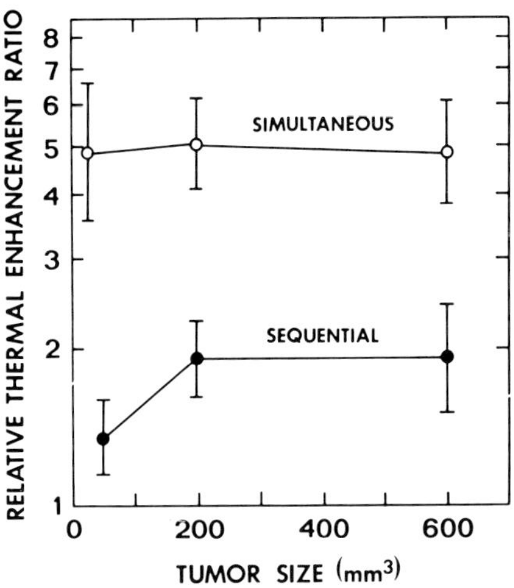

Fig. 8. Relative thermal enhancement ratios as a function of the size of tumours given a combined heat and radiation treatment. C3H mouse mammary carcinomas were treated with heat (43.5°C; 60 min) and radiation either simultaneously or sequentially (heat 4 h after radiation). Thermal enhancement ratios are means (±95% confidence intervals) and were calculated from the ratios of the radiation doses for radiation alone and radiation + heat, necessary to produce local tumour control in 50% of treated animals. (Redrawn from OVERGAARD, 1987.)

those which benefit most from adjuvant hyperthermia has also been reported in several clinical studies (KIM et al, 1982; OVERGAARD, 1989b).

The tumour vascular supply is also influenced by the heat itself. It has been shown that during heating tumour blood flow can increase (SONG et al, 1987; HORSMAN et al, 1990), but after heating vascular collapse is generally apparent at temperatures which can cause a substantial increase in blood flow in certain normal tissues (SONG, 1984). Such vascular changes will have a critical effect on sequencing between hyperthermia and radiation. Any decrease in blood flow might be expected to lead to a reduction in available oxygen and a subsequent increase in hypoxia and radioresistance, while with an increased blood flow the reverse should be true. A correlation between a change in tumour blood flow and oxygenation status following hyperthermia, has been documented (VAUPEL et al, 1983). Administration of radiation after heating might therefore be expected to radioprotect the tumour yet radiosensitize the normal tissue, although in the latter case these effects could be expected to be small because of their already high level of oxygenation.

Clinically relevant problems

Thermotolerance

The combined use of radiation and heat as a clinical regime is most likely to be in fractionated schedules. This may be a problem since there are many studies in both tumours and normal tissues showing that hyperthermia may induce a temporary resistance to a subsequent heat treatment (for review, see NIELSEN, 1984). The phenomenon is often referred to as thermotolerance and is illustrated in Fig. 9A. Here a C3H mouse mammary carcinoma was locally heated at 43.5°C for various times following a preheating at 43.5°C for 30 minutes. The thermotolerance ratio represents the ratios of the slopes of the resulting curves of tumour growth versus heating time for single

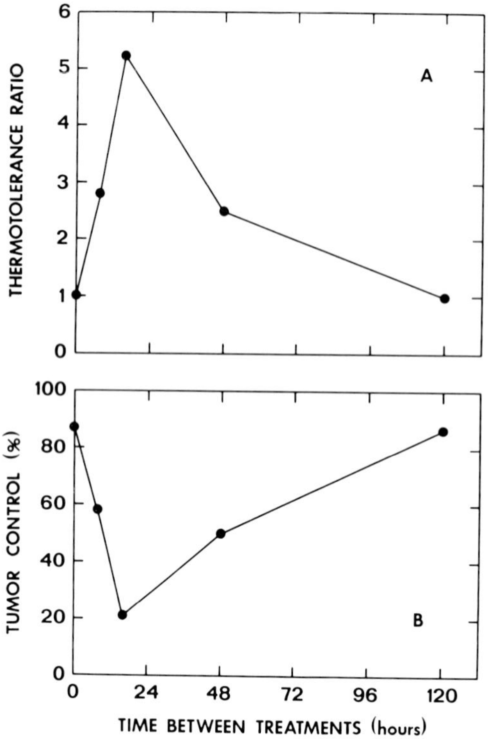

Fig. 9. Time course for the development of resistance to either heat alone or a simultaneous heat and radiation treatment in a C3H mouse mammary carcinoma, following prior exposure to 43.5°C for 30 minutes. (A) Tumours were heated (43.5°C; 30 min) and then a time interval allowed before a second heating at 43.5°C for various times. The thermotolerance ratio represents the ratios of the slopes from the resulting curves for tumour growth versus heating time for single heated tumours compared to tumours exposed to a prior heating. (B) Percentage local tumour control measured 120 days after tumours were heated (43.5°C; 30 min) at various time intervals prior to a simultaneous treatment with radiation (15 Gy) and heat (43.5°C; 60 min). Tumours at the 0 h time interval received no prior heating before the simultaneous treatment. (Redrawn from NIELSEN et al, 1983.)

heated tumours relative to pre-heated tumours. It is obvious that thermotolerance develops rapidly, reaching a maximum after a 16 hour interval between the two heat treatments and then decaying, being lost when the heat treatments are separated by a gap of 120 hours.

The influence of thermotolerance on a simultaneous heat and radiation treatment is shown in Fig. 9B. Pretreatment at 43.5°C for 30 minutes clearly alters the response of this C3H mouse mammary carcinoma. Moreover, the response is identical to that seen for the kinetics of thermotolerance with heat alone, with the maximum effect occurring after 16 hours, then decreasing and finally disappearing by 120 hours. This effect of thermotolerance on the interaction between heat and radiation is even more pronounced when heat is given 4 hours after radiation in a sequential regime (NIELSEN et al, 1983). A similar reduction in TER for radiation and heat by a prior heat treatment has been reported for tumours both *in vitro* and *in vivo* (STEWART and DENEKAMP, 1982; HARTSON-EATON et al, 1984; OVERGAARD and NIELSEN, 1984). While in normal tissues a pretreatment with hyperthermia has been reported to both have no effect on the heat and radiation TER as well as to decrease it (LAW et al, 1979; LAW and AHIER, 1982; MARIGOLD and HUME, 1982; STEWART and DENEKAMP, 1982; WONDERGEM and HAVEMAN, 1984).

Clinically, multifractional heat treatments are likely. OVERGAARD and NIELSEN (1983) in an experimental system reported that if hyperthermia and radiation were combined in a fractionated treat-

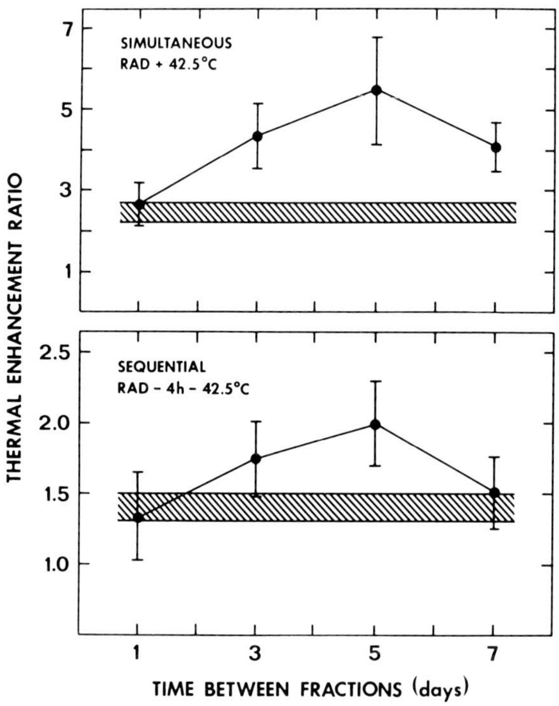

Fig. 10. Thermal enhancement ratios after five fractions of a combined heat and radiation treatment as a function of the time interval between the fractions. C3H mouse mammary carcinomas were given radiation and heat (42.5°C; 60 min) either simultaneously or sequentially (heat 4 h after radiation) at each fraction. Thermal enhancement ratios were calculated from the ratios of the radiation doses for radiation alone and radiation + heat, necessary to produce local tumour control in 50% of treated animals. Values represent means ±95% confidence intervals. The shaded area shows the 95% confidence intervals for single heat and radiation treatment. (Redrawn from OVERGAARD and NIELSEN, 1983.)

ment of five daily fractions, then the observed TER was not significantly different from that obtained with a single fraction (Fig. 10) regardless of whether the heat was given simultaneously with radiation or 4 hours later in a sequential regime. Moreover, if the intervals between fractions was extended to allow for thermotolerance to disappear then the TER actually increased above that obtained with a single dose, reaching a maximum when a 5-day interval was used, a time when thermotolerance has disappeared (Fig. 9). This should not be considered as an improved response, because although the TER has increased the radiation effect with a 5-day interval is actually reduced. At time intervals greater than 5 days the TER decreased, probably as a consequence of the length of the time interval allowing for the tumours to regrow between fractions.

These results contrast with those of Stewart and Denekamp (1982) who found that thermal sensitization was reduced by giving 1 or 4 pretreatments with hyperthermia. These same workers showed that the TER for skin was unchanged when heat and radiation were given in 2 or 5 fractions, regardless of whether the heat followed immediately after irradiating or 3 hours later (Stewart and Denekamp, 1980, 1982). Similar results were seen with fractionated heat and radiation in mouse ear provided the heat was administered after irradiating (Law, 1979), but if the heat proceeded the radiation in each combined treatment, a large reduction in TER was observed with increasing number of fractions.

Step-down and step-up heating

Another clinical problem that needs to be considered is that during heat treatment considerable fluctuations in tissue tem-

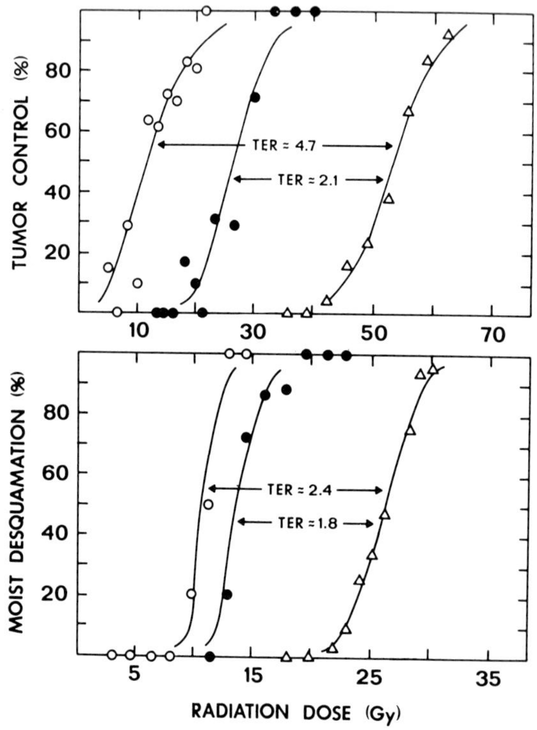

Fig. 11. The effect of step-down and step-up heating on the response of a C3H mouse mammary carcinoma and normal skin to radiation. Tissues were locally given either radiation alone (△) or simultaneously irradiated with step-up heating (●; 41.5°C for 60 min followed immediately by 44.5°C for 10 min) or step-down heating (○; 44.5°C for 10 min followed immediately by 41.5°C for 60 min). Thermal enhancement ratios were calculated from the ratios of the doses to produce tumour control or moist desquamation in 50% of treated animals (Redrawn from Lindegaard and Overgaard, 1988.)

perature are often observed (HAHN, 1982; OVERGAARD et al, 1987). Experimentally this phenomenon has been examined by subjecting tumours or normal tissues to 2 consecutive heat treatments, one higher than the other. Exposure of the tissue to the higher temperature followed by the lower is referred to as step-down heating (SDH), whereas the reverse treatment order is called step-up heating (SUH). From the data accumulated to date (for review see HORSMAN and OVERGAARD, 1989) it has been found that with SUH the tumour response is the result of an additive effect of the two heat treatments. With SDH not only is there additional cell killing from the higher temperature, but significant sensitization to the second heat treatment is also observed. The effects of SDH and to a lesser extent SUH on a combined heat and radiation treatment have been studied both *in vitro* (HENLE and LEEPER, 1976, 1977, 1979; MIYAKOSHI et al, 1979) and *in vivo* (PADOVANI et al, 1987; LINDEGAARD and OVERGAARD, 1988; LINDEGAARD et al, 1991). A comparison of the ability of SDH and SUH to enhance a simultaneous radiation treatment in a C3H mouse mammary carcinoma and normal foot skin is made

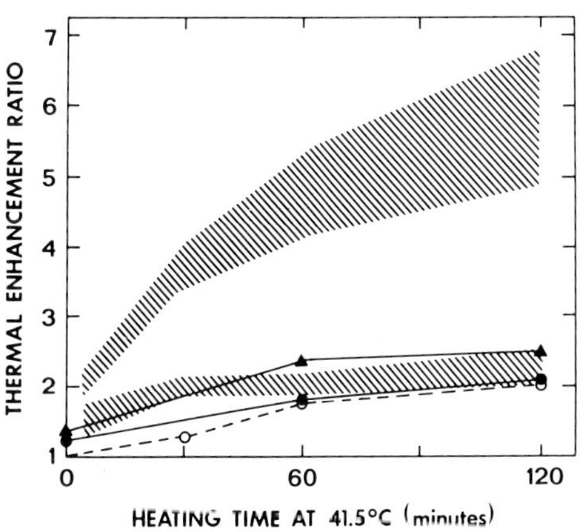

Fig. 12. Step-down (SDH) and step-up heating (SUH) induced changes in thermal enhancement ratios in a C3H mouse mammary carcinoma and normal skin as a function of the lower temperature treatment time. The tumour and normal tissues were irradiated simultaneously with either SUH (41.5°C for various times + 44.5°C for 10 min) or SDH (44.5°C for 10 min + 41.5°C for various times). Radiation + single heating in skin (○); radiation + SDH in skin (▲); radiation + SUH in skin (●); radiation + SUH in tumours (lower shaded area); radiation + SDH in tumours (upper shaded area). Thermal enhancement ratios were calculated from data similar to that shown in Fig. 11. (Redrawn from LINDEGAARD and OVERGAARD, 1988.)

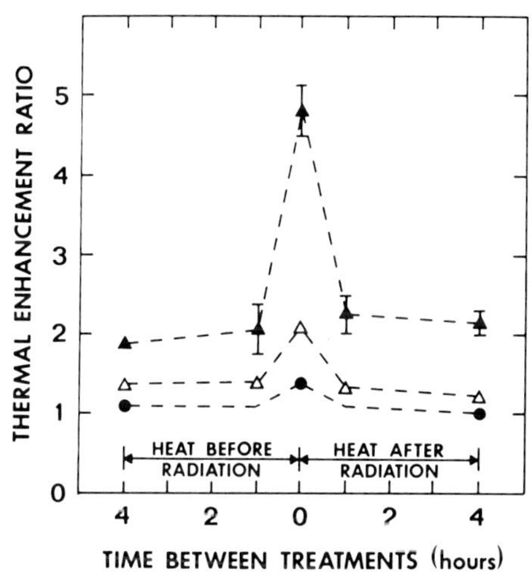

Fig. 13. The effect of step-down and step-up heating on the response of a C3H mouse mammary carcinoma to radiation and heat. Tumours were locally irradiated either simultaneously with heating or with a time interval between the heat and radiation. Heat treatments were either heat alone (●; 41.5°C; 60 min), step-up heating (△; 41.5°C for 60 min followed immediately by 44.5°C for 10 min) or step-down heating (▲; 44.5°C for 10 min followed immediately by 41.5°C for 60 min). The thermal enhancement ratios were calculated from data similar to that shown in Fig. 11. (Redrawn from LINDEGAARD et al, 1991.)

in Fig. 11. The heat treatments were 44.5°C for 10 minutes and 41.5°C for 60 minutes. It is obvious that both SUH and SDH radiosensitize the tumour and skin. Furthermore, SDH produces a greater effect than SUH and appears to be more prominent in the tumour. This is clearly shown in Fig. 12, in which the skin and tumour data at several different test treatment times are summarized. In both tissues, SUH produced only a small increase in radiation response above that found with a single heat treatment. A slightly larger enhancement was obtained with SDH in the skin, but the TER was much less than that found in tumours, suggesting that the phenomenon of SDH may actually result in a potential clinical benefit.

The tumour enhancements produced by both SDH and SUH when combined with a simultaneous radiation treatment are significantly reduced with an introduction of a time interval between the heat and radiation (Fig. 13). This reduction in TER is the same regardless of whether the interval is for 1 or 4 hours and is also independent of the heat and radiation sequence.

Clinical implications

The abundant evidence from *in vitro* and *in vivo* studies clearly shows that hyperthermia has a role to play in combination with radiation therapy (Raaphorst, 1989; Horsman and Overgaard, 1989). This suggestion has now been confirmed from early clinical studies in which heat has been shown to significantly enhance the effect of radiation (Overgaard, 1989a). However, it is still not entirely clear as to how heat and radiation should be combined to produce the maximum response. As illustrated in Fig. 14, the results from experimental studies of single dose treatments show that the greatest damage to tumours occurs with a simultaneous application of heat and radiation, a schedule which utilizes the hyperthermic radiosensitization mechanism. However, a therapeutic advantage will only be achieved if preferential tumour heating can be obtained. With such a schedule the highest possible heat treatment should be given, the only limitation being the damage induced by the heat in the critical surrounding normal tissue. If a preferential tumour heating cannot be obtained, then the treatment rationale should be based on a sequential application of radiation and hyperthermia, thus involving the hyperthermic cytotoxic destruction of chronically hypoxic radioresistant tumour cells. Such a treatment should be given with a sequence where hyperthermia is applied at least 3–4 hours after radiation. Although a sequential treatment will result in a smaller thermal enhancement in the tumour, than seen with a simultaneous heat and radiation schedule, an improvement in therapeutic gain should be possible because of the minimal enhancement of radiation response in the normal tissues. The validity of this biological rationale has been demonstrated in a few clinical trials (Overgaard, 1981; Overgaard and Overgaard, 1987; Arcangeli et al, 1984) and is shown in Fig. 15. Although a TER of 1.4 was observed in this malignant melanoma after a simultaneous treatment, a similar enhancement occurred in the heated overlaying skin, resulting in no therapeutic gain. Heating tumours 3–4 hours after irradiating, in a sequential

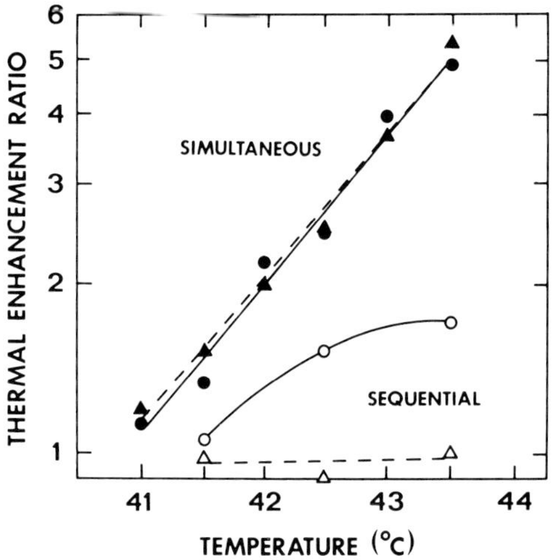

Fig. 14. The effect of a simultaneous or sequential radiation and heat treatment on the thermal enhancement ratio in a C3H mouse mammary carcinoma and its surrounding skin. Tissues were locally heated at different temperatures for 60 minutes either at the same time as irradiation (closed symbols) or 4 h later (open symbols). The thermal enhancement ratios for tumours (○ ●) were calculated from tumour control data and for skin (△ ▲) from moist desquamation results, similar to those shown in Fig. 11. (OVERGAARD, unpublished observations.)

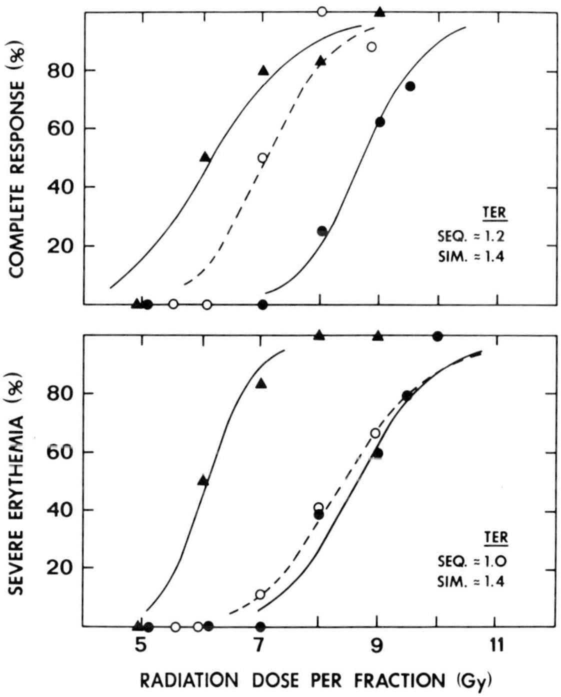

Fig. 15. Dose-response relationship for radiation alone or combined radiation and hyperthermia in malignant melanomas and surrounding skin. One hundred and eighteen cutaneous or lymph node metastases or recurrent primary tumours were treated with three fractions of radiation in 8 days either alone (●), with heat given immediately after irradiation (▲) or 3–4 h later (○). Thermal enhancement ratios (TER) were calculated from the ratio of the radiation doese for radiation alone and radiation + heat, necessary to produce tumour control or severe erythema in 50% of treated fields. (Redrawn from OVERGAARD and OVERGAARD, 1987.)

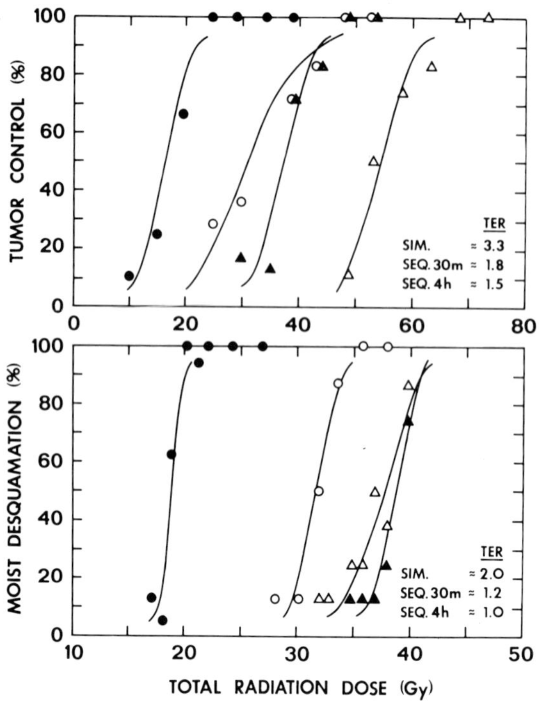

Fig. 16. The effect of varying the interval between radiation and heat on the response of a C3H mouse mammary carcinoma and normal skin. Radiation and heat (43.5°C; 30 min) were given together as 3 fractions in 8 days. Tissues were locally irradiated (△); irradiated simultaneously with heating (●); heated 30 minutes after radiation (○); heated 4 hours after radiation (▲). The thermal enhancement ratios (TER) were calculated from the ratios of the doses to produce tumour control or moist desquamation in 50% of treated animals. (Redrawn from Overgaard et al, 1987.)

protocol, produced a smaller TER of 1.2 in the tumour but a therapeutic gain was observed because there was no significant increase in heat-induced radiation damage to the skin. In this clinical study the simultaneous radiation and heat treatment was not truly simultaneous, since a 30 minutes time interval elapsed between irradiation and subsequent heating. As was mentioned earlier, heating even immediately after irradiation can substantially reduce the TER observed when radiation was given in the middle of the heat sequence. The significance of this is illustrated in Fig. 16, in which the malignant melanoma study was simulated in a C3H mouse mammary carcinoma and normal skin. It is obvious that there is a significant improvement in the TER for both skin and tumour when one compares a true simultaneous treatment with a 30 minute interval between radiation and heat.

One of the potential clinical advantages of simultaneous heat and radiation treatments over sequential procedures concerns the temperature fluctuations observed during the heating of tissues (HAHN, 1982; OVERGAARD et al, 1987). Experimentally it has been shown that these temperature changes can actually enhance the TER for heat and radiation (LINDEGAARD and OVERGAARD, 1988; LINDEGAARD et al, 1991). For a simultaneous treatment the TER in tumours is much greater than with a sequential protocol (Fig. 13), especially if a high temperature is followed by a lower temperature heating. Moreover, this enhancement of the TER by SDH in a simultaneous regime was minimal in at least one normal tissue (Fig. 12), suggesting a possible clinical benefit of such a treatment.

Clinically, heat is going to be given with radiation in a fractionated schedule. Table 1 shows the results of an experiment in which fractionated treatments were administered to a C3H mouse mammary carcinoma. Heating tumours 4 hours after each radiation treatment did not improve the TER above that seen when tumours were heated after only one of the 5 radiation treatments. On the other hand, a single simultaneous heat and radiation exposure in this fractionated radiation schedule produced a slightly larger TER than observed with either sequential treatment, but this TER was substantially increased when the heat was given with every radiation fraction.

In conclusion it would appear that a simultaneous heat and radiation treatment does have an advantage over a sequential treatment protocol especially if a preferential tumour heating can be obtained. Such a situation should be possible with improvements in technology. Another approach may be by the use of interstitial hyperthermia (URANO and DOUPLE, 1989). Two of the procedures which show the greatest potential

Table 1. The effect of a fractionated heat (42.5°C; 60 min) and radiation treatment on the response of a C3H mouse mammary carcinoma[a]

Treatment[b]	TCD-50[c]	TER[d]
Rad alone		
R+R+R+R+R	60 Gy	—
Simultaneous		
RH+RH+RH+RH+RH	23 Gy	2.59
R+R+R+R+RH	41 Gy	1.46
Sequential		
RH+RH+RH+RH+RH	45 Gy	1.34
R+R+R+R+RH	46 Gy	1.31

[a] Overgaard, unpublished observations.
[b] Tumours were irradiated (R) and/or heated (H) as 5 fractions in 4 days. Combined treatments were given either simultaneously or sequentially (heat 4 hours after radiation).
[c] TCD-50 represents the radiation dose required to produce local tumour control in 50% of treated animals 90 days after treatment.
[d] Thermal enhancement ratios (TER) are the ratios of the radiation dose for radiation alone to that for radiation + heat.

in this respect involve either the use of hot water (SCHREIER et al, 1990) or ferromagnetic thermoseeds (BREZOVICH et al, 1990). In the former study, hot water was passed through 1.6 mm diameter stainless steel tubes implanted 10 or 14 mm apart in normal tissues of rabbits and pigs. With a water temperature of 48°C, tissue temperatures exceeding 42.5°C were possible. The thermoseed implantation procedure involves using ferromagnetic materials and implanting them in the tissue to be heated. The thermoseeds then heat the tissue as a result of the absorbed power from an externally applied electromagnetic induction field. This heat production by thermoseeds is strongly dependent on their magnetic properties and they lose their magnetic properties as a characteristic temperature, commonly referred to as the "Curie point", is approached. Thus, if the thermoseeds are made from a material having the appropriate Curie point one can control the temperature at the required level. With both the hot water and ferromagnetic thermoseed procedures preferential tumour heating should be possible and the heat administered at the same time as the radiation.

References

Arcangeli G, Nervi C, Cividalli A, Lovisolo GA, Mauro F (1984) The clinical use of experimental parameters to evaluate the response of combined heat (HT) and radiation (RT). In: Overgaard J (ed) Hyperthermic Oncology 1984, vol 1. Summary papers. Taylor & Francis, London, New York, Philadelphia, pp 329–332

Bowden GT, Kasunic M, Cress AE (1982) Thermal enhancement of X-ray-induced DNA crosslinking. Radiat Res 89: 203–208

Brezovich IA, Lilly MB, Meredith RF, Weppelmann B, Henderson RA, Brawner J, Salter MM (1990) Hyperthermia of pet animal tumours with self-regulating ferromagnetic thermoseeds. Int J Hyperthermia 6: 117–130

Clark EP, Dewey WC, Lett JT (1981) Recovery of CHO cells from hyperthermic potentiation to X rays: Repair of DNA and chromatin. Radiat Res 85: 302–313

Corry PM, Robinson S, Getz S (1977) Hyperthermic effects on DNA repair mechanisms. Radiology 123: 475–482

Dewey WC, Freeman ML, Raaphorst GP, Clark EP, Wong RSL, Highfield DP, Spiro IJ, Tomasovic SP, Denman DL, Coss RA (1980) Cell biology of hyperthermia and radiation. In: Meyn RE, Withers HR (eds) Radiation Biology in Cancer Research. Raven Press, New York, pp 589–621

Dewey WC, Thrall DE, Gillette EL (1977) Hyperthermia and radiation – a selective thermal effect on chronically hypoxic tumor cells *in vivo*. Int J Radiat Oncol Biol Phys 2: 99–103

Eddy HA (1980) Alterations in tumor microvasculature during hyperthermia. Radiology 137: 515–521

Field SB, Bleehen NM (1979) Hyperthermia in the treatment of cancer. Cancer Treat Rev 6: 63–94

Folkman J (1976) The vascularization of tumors. Sci Am 234: 58–73

Gerweck LE, Gillette EL, Dewey WC (1974) Killing of Chinese hamster cells *in vitro* by heating under hypoxic or aerobic conditions. Eur J Cancer 10: 691–693

Gerweck LE, Nygaard TG, Burlett M (1979) Response of cells to hyperthermia under acute and chronic hypoxic conditions. Cancer Res 39: 966–972

Gillette EL, Ensley BA (1979) Effect of heating order on radiation response of mouse tumor and skin. Int J Radiat Oncol Biol Phys 5: 209–213

Hahn GM (1974) Metabolic aspects of the role of hyperthermia in mammalian cell inactivation and their possible relevance to cancer treatment. Cancer Res 34: 3117–3123

Hahn GM (1982) Hyperthermia and Cancer. Plenum Press, New York

Hartson-Eaton M, Malcolm AW, Hahn GM (1984) Radiosensitivity and thermosensitization of thermotolerant Chinese hamster cells and RIF-1 tumors. Radiat Res 99: 175–184

Henderson BW, Waldow SM, Potter WR, Dougherty TJ (1985) Interaction of photodynamic therapy and hyperthermia: Tumor response and cell survival studies after treatment of mice *in vivo*. Cancer Res 45: 6071–6077

Henle KJ, Leeper DB (1976) Combinations of hyperthermia (40°, 45°C) with radiation. Radiology 121: 451–454

Henle KJ, Leeper DB (1977) The modification of radiation damage in CHO cells by hyperthermia at 40 and 45°C. Radiat Res 70: 415–424

Henle KJ, Leeper DB (1979) Interaction of sublethal and potentially lethal 45° – hyperthermia and radiation damage at 0, 20, 37 or 40°C. Eur J Cancer 15: 1387–1394

Hill RP (1987) Cellular basis of radiotherapy. In: Tannock IF, Hill RP (eds) The Basic Science of Oncology. Pergamon Press, New York, pp 237–255

Hill SA, Denekamp J (1978) The effect of vascular occlusion on the thermal sensitization of a mouse tumour. Br J Radiol 51: 997–1002

Hill SA, Denekamp J (1979) The response of six mouse tumours to combined heat and X-rays: Implications for therapy. Br J Radiol 52: 209–218

Hiraoka M, Hahn GM (1990) Changes in pH and blood flow induced by glucose, and their effects on hyperthermia with or without BCNU in RIF-1 tumours. Int J Hyperthermia 6: 97–103

Horsman MR, Chaplin DJ, Overgaard J (1991) The effect of combining flavone acetic acid and hyperthermia on the growth of a C3H mammary carcinoma *in vivo*. Int J Radiat Biol (in press)

Horsman MR, Christensen KL, Chaplin DJ, Overgaard J (1991) Improved treatment of tumours *in vivo* by combining the bioreductive drug RSU-1069, hydralazine and hyperthermia. In: Adams GE, Breccia A, Fielden EM, Wardman P (eds) Selective Activation of Drugs by Redox Processes. Nato ASI Series. Plenum Press, New York, pp 193–202

Horsman MR, Christensen KL, Overgaard J (1989) Hydralazine induced enhancement of hyperthermic damage in a C3H mammary carcinoma *in vivo*. Int J Hyperthermia 5: 123–136

Horsman MR, Overgaard J (1989) Thermal radiosensitization in animal tumors: The potential for therapeutic gain. In: Urano M, Douple EB (eds) Hyperthermia and Oncology, vol 2. VSP, The Netherlands, pp 113–145

Horsman MR, Overgaard J, Chaplin DJ (1988) The interaction between RSU-1069, hydralazine and hyperthermia in a C3H mammary carcinoma as assessed by tumour growth delay. Acta Oncol 27: 861–862

Hume SP, Field SB (1978) Hyperthermic sensitization of mouse intestine to damage by X-rays: The effect of sequence and temporal separation of the two treatments. Br J Radiol 51: 302–307

Jorritsma JBM, Konings AWT (1983) Inhibition of repair of radiation-induced strand breaks by hyperthermia, and its relationship to cell survival after hyperthermia alone. Int J Radiat Biol 43: 505–516

Kallinowsky F, Moehle R, Vaupel P (1989) Substantial enhancement of tumor hyperthermic response by tumor necrosis factor. In: Sugahara T, Saito M (eds) Hyperthermic Oncology 1988, vol 1. Taylor & Francis, London, pp 258–259

Kalmus J, Okunieff P, Vaupel P (1990) Dose-dependent effects of hydralazine on microcirculatory function and hyperthermic response of murine FSaII tumors. Cancer Res 50: 15–19

Kim JH, Hahn EW, Ahmed SA (1982) Combined hyperthermia and radiation therapy for malignant melanoma. Cancer 50: 478–482

Law MP (1979) Some effects of fractionation on the response of the mouse ear to combined heat and X rays. Radiat Res 80: 360–368

Law MP, Ahier RG (1982) A differential effect of prior heat treatment on the thermal enhancement of radiation damage in the ear of the mouse. Radiat Res 90: 628–637

Law MP, Ahier RG, Field SB (1977) The response of mouse skin to combined hyperthermia and X-rays. Int J Radiat Biol 32: 153–163

Law MP, Ahier RG, Field SB (1979) The effect of prior heat treatment on the thermal enhancement of radiation damage in the mouse ear. Br J Radiol 52: 315–321

Leeper D (1985) Molecular and cellular mechanisms of hyperthermia alone or combined with other modalities. In: Overgaard J (ed) Hyperthermic Oncology 1984, vol 2. Review Lectures, Symposium Summaries and Workshop Summaries. Taylor & Francis, London, pp 9–40

Levendag PD, Marijnissen HPA, de Ru VJ, Versteeg JAC, van Roon GC, Star WM (1988) Interaction of interstitial photodynamic therapy and interstitial hyperthermia in a rat rhabdomyosarcoma – a pilot study. Int J Radiat Oncol Biol Phys 14: 139–145

Lindegaard JC, Grau C, Overgaard J (1991) Effect of step-down heating on the interaction between heat and radiation in a C3H mammary carcinoma *in vivo*. Int J Radiat Biol (in press)

Lindegaard JC, Overgaard J (1987) Factors of importance for the development of the step-down heating effect in a C3H mammary carcinoma *in vivo*. Int J Hyperthermia 3: 79–92

Lindegaard JC, Overgaard J (1988) Effect of step-down heating on hyperthermic radiosensitization in an experimental tumor and a normal tissue *in vivo*. Radiother Oncol 11: 143–151

Lunec J, Hesselwood IP, Parker R, Leaper S (1981) Hyperthermic enhancement of radiation cell killing in HeLa S3 cells and its effect on the production and repair of DNA strand breaks. Radiat Res 85: 116–125

Marigold JCL, Hume SP (1982) Effect of prior hyperthermia on subsequent thermal enhancement of radiation damage in mouse intestine. Int J Radiat Biol 42: 509–516

Mills MD, Meyn RE (1981) Effects of hyperthermia on repair of radiation-induced DNA strand breaks. Radiat Res 87: 314–328

Mills MD, Meyn RE (1983) Hyperthermic potentiation of unrejoined DNA strand breaks following irradiation. Radiat Res 95: 327–338

Mitchel REJ, Birnboim HC (1985) Triggering of DNA strand breaks by 45°C hyperthermia and its influence on the repair of gamma-radiation damage in human white blood cells. Cancer Res 45: 2040–2045

Mittler S (1986) Effects of hyperthermia on radiation-induced chromosome breakage and loss in excision repair deficient Drosophila melanogaster. Int J Radiat Biol 50: 225–230

Miyakoshi J, Ikebuchi M, Furukawa M, Yamagata K, Sugahara T, Kano E (1979) Combined effects of X irradiation and hyperthermia (42 and 44°C) on Chinese hamster V-79 cells *in vitro*. Radiat Res 79: 77–88

Moulder JE, Rockwell S (1984) Hypoxic fractions of solid tumors. Int J Radiat Oncol Biol Phys 10: 695–712

Myers R, Field SB (1977) The response of the rat tail to combined heat and X-rays. Br J Radiol 50: 581–586

Nielsen OS (1981) Effect of fractionated hyperthermia on hypoxic cells *in vitro*. Int J Radiat Biol 39: 73–80

Nielsen OS (1984) Fractionated hyperthermia and thermotolerance. Danish Med Bull 31: 376–390

Nielsen OS, Overgaard J, Kamura T (1983) Influence of thermotolerance on the interaction between hyperthermia and radiation in a solid tumour *in vivo*. Br J Radiol 56: 267–273

Overgaard J (1980) Simultaneous and sequential hyperthermia and radiation treatment of an experimental tumor and its surrounding normal tissue *in vivo*. Int J Radiat Oncol Biol Phys 6: 1507–1515

Overgaard J (1981) Fractionated radiation and hyperthermia experimental and clinical studies. Cancer 48: 1116–1123

Overgaard J (1982) Influence of sequence and interval on the biological response to combined hyperthermia and radiation. NCI Mono 61: 325–332

Overgaard J (1984) Time-temperature relationship for hyperthermic cytotoxicity and radiosensitization implications for a thermal dose unit. In: Overgaard J (ed), Hyperthermic Oncology 1984, vol 1. Taylor & Francis, London, pp 191–194

Overgaard J (1985) Rationale and problems in the design of clinical trials. In: Overgaard J (ed) Hyperthermic Oncology 1984, vol 2. Review Lectures, Symposium Summaries and Workshop Summaries. Taylor & Francis, London, pp 325–338

Overgaard J (1987) The design of clinical trials in hyperthermia. In: Field SB, Franconi C (eds) Physics and Technology of Hyperthermia. Martinus Nijhoff, Amsterdam, pp 598–620

Overgaard J (1989a) The current and potential role of hyperthermia in radiotherapy. Int J Radiat Oncol Biol Phys 16: 535–549

Overgaard J (1989b) Combined hyperthermia and radiation treatment of malignant melanoma. In: Sugahara T (ed) Hyperthermic Oncology 1988, vol 2. Special Plenary Lectures, Plenary Lectures, and Symposium and Workshop Summaries, Taylor & Francis, London, pp 464–467

Overgaard J (1989c) Sensitization of hypoxic tumour cells – clinical experience. Int J Radiat Biol 56: 801–811

Overgaard J, Bichel P (1977) The influence of hypoxia and acidity on the hyperthermic response of malignant cells *in vitro*. Radiology 123: 511–514

Overgaard J, Nielsen OS (1980) The role of tissue environmental factors on the kinetics and morphology of tumor cells exposed to hyperthermia. Ann NY Acad Sci 335: 254–280

Overgaard J, Nielsen OS (1983) The importance of thermotolerance for the clinical treatment with hyperthermia. Radiother Oncol 1: 167–178

Overgaard J, Nielsen OS (1984) Influence of thermotolerance on the effect of combined hyperthermia and radiation in a C3H mammary carcinoma *in vivo*. In: Overgaard J (ed) Hyperthermic Oncology 1984, vol 1. Summary papers, Taylor & Francis, London, pp 227–230

Overgaard J, Nielsen OS, Lindegaard JC (1987) Biological basis for rational design of clinical treatment with combined hyperthermia and radiation. In: Field SB, Franconi C (eds) Physics and Technology of Hyperthermia. Martinus Nijhoff, Amsterdam, pp 54–79

Overgaard J, Overgaard M (1987) Hyperthermia as an adjuvant to radiotherapy in the treatment of malignant melanoma. Int J Hyperthermia 3: 483–501

Padovani A, Cividalli A, Della Torre A, Galloni L, Mauro F (1987) The effect of step-down heating on murine tumour tissue after fractionated X-ray treatments. Int J Hyperthermia 3: 585–586

Peterson HI (1979) Tumor blood flow compared with normal tissue blood flow. In: Peterson HI (ed) Tumor Blood Circulation: Angiogenesis Vascular Morphology and Blood Flow of Experimental and Human Tumors. CRC Press Inc., Boca Raton, Florida, USA, pp 103–114

Power JA, Harris JW (1977) Response of extremely hypoxic cells to hyperthermia: Survival and oxygen enhancement ratios. Radiat Biol 123: 767–770

Raaphorst GP (1989) Thermal radiosensitization *in vitro*. In: Urano M, Douple EB (eds) Hyperthermia and Oncology, vol. 2. VSP, The Netherlands, pp 17–51

Raaphorst GP, Azzam EI (1984) A comparative study of heat and/or radiation sensitivity of V79 cells synchronized by three different methods. In: Overgaard J (ed) Hyperthermic Oncology 1984, vol 1. Summary papers. Taylor & Francis, London, pp 301–304

Radford IR (1983) Effects of hyperthermia on the repair of X-ray induced DNA double strand breaks in mouse L cells. Int J Radiat Biol 43: 551–557

Reinhold HS (1988) Physiological effects of hyperthermia. In: Issels RD, Wilmanns W (eds) Recent Results in Cancer Research: Application of Hyperthermia in the Treatment of Cancer, vol 107. Springer, Berlin, Heidelberg, New York, Tokyo, pp 32–43

Reinhold HS, Blackiewicz B, Berg-Blok A (1978) Decrease in tumor microcirculation during hyperthermia. In: Streffer C, van Beuningen D, Dietzel F (eds) Cancer Therapy by Hyperthermia and Radiation. Urban Schwarzenberg, Baltimore, pp 231–232

Rhee JG, Song CW, Lewitt SH (1984) Thermosensitizing effect of heat-induced vascular damage. In: Overgaard J (ed) Hyperthermic Oncology 1984, vol 1. Summary papers. Taylor & Francis, London, pp 153–156

Schreier K, Budihna M, Lesnicar H, Handl-Zeller L, Hand JW, Prior MV, Clegg ST, Brezovich IA (1990) Preliminary studies of interstitial hyperthermia using hot water. Int J Hyperthermia 6: 431–444

Song CW (1984) Effect of local hyperthermia on blood flow and microenvironment: A review. Cancer Res 44: 4721–4730

Song CW, Kang MS, Rhee JG, Levitt SH (1980) The effect of hyperthermia on vascular function, pH, and cell survival. Radiology 137: 795–803

Song CW, Patten MS, Chelstrom LM, Rhee JG, Levitt SM (1987) Effect of multiple heatings on the blood flow in RIF-1 tumours, skin and muscle of C3H mice. Int J Hyperthermia 3: 535–545

Stewart FA, Denekamp J (1977) Sensitization of mouse skin to X-irradiation by moderate heating. Radiology 123: 195–200

Stewart FA, Denekamp J (1978) The therapeutic advantage of combined heat and X-rays on a mouse fibrosarcoma. Br J Radiol 51: 307–316

Stewart FA, Denekamp J (1980) Fractionation studies with combined X-rays and hyperthermia *in vivo*. Br J Radiol 53: 346–356

Stewart FA, Denekamp J (1982) Loss of therapeutic advantage for combined heat and X-rays with fractionation. NCI mono 61: 291–293

Suit HD (1975) Hyperthermia in the treatment of tumours. In: Proceedings of the International Symposium on Cancer Therapy by Hyperthermia and Radiation. April 28–30, American College of Radiology, Washington, pp 107–114

Suit HD, Gerweck LE (1979) Potential for hyperthermia and radiation therapy. Cancer Res 39: 2290–2298

Thrall DE, Gillette EL, Dewey WC (1975) Effect of heat and ionizing radiation on normal and neoplastic tissue of the C3H mouse. Radiat Res 63: 363–377

Urano M, Douple EB (1989) Hyperthermia and Oncology, vol 3, Interstitial Hyperthermia. VSP, The Netherlands

Urano M, Gerweck LE, Epstein R, Cunningham M, Suit, HD (1980) Response of a spontaneous murine tumor to hyperthermia: Factors which modify the thermal response *in vivo*. Radiat Res 83: 312–322

Urano M, Maher J, Rice LC, Kahn J (1982) Response of spontaneous murine tumors to hyperthermia: Temperature dependence in two different-sized tumors. NCI mono 61: 299–301

Urano M, Montoya V, Booth A (1983) Effect of hyperglycemia on the thermal response of murine normal and tumor tissue. Cancer Res 43: 453–455

Vaupel P (1979) Oxygen supply to malignant tumors. In: Peterson HI (ed) Tumor Blood Circulation: Angiogenesis, Vascular Morphology and Blood Flow of Experimental and Human Tumors. CRC Press Inc, Boca Raton, Florida, USA, pp 143–168

Vaupel P, Kallinowski F (1987) Physiological effects of hyperthermia. In: Streffer C (ed) Hyperthermia and the Therapy of Malignant Tumors. Springer, Berlin, Heidelberg, New York, Tokyo, pp 71–109

Vaupel P, Kallinowski F, Okunieff P (1989) Blood flow, oxygen and nutrient supply, and metabolic micro-environment of human tumors: a review. Cancer Res 49: 6449–6465

Vaupel P, Müller-Kliesser W, Otte J, Manz R, Kallinowski F (1983) Blood flow, tissue oxygenation, and pH-distribution in malignant tumors upon localized hyperthermia. Basic pathophysiological aspects and the role of various thermal doses. Strahlentherapie 159: 73–81

Waldow SM, Dougherty TJ (1984) Interaction of hyperthermia and photoradiation therapy. Radiat Res 97: 380–385

Wallen CA, Colby TV, Stewart JR (1986) Cell kill and tumour control after heat treatment with and without vascular occlusion in RIF-1 tumours. Radiat Res 106: 215–223

Watanabe N, Niitsu Y, Umeno H, Kuriyama H, Neda H, Yamauchi N, Maeda M, Urushizaki I (1988) Toxic effect of tumor necrosis factor on tumor vasculature in mice. Cancer Res 48: 2179–2183

Westra A, Dewey WC (1971) Variation in sensitivity to heat shock during the cell-cycle of Chinese hamster cells *in vitro*. Int J Radiat Biol 19: 467–477

Wike-Hooley JL, Haveman J, Reinhold HS (1984) The relevance of tumor pH to the treatment of malignant disease. Radiother Oncol 2: 343–366

Wondergem J, Haveman J (1984) A study of the effects of prior heat treatment on the skin reaction of mouse feet after heat alone or combined with X-rays: Influence of misonidazole. Radiother Oncol 2: 159–170

3

Local Hyperthermia in Combination with Chemotherapeutic Agents*

M. Urano[1], *J. Kahn*[2], and *H. Majima*[1]

[1] Department of Radiation Medicine, University of Kentucky Medical Center, Kentucky, U.S.A.
[2] Department of Radiation Medicine, Massachusetts General Hospital, Boston, Massachusetts, U.S.A.

Introduction

It has been demonstrated that the cytotoxic effect of some chemotherapeutic agents is enhanced at elevated temperatures (JOHNSON and PAVELEC, 1973, HAHN, 1978). As early as 1960 a clinical trial of combined hyperthermia and drug perfusions was performed on the patients with head and neck tumors (WOODHALL et al, 1960). The combined use of hyperthermia and chemotherapeutic agents has been extensively studied since the early 1970s. JOHNSON and PAVELEC (1973) demonstrated that the effect of an alkylating agent, thio-TEPA, on Chinese hamster fibroblasts was enhanced at elevated temperatures *in vitro*. The mechanism of this enhancement appeared to be due to an increased rate constant of alkylation at elevated temperatures. HAHN and his colleagues (1975) have demonstrated thermal enhancement of cytotoxicity of various agents and proposed additional mechanisms of thermal enhancement.

Thermal enhancement of the cytotoxic effect of various agents has been shown in animal tumors by many investigators following systemic or local hyperthermia (MARMAR et al, 1979; ROSE et al, 1979; ALBERTS et al, 1980; DAHL and MELLA, 1982; HERMAN and TEICHER, 1988). Investigations of the mechanism of action have provided the biological basis to the thermochemotherapy. In addition to these studies, critical factors for its clinical trials may include (a) type of administration: systemic or local, (b) timing of administration: which should be given first or simultaneous, (c) concentration of the agent, (d) temperature and treatment time of hyperthermia, and (e) speed of drug administration: quick *iv* shot or continuous infusion. This review paper will discuss these critical factors as well as the mechanisms of thermal chemosensitization.

* This study was partially supported by a grant CA26350 awarded by National Cancer Institute, DHHS.

Mechanism of thermal enhancement

Several mechanisms for the thermal enhancement of cytotoxicity of chemotherapeutic agents have been proposed, including increased rate constant, increased uptake of drugs and inhibition of repair of chemically induced potentially lethal or sublethal damage at elevated temperatures (HAHN et al, 1975). In addition, membrane-acting agents may share the target with hyperthemia which might cause damage to membrane-proteins with a resultant increase in cell-death (HAHN et al, 1977; GEORGE and SINGH, 1982).

The increased rate constant at elevated temperatures was first shown by JOHNSON and PAVELEC (1973) in the thermal enhancement of thio-TEPA, an alkylating agent. He obtained cell survival curves as a function of treatment time with thio-TEPA at various temperatures. An Arrhenius plot between the reciprocal of the D_0 value (min^{-1}) and the reciprocal of the absolute treatment temperature (T^{-1}) was analysed. The D_0 value was the treatment time to reduce survival from s to s/e in the exponential portion of the survival curve and was considered to be proportional to the rate constant of chemical reactions involved in drug cytotoxicity. Accordingly, the slope of the Arrhenius plot gave the activation energy which was found to be approximately 35 kcal/M for thio-TEPA at the temperature below 41°C. Above 41°C, hyperthermia *per se* can cause lethal damage to mammalian cells and the activation energy increases as a result of the addition of direct thermal cell killing on the thermal enhancement of drug cytotoxicity.

HAHN (1978) analysed activation energies for three nitrosoureas, which were slightly greater than the activation energy for alkylation at temperatures between 37 and 43°C. These activation energies were constant in the temperature range from 37 to 43°C.

A biochemical study on the action of an alkylating agent at 37 and 42°C demonstrated that the average number of DNA single-strand breaks (SSB) induced by an alkylating agent, methyl methanesulfonate, was increased at 42°C compared to that at 37°C (BRONK et al, 1973). These authors also investigated rejoining of SSB after heating at 37 or 42°C. Substantial rejoining of SSB was observed after 37°C treatment, while the rejoining was insignificant after 42°C treatment. This result suggested that hyperthermia at 42°C induced more SSB than the treatment at 37°C and inhibited the rejoining of DNA-SSB. It is likely that 42°C induces protein denaturation, thus inactivating the repair enzymes. Inhibition of repair is also reported by LONGO et al (1983). However, it is unknown if this type of repair inhibition can be observed at temperatures below 42°C.

MURRAY et al (1984) studied the induction of cross-links in a murine fibrosarcoma treated with cyclophosphamide (CY), an alkylating agent, which must be activated *in vivo*. Tumors which were treated with CY at 41.5°C were used for alkaline elution studies. They observed an increased production of DNA-DNA cross-links after treatment with CY at 41.5°C, with no significant repair of DNA damage. Increased production of interstrand cross-links was also demonstrated following nitrosourea treatment (TOFILON et al, 1985).

Recently, URANO et al (1988, 1989, 1990a) performed an Arrhenius plot analysis for four different agents (cis-diamminedichloroplatinum (II); cis-DDP, Bleomycin; BLM, 1,3 bis(2-chloroethyl)-N-nitrosourea; BCNU, and

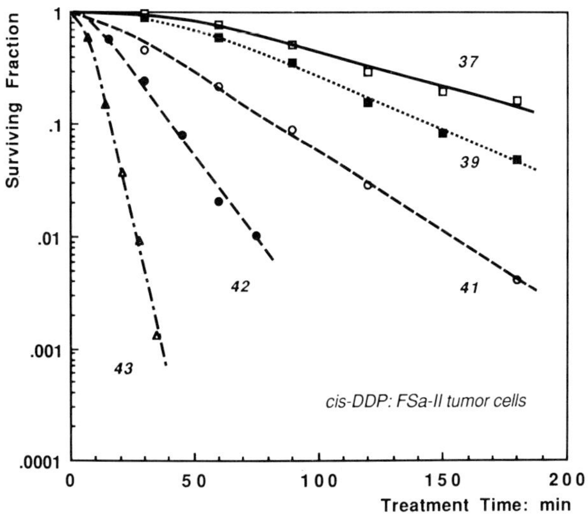

Fig. 1. Cell survival curves for FSa-II tumor cells treated *in vitro* with 2μM cis-DDP at various temperatures. Cell survival is plotted as a function of treatment time. Treatment temperatures (°C) are indicated in the figure

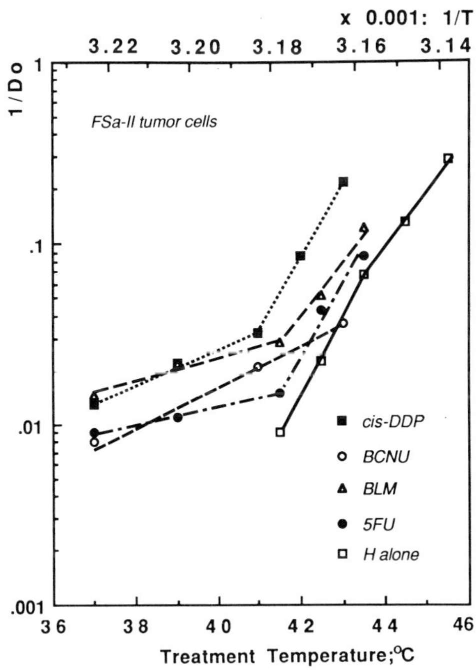

Fig. 2. Arrhenius plots for various chemotherapeutic agents (cis-DDP, BCNU, BLM and 5FU) and for hyperthermia alone. Cells are FSa-II tumor cells treated at pH 7.4. Activation energies are listed in Table 1

5 fluorouracil; 5FU) using a mouse fibrosarcoma cell line, FSa-II. An increased rate constant has been observed for all agents tested. Cell survival curves as a function of treatment time with cis-DDP at elevated temperatures are shown in Fig. 1. It indicates a decrease in the D_0 values with increasing temperatures. Arrhenius plots for these four agents, together with that for heat alone, are

shown in Fig. 2 which indicates various activation energies at temperatures between 37.0 and 41 (or 41.5)°C and a presence of a breaking point at 41 (or 41.5)°C with an exception of BCNU. At temperatures above 41 (or 41.5)°C, the slopes of the Arrhenius plots were almost parallel to the slope for hyperthermia alone. Although the Arrhenius plot may be modified by other factors, such as altered drug uptake or repair inhibition by heat, these results suggest that the increased rate constant at elevated temperatures might be one of the significant mechanisms not only for alkylating agents but also for some antibiotics (BLM), antimetabolites (5FU) and platinum compounds (cis-DDP).

The mechanism of action of cis-DDP is the binding of the agent to DNA with a formation of *intra*strand cross-links, unlike alkylating agents which form *inter*strand cross-links (Pinto and Lippard, 1985; Reed et al, 1987). An investigation of molecular mechanisms responsible for the thermal enhancement of cis-DDP cytotoxicity demonstrated that a greater amount of DNA cross-links was observed in cells treated at 43°C compared to cells treated at 37°C (Meyn et al, 1980). Their comparison of the amount of cross-links with thermal enhancement of cell survival showed that the cytotoxicity of cis-DDP was enhanced by a factor of 10 at 43°C over 37°C, whereas the increase of cross-links was by a factor of 6.5. These results may indicate that an increased rate constant at elevated temperatures is not a single mechanism of thermal enhancement. It is also likely that, as these authors postulated, the increased drug uptake is the major mechanism of thermal enhancement of cis-DDP cytotoxicity (Eichholtz-Wirth and Hietel, 1986). The repair of cross-links was not observed in this study. Furthermore, a difference in the enhancement factors between cell survival and cross-links may suggest an involvement of two or more different mechanisms in the thermal enhancement. Brouwer et al (1982) demonstrated that the amount of platinum bound to DNA increased with increasing temperatures. This is also supported by Herman et al (1989). Albert et al (1980) indicated an increased uptake of cis-DDP at elevated temperatures, which might have resulted in a greater observed activation energy than the activation energy which is solely due to the increased rate constant. It has been shown at 37°C that the uptake of cis-DDP is well correlated with cellular drug sensitivity (Eichholtz-Wirth and Hietel, 1986). These studies suggest that at least both increased rate constant for cross-links and increased drug uptake are involved in the thermal enhancement of cis-DDP cytotoxicity.

It was postulated that thermal enhancement of BLM cytotoxicity is due to the inhibition of BLM-induced potentially lethal damage (Braun and Hahn, 1975). It has been shown that BLM induces strand breaks in DNA (Terasima et al, 1970). Meyn et al (1979) investigated the relationship between the production of strand breaks and cell survival, and reported that strand breaks produced at 43°C were more effective on cell-killing compared to those produced at 37°C. They further observed inhibition of the repair of strand breaks at 43°C while strand breaks produced at 37°C were rapidly repaired. Chapman et al (1983) reported that DNA-BLM interaction was significantly higher at 43°C than at 37°C. Smith et al (1986) demonstrated inhibition of the repair of DNA damage at 44°C. These experiments suggest that the repair inhibition of DNA damage and increased rate constant in the DNA-BLM interaction at 43°C may be significant factors for the thermal enhancement of BLM cytotoxicity.

It must be pointed out that biochemical studies on the mechanism of thermal enhancement were performed at temperatures above 42.0°C at which hyperthermia *per se* can produce lethal damage in mammalian cells. It must be asked if the same mechanisms operate at temperatures below 41.0°C which gives no lethal damage to mammalian cells.

A single activation energy was found for BCNU at temperatures between 37.0 and 43.0°C (HAHN, 1978; URANO et al, in press), while Arrhenius plots for other agents showed a breaking point at 41 or 41.5°C. This may be due to a specific mechanism of BCNU alkylation; namely, nitrosoureas are decomposed in aqueous media (WEINKAN and DEEN, 1982) and highly reactive intermediates lead to bifunctional alkylation (KAHN et al, 1981). Our study suggests that the rate of decomposition increases with increasing temperatures. It is likely that the two-steps in the mechanism of action, decomposition of this agent and alkylation or DNA cross-links, lead to a constant activation energy between 37 and 43°C for BCNU.

Limited studies have been performed on the mechanism of thermal enhancement of various chemotherapeutic agents. Several studies have focused on the uptake and cytotoxicity of adriamycin at elevated temperatures. Studies by HAHN et al (1975) demonstrated that cells exposed to 43°C contained a higher average amount of adriamycin/cell compared to cells exposed to 37°C. BATES and MACKILLOP (1986) observed that the magnitude of the increase in intracellular drug level at elevated temperatures was insufficient to account for increased cytotoxicity at these temperatures. This study also suggests an involvement of multiple mechanisms in thermal chemosensitization. Furthermore, a question is whether this increased uptake can be observed at temperatures below 43.0°C.

Effect of thermochemotherapy on animal tumors

Many investigations have been performed on the anti-tumor effect of combined chemotherapy and hyperthermia in various animal-tumor systems (see ENGELHARDT, 1987 for summary). Table 2 summarizes drugs which are significantly or not significantly enhanced at elevated temperatures *in vitro* and/or *in vivo*. In this section we will focus on our studies using C3Hf/Sed mouse FSa-II tumors which originated from a spontaneous fibrosarcoma in the same strain of mouse (URANO and KIM, 1983; URANO et al, 1985, 1988, 1989, 1990a) since it is extremely difficult to gather data derived from experiments using numerous animal-tumor systems in a limited space.

CY, an alkylating agent, was first selected because thermal enhancement of many alkylating agents had been demonstrated and the plasma half time of this agent was longer compared to other agents. Tumors were transplanted into the subcutaneous tissue of the murine foot and treated in a constant temperature water bath when they reached an average diameter of 4 mm (35 mm^3). TG (tumor growth) time, i.e., the time required for one-half of the treated tumors to reach 1000 mm^3 from the initial treatment day was used as

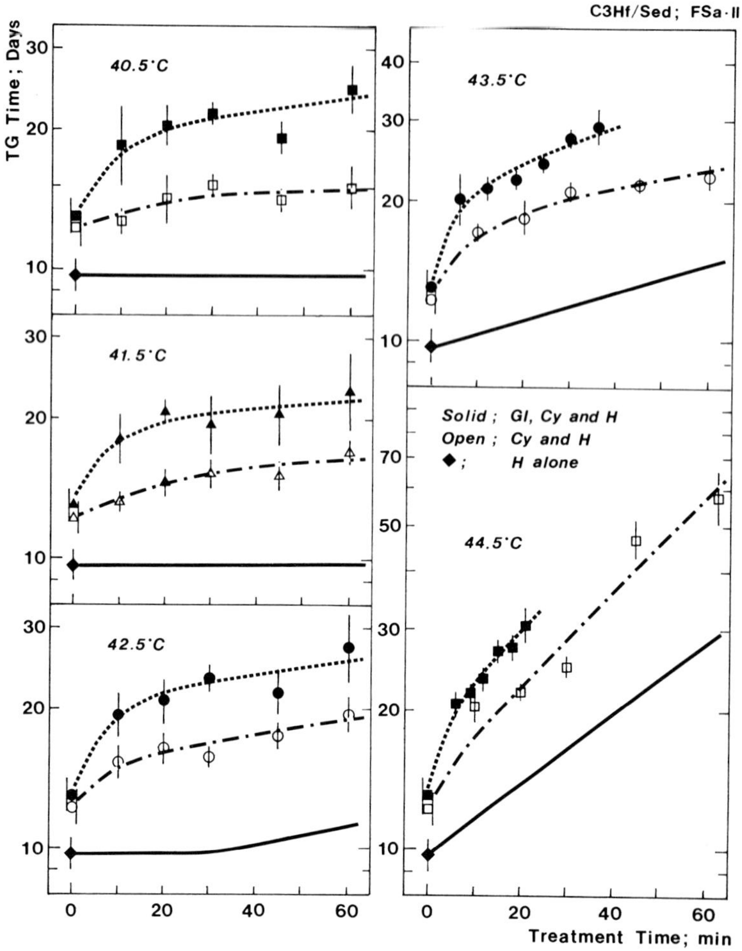

Fig. 3. Tumor response to combined CY (200 mg/kg) and heat treatments. TG (tumor growth) time of FSa-II tumors from treatment day to reach 1000 mm^3 is plotted as a function of treatment time at elevated temperatures. Solid symbols indicate that glucose (5 g/kg) was administered before combined CY and heat treatments

an endpoint. In an experiment shown in Fig. 3, animals with a tumor received an ip injection of 200 mg/kg CY 30 minutes before hyperthermia given at temperatures between 40.5 and 44.5°C, and the TG time was plotted as a function of treatment time at elevated temperatures (URANO et al, 1985). Solid lines indicate the effect of hyperthermia alone. A CY dose of 200 mg/kg prolonged the TG time from 9.8 to 13 days. Further prolongation was observed with increasing treatment time, but it reached a maximum at 40.5 and 41.5°C after 30 minutes treatment. At temperatures above 42.5°C, heat itself prolonged the TG time and the magnitude of this prolongation increased with increasing temperatures. In spite of this prolongation, the magnitude of thermal enhancement appeared to be identical at temperatures above 41.5°C. These results indicated that the effect of CY was enhanced at temperatures between 40.5 and 44.5°C, but the anti-tumor effect of heat itself contributed to this combined effect at temperatures above 42.5°C.

Solid symbols with dotted lines indicate that a glucose dose of 5 g/kg was administered *ip* 60 minutes before hyperthermia. An *ip* injection of glucose increases synthesis and release of insulin which facilitates all pathways of glycolysis. Tumors undergo active glycolysis and further addition of glucose facilitates glycolysis, resulting in an accumulation of lactic acid which reduces tumor tissue pH (GULLINO et al, 1965). Another effect of an *ip* administration of glucose is to increase blood viscosity and to decrease blood flow (CALDERWOOD and DICKSON, 1980; VON ARDEN and REITNAUER, 1980; WARD and JAIN, 1988). This effect may contribute to prolonged accumulation of the drug in the tumor tissue. As a result, a further prolongation of the TG time was observed. These studies on CY suggested that cytotoxic effect of some chemotherapeutic agents could be enhanced at relatively low temperatures and that of some chemotherapeutic agents might be more substantially enhanced at low tissue pH.

Fig. 4 summarizes the tumor response curves of our FSa-II tumors treated with five different drugs. The TG time is plotted as a function of drug dose. Animals received an *ip* injection of each drug at room temperature (RT) or animal tumors were immersed into a 41.5°C water bath for 60 minutes immediately after *ip* injection of each drug. The treatment temperature of 41.5°C was selected because (a) the experiment of CY and the cell survival curves at various temperatures (shown in Figs. 1 and 3) indicated that the cytotoxicity of many chemotherapeutic agents was enhanced at relatively low temperatures, (b) this treatment at 41.5°C for 60 minutes *per se* does not cause thermal cell killing and (c) this temperature was acceptable for whole body hyperthermia. Maximum drug dose used in each drug experiment was the highest tolerable dose in animals (approximately LD_5).

Anti-tumor effects of cis-DDP, CY, BLM, 5FU, and BCNU were investigated. The activation energies of these agents, with an exception of CY, have been investigated using the same tumor cell line *in vitro* as shown in Fig. 2. These two series of experiments allowed a comparison between *in vitro* and *in vivo* data. Sensitivity to a chemotherapeutic agent depends on cell lines. For example, 6μM cis-DDP to our Chinese hamster ovary (CHO) cells induced a similar cell killing effect as 2μM dose to our FSa-II tumor cells (URANO et al, 1990a, 1990b). FSa-II tumor cells showed a strong sensitivity to cis-DDP and 5-FU, moderate sensitivity to CY and BCNU at room temperature (no hyperthermia). The tumor response to BLM reached a maximum at a BLM dose of ~10 mg/kg. The tumor response to these agents were enhanced when animal tumors were treated at 41.5°C for 60 minutes immediately after drug injection. The thermal enhancement ratio (TER), if expressed as a ratio of the slope of the dose response curve at 41.5°C to the slope at room temperature (RT) of dose-response curves, was largest for CY followed by BCNU, cis-DDP, BLM, and 5FU. The TER values were 2.4, 2.0, 1.7, 1.5, and 1.0 for CY, BCNU, cis-DDP, BLM, and 5FU, respectively. It is of interest that the order of the magnitude of thermal chemosensitization for these agents (with an exception of CY) is well

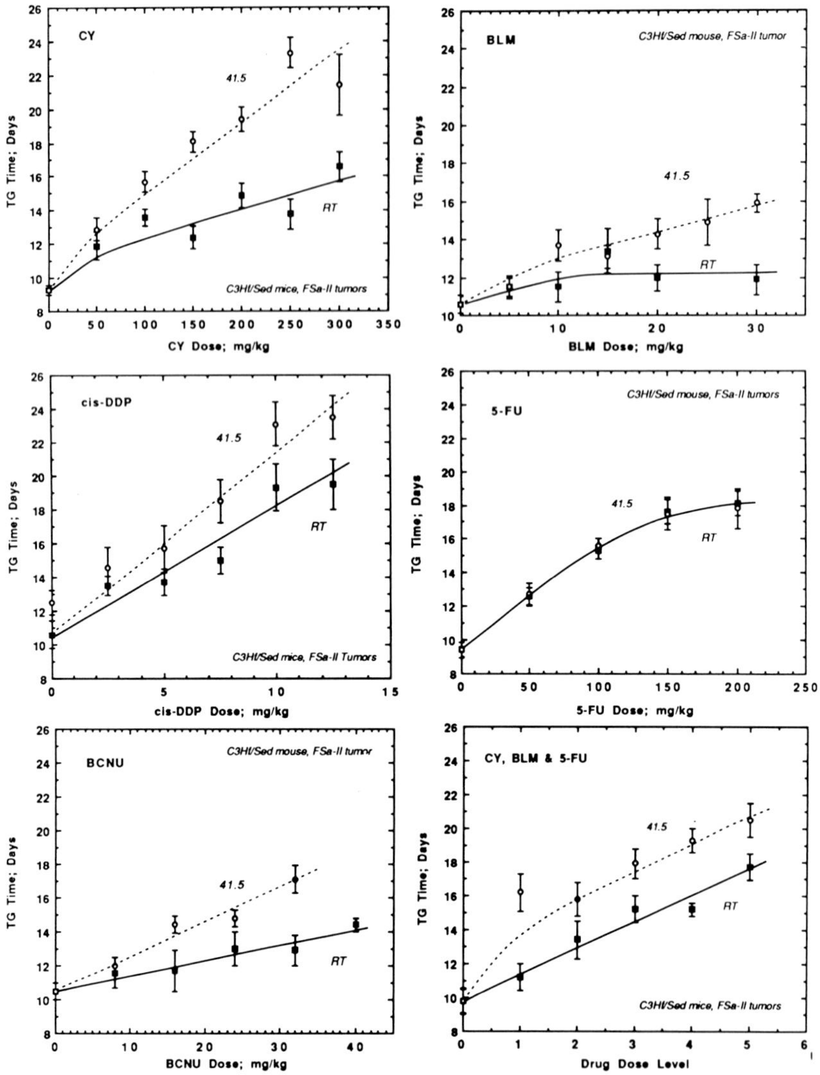

Fig. 4. Response of FSa-II tumors to combined chemotherapy and hyperthermia (at 41.5°C). The TG time is plotted as a function of drug dose. RT indicates that animals received drug alone at room temperature. Drugs are CY, cis-DDP, BCNU, BLM and 5FU. Right bottom panel indicates multiple drugs (CY, BLM + 5FU)

correlated with the order of the magnitude of activation energies for these agents, including 5FU which showed a minimum activation energy and insignificant sensitization (see Table 1).

On the bottom panel of the right-hand side in the figure, results of a trial with multi-drug treatment are shown. Maximum doses used were 100 mg/kg CY, 15 mg/kg BLM and 75 mg/kg 5FU. Strong

Table 1. Activation energies reported for various chemotherapeutic agents at pH 7.4

<table>
<tr><th rowspan="2">Drug</th><th rowspan="2">Cell Line</th><th colspan="2">Activation Energies (kcal/M)</th></tr>
<tr><th>37–41 (or 41.5)°C</th><th>41(41.5)–43 (or 43.5)°C</th></tr>
<tr><td>Thio-TEPA</td><td>C.H. V strain</td><td>33–37</td><td>185</td></tr>
<tr><td>BCNU</td><td>HA</td><td colspan="2">40</td></tr>
<tr><td>BCNU</td><td>FSa-II</td><td colspan="2">51 ± 5</td></tr>
<tr><td>Bleomycin</td><td>FSa-II</td><td>35 ± 6</td><td>165 ± 15</td></tr>
<tr><td>5-Fluorouracil</td><td>FSa-II</td><td>23 ± 3</td><td>175 ± 21</td></tr>
<tr><td>cis-DDP</td><td>FSa-II</td><td>44 ± 5</td><td>191 ± 0</td></tr>
<tr><td>Heat alone</td><td>FSa-II</td><td>—</td><td>200 ± 10</td></tr>
</table>

enhancement was observed with the combination of low doses. The maximum enhancement due to combined treatment appeared to be the sum of the effects of these three agents. However, further studies are needed to obtain an advantage of multi-drug treatments over the single agent.

For *in vivo* thermochemotherapy, a critical factor may be the biological half-life in plasma and/or tumor tissue of each agent. Most chemotherapeutic agents show a short plasma half-life, mostly 10–15 minutes or less. Our experiment (URANO et al, 1990a) showed that no thermal enhancement of cis-DDP was obtained by continuous infusion, although a single quick injection and multiple quick injections resulted in thermal chemosensitization. This experiment indicates that high peak drug concentration in plasma or tissue drug concentration is essential for thermal chemosensitization. This is in agreement with an *in vitro* study by WALLNER and LI (1987).

The effect of treatment intervals between drug administration and hyperthermia has been studied by several investigators. In general, a drug given immediately before hyperthermia is most effective and the thermal enhancement of the drug cytotoxicity decreases rapidly with increasing intervals between drug administration and hyperthermia. If a drug is administered after hyperthermia (even given immediately after hyperthermia), no thermal enhancement is usually observed except for cis-DDP (DAHL and MELLA, 1983; URANO et al, 1985, 1990a). These results indicate that drug(s) except cis-DDP must be present during the time of hyperthermia. It is unknown whether the synergistic effect observed for cis-DDP given immediately after hyperthermia is due to thermal enhancement of cis-DDP cytotoxicity or cis-DDP enhancement of thermal damage. It is likely that the repair process of heat-induced damage interacts with cis-DDP-induced damage. Synergistic action of post-hyperthermic administration has not been reported for any other chemotherapeutic agents *in vivo*, although experiments *in vitro* show post-hyperthermic sensitization of the cytotoxicity of BLM and BCNU (MORGAN et al, 1979). On the other hand, OSBORNE and MACKILLOP (1987) observed that membrane permeability to adriamycin was significantly decreased after hyperthermia.

Interaction between thermotolerance and thermal chemosensitization

Thermotolerance is a phenomenon which cells or tissues treated with hyperthermia become resistant to subsequent heat treatment. It develops very rapidly, reaches a maximum within 8–24 hours and decays slowly over 72 hours or longer. The kinetics of thermotolerance has been studied in cultured cells, and in animal tumors and normal tissues (see review papers: HENLE and DETHLEFSEN, 1978; URANO, 1986). Questions are (a) if thermotolerant cells are also resistant to chemotherapeutic agents and (b) if the cytotoxic effect of chemotherapeutic agents to thermotolerant cells is equally enhanced by subsequent hyperthermia. MAJIMA et al (1988a, 1988b) tested the effect of treatment interval between hyperthermia and cis-DDP or BLM. Simultaneous administrations showed, as expected, a thermal chemosensitization. With increasing treatment intervals, this sensitization was lost, and the effect of both agents became additive. In other words, thermotolerant cells are not resistant to chemotherapeutic agents. If thermotolerant cells were treated with combined heat and drug treatments, the

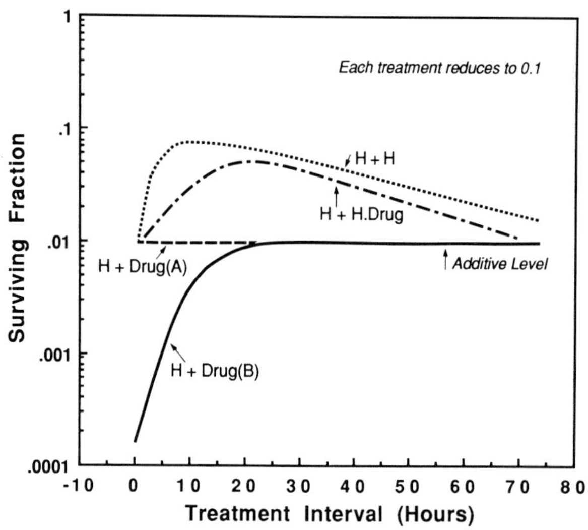

Fig. 5. Schematic illustrations of the effect of preheating on the subsequent treatments given with various treatment intervals. It is assumed that each treatment reduces survival to 0.1. Preheating followed by second heat (H + H) shows a development and decay of thermotolerance. If the preheating is followed by simultaneous treatment of drug and heat (H + H.Drug), cells show resistance to second treatment and the kinetics of this resistance may be similar to the kinetics of thermotolerance. If the preheating is followed by drug alone, most drugs show additive effect (H + Drug (A)). Cytotoxicity of some drugs such as cis-DDP may be enhanced by preheating, although this enhancement may rapidly decay to additive level (H + Drug (B)). There may be another type which shows a resistance when a drug was given immediately following hyperthermia and soon follows an additive line. If drugs shown as Drug (B) are combined with second heat, some enhanced cell killing may be observed at time 0 which soon follows the "H + H.Drug" curve

Table 2. Drugs which are significantly or not significantly enhanced at elevated temperatures

A. Drugs which are enhanced at elevated temperatures
  a. Alkylating agents (probably all)
    Cyclophospamide (Cytoxan)
    Thio-TEPA [tris (1-aziridinyl)-phosphine sulfide]
    Melphalan (phenylalanine mustard, L-PAM)
    Nitrosourea [1,3-bis(-2-chloroethyl)-N-nitrosourea; BCNU (carmustine), CCNU (domustin), methy-CCNU]
    Chlorambucil
    (Mitomycin C – this is an antibiotic, but the mechanism is alkylation)
  b. Antimetabolites (probably none)
  c. Antibiotics
    Bleomycin
    Actinomycin D
    Adriamycin
    Daunorubicin
    Mitoxantrone
    Quelamycin
    Mitomycin C
  d. Vinca Alkaloids
    Vincristine
  e. Others
    Cis-diamminedichloroplatinum (cis-DDP) and related compounds
    Misonidazole (Nitroimidazole group: hypoxic cell sensitizers)
    Hydralazine (decreases blood flow)

B. Drugs which show synergistic effect with hyperthermia
  a. Membrane-acting agents
    Amphotericin B
    Chlorpromazine
    Polyamines
  b. Some biological response modifiers

C. Drugs which are not significantly enhanced at elevated temperatures
  a. Alkylating agents (probably none)
  b. Antimetabolites (probably most)
    5-fluorouracil (5FU)
    Methotrexate (MTX)
    Flurordeoxyuridine (FUdR)
  c. Antibiotics
    Aclocinomycin
  d. Vinka alkaloid
    Vinblastine (may be slightly enhanced)
  e. Others
    Hydroxyurea
    Steroid hormones

cytotoxicity of the drug was enhanced by the 2nd heat treatment. However, the treatment interval between the 1st heat and combined 2nd treatment (2nd heat and drug) was critical for overall effectiveness. If 1st and 2nd treatments are given simultaneously, a complete sensitization is observed. With increasing intervals, thermotolerance developed and the magnitude of thermal chemosensitization decreased. With the decay of thermotolerance, the thermal chemosensitization was again observed. These results are illustrated in Fig. 5.

Studies performed in other laboratories showed some controversial results. The effect of preheating may depend on the choice of drugs as well as the timing of drug administration. At 37°C or elevated temperatures Morgan et al (1979) observed that preheating for 1 hour at 43°C sensitized EMT6 cells to a BLM and BCNU treatment at 37°C, but protected against subsequent Adriamycin cytotoxicity. These sensitization and protection effects were eliminated after 12 hours incubation at 37°C after the 1st heating. These authors also reported that preheating at 40°C did not alter the cytotoxicity of these agents. The protective effect of preheating against Adriamycin is also reported by Donaldson et al (1978). Hahn and STRANDE (1976) and OSBORNE and MACKILLOP (1987) reported reduced uptake of Adriamycin by preheated cells. MORGAN et al (1979) also demonstrated that the 1st heating at 40°C for 3 hours reduced the thermal sensitization of BLM and BCNU cytotoxicity at 43°C. However, no experiments on the treatment interval between the 2 treatments are reported.

It is likely that hyperthermia damages the cell membrane and leads to an alteration in drug uptake and/or efflux. Heat shock proteins may interact with drug cytotoxicity. In animal tumors and normal tissues, additional factors, including a change in blood flow and tissue pH (SONG et al, 1980), may be involved. A study on repeated administrations of CY alone or combined CY and heat at 41.5°C demonstrated that CY treated cells showed resistance to subsequent drug treatments. As a result, combined treatment induced resistance to subsequent combined treatments (URANO et al, 1988). To our knowledge, no other drugs have been studied in animal tumors. Further studies on these questions are needed and must be encouraged.

Future questions

Studies on the mechanisms of thermal chemosensitization are very limited. Most studies are performed above 42°C at which hyperthermia *per se* can give lethal damage to mammalian cells or some damage to macromolecules (most likely, protein denaturation). It is a critical question if the mechanism at these high temperatures can be also observed at temperatures below 42°C at which heat itself gives insignificant damage to mammalian cells. It appears to be important to investigate the mechanism at low temperatures, since thermochemotherapy can be performed at low temperatures, particularly when it is applied with whole body hyperthermia.

For the treatment of human cancer, combinations of different types of chemotherapeutic agents are frequently used. The rationale of the use of multiple drugs might be that (a) combination of some agents may be synergistic and (b) the use of drugs which have toxicity to different organs can minimize the side-effects and allow an administration of more drug doses than a single agent. The same principle can be applied to thermochemotherapy, particularly to chemotherapy given in combination with whole body hyperthermia. It has been shown that when a single agent was combined with whole body hyperthermia no therapeutic gain was obtained with a few exceptions (HONESS and BLEEHEN, 1982 and 1985). In addition, it may be significant to use agents which show synergistic effects or to use agents which potentiate the cytotoxicity of some chemotherapeutic agents either biochemically or physiologically (YATVIN et al, 1981; JAIN and WARD-HARTLEY, 1984; ADWANKAR and CHITNIS, 1986). These questions must receive further attention.

A critical factor for hyperthermia treatments is that the tumor tissue pH is lower compared to the normal tissue pH (summarized by WIKE-HOOLEY, 1984). Some agents are more effective at low pH than normal pH (HAHN and SHIU, 1983; URANO and KIM, 1983; GROOS et al, 1986; ROTIN et al, 1987). Some agents are also oxygen-dependent (TEICHER et al, 1981; HERMAN et al, 1988). The combination of these agents could result in an increased anti-tumor effect with limited toxicities to normal tissues. Recent studies have shown a synergistic action between biological response modifiers and hyperthermia (URANO, 1988). Limited space does not allow detailed discussion on this topic. Finally, it must be mentioned that thermotolerance is a critical factor for hyperthermic treatments of human cancer. Studies on the interaction between thermotolerance and drug cytotoxicity or between thermotolerance and thermal chemosensitization are very scattered. The best treatment may be to avoid this complexity. Further studies on these topics should be encouraged.

References

Adwankar MK, Chitnis MP (1986) Modification of tumor cell sensitivity to antineoplastic agents lonidamine and bouvardin (NSC 259968) at elevated temperatures. Neoplasma 33: 217–223

Alberts DS, Peng Y-M, Chen HSG, Moon TE, Cetas TC, Hoeschele JD (1980) Therapeutic synergism of hyperthermia-cisplatinum in a mouse tumor model. Natl Cancer Inst 65: 455–461

Bates DA, MacKillop WJ (1986) Hyperthermia, adriamycin transport, and cytotoxicity in drug-sensitive and -resistant Chinese hamster ovary cells. Cancer Res 46: 5477–5481

Braun J, Hahn GM (1975) Enhanced cell killing by bleomycin and 43°C hyperthermia and the inhibition of recovery from potentially lethal damage. Cancer Res 35: 2921–2927

Bronk BV, Wilkins RJ, Regan JD (1973) Thermal enhancement of DNA damage by an alkylating agent in human cells. Biochem Biophys Res Commun 52: 1064–1070

Brouwer J, Fichtinger-Schepman AMS, van de Putten P, Reedijk J (1982) Influence of temperature on platinum binding to DNA, cell killing, and mutation induction in Escherichia coli K-12 cells treated with *cis*-diamminedichloroplatinum. Cancer Res 42: 2416–2419

Calderwood SK, Dickson JA (1980) Effect of hyperglycemia on blood flow, pH and response to hyperthermia (42°) of the Yoshida sarcoma in the rat. Cancer Res 40: 4728–4733

Chapman IV, Leyko W, Gaozdzinski K, Koter M, Grzelinska E, Bartosz G (1983) Hyperthermia modification of bleomycin-DNA interaction detected by electron spine response. Radiat Res 96: 518–522

Dahl O, Mella O (1982) Enhanced effect of combined hyperthermia and chemotherapy (bleomycin, BCNU) in a neurogenic rat tumour (BT_4A) *in vivo*. Anticancer Res 2: 359–364

Dahl O, Mella O (1983) Effect of timing and sequence of hyperthermia and cyclophosphamide on a neurogenic rat tumor (BT_4A) *in vivo*. Cancer 52: 983–987

Donaldson SS, Gordon LF, Hahn GM (1978) Protective effect of hyperthermia against the cytotoxicity of actinomycin D on Chinese hamster cells. Cancer Treat Rep 62: 1489–1495

Eichholtz-Wirth H, Hietel B (1986) The relationship between cisplatin sensitivity and drug uptake into mammalian cells *in vitro*. Br J Cancer 54: 239–243

Engelhardt R (1987) Hyperthermia and drugs. Recent Results Cancer Res 104: 136–203

George KC, Singh BB (1982) Synergism of chlorpromazine and hyperthermia in two mouse solid tumours. Br J Cancer 45: 309–313

Groos E, Walker L, Masters JRW (1986) Intravesical chemotherapy. Studies on the relationship beween pH and cytotoxicity. Cancer 58: 1199–1203

Gullino PM, Grantham FH, Smith SH, Haggerty AC (1965) Modification of the acid-base status of the internal milieu of tumors. J Natl Cancer Inst 34: 857–869

Hahn GM (1975) Thermochemotherapy: Interactions between hyperthermia and chemotherapeutic agents. Proceedings of International Symposium on Cancer Therapy by Hyperthermia and Radiation, 28–30 April 1975. Washington, DC.

Hahn GM (1978) Interactions of drugs and hyperthermia *in vitro* and *in vivo*. In: Streffer E, van Beuningen D, Dietzel F, Rötinger E, Robinson JE, Scherer E, Seeber S, Trott K-R (eds) Cancer Therapy by Hyperthermia and Radiation. Urban & Schwarzenberg, Baltimore-Munich, pp 72–79

Hahn GM, Braun J, Har-Kedar I (1975) Thermochemotherapy: Synergism between hyperthermia (42–43°) and adriamycin (or bleomycin) in mammalian cell inactivation. Proc Natl Acad Sci USA 72: 937–940

Hahn GM, Li GG, Shiu E (1977) Interaction of amphotericin B and 43° hyperthermia. Cancer Res 37: 761–764

Hahn GM, Shiu EC (1983) Effect of pH and elevated temperatures on the cytotoxicity of some chemotherapeutic agents on Chinese hamster cells *in vitro*. Cancer Res 43: 5789–5791

Henle KS, Dethlefsen LA (1978) Heat fractionation and thermotolerance: A review. Cancer Res 38: 1843–1851

Herman TS, Teicher BA (1988) Sequencing of trimodality therapies: cis-diamminedichloroplatinum (II)/hyperthermia/radiation by tumor growth delay and human cell survival in the FSaIIC fibrosarcoma. Cancer Res 48: 2693–2697

Herman TS, Teicher BA, Chan V, Collins LS, Abrams MJ (1989) Effect of heat on the cytotoxicity and interaction with DNA of a series of platinum complexes. Int J Radiat Oncol Biol Phys 16: 443–449

Herman TS, Teicher BA, Collins LS (1988) Effect of hypoxia and acidosis on the cytotoxicity of four platinum complexes at normal and hyperthermic temperatures. Cancer Res 48: 2342–2347

Honess DJ, Bleehen NM (1982) Sensitivity of normal mouse marrow and RIF-1 tumour to hyperthermia combined with cyclophosphamide or BCNU: A lack of therapeutic gain. Br J Cancer 46: 236–246

Honess DJ, Bleehen NM (1985) Thermochemotherapy with cis-platinum, CCNU, BCNU, chlorambucil and melphalan on murine marrow and two tumours: Therapeutic gain for melphalan only. Br J Radiol 58: 63–72

Jain RK, Ward-Hartley K (1984) Tumor blood flow-characterization, modifications and role in hyperthermia. IEEE Trans Sonics Ultrasonics 54/31: 504–526

Johnson HA, Pavelec M (1973) Thermal enhancement of thio-TEPA cytotoxicity. Natl Cancer Inst 50: 903–908

Kohn KW, Erickson LC, Laurent G, Ducore J, Sharkey N, Ewing RA (1981) DNA crosslinking and the origin of sensitivity to chloroethylnitrosourea. In: PresTaylo AW, Baker LH, Crooke ST, Carter SK, Schein PS, Alder NA (eds) Nitrosourea: Current Status and New Developments. Academic Press, New York, pp 69–83

Longo FW, Tomashefsky P, Rivin BD, Tannenbaum M (1983) Interaction of ultrasonic hyperthermia with two alkylating agents in a murine bladder tumor. Cancer Res 43: 3231–3235

Majima H (1988) Thermotolerance and thermochemotherapy. Hyperthermic Oncology 2: 160–162

Majima H, Urano M, Kahn J (1988) Effect of previous treatment with hyperthermia or bleomycin on the subsequent thermobleomycin treatment. Hyperthermic Oncology 1: 68–70

Marmor JB, Kozak D, Hahn GM (1979) Effects of systemically administered bleomycin or adriamycin with local hyperthermia on primary tumor and lung metastases. Cancer Treatment Reports 63: 1279–1290

Meyn RE, Corry PM, Fletcher SE, Demetriades M (1979) Thermal enhancement of DNA strand breakage in mammalian cells treated with bleomycin. Int J Radiat Oncol Biol Phys 5: 1487–1489

Meyn RE, Corry PM, Fletcher SE, Demetriades M (1980) Thermal enhancement of DNA damage in mammalian cells treated with cis-diamminedichloroplatinum (II). Cancer Res 40: 1136–1139

Morgan JE, Bleehen, NM (1981) Response of EMT6 multicellular tumour spheroids to hyperthermia and cytotoxic drugs. Br J Cancer 43: 384–391

Murray D, Milas L, Meyn RE (1984) DNA damage produced by combined hyperglycemia and hyperthermia in two mouse fibrosarcoma tumors *in vivo*. Int J Radiat Oncol Biol Phys 10: 1679–1682

Osborne HJ, MacKillop WJ (1987) The effect of exposure to elevated temperatures on membrane permeability to adriamycin in Chinese hamster ovary cells *in vitro*. Cancer Lett 37: 213–224

Pinto AL, Lippard SJ (1985) Binding of the antitumor drug cis-diamminedichloroplatinum (II) (cisplatin) to DNA. Biochem Biophys Acta 780: 167–180

Reed E, Ozols RF, Tarone R, Yuspa SH, Poirier MC (1987) Platinum-DNA adducts in leukocyte DNA correlate with disease response in ovarian cancer patients receiving platinum-based chemotherapy. Proc Natl Acad Sci [USA] 84: 5024–5028

Rose WC, Veras GH, Laster WR, Schabel FM Jr (1979) Evaluation of whole-body hyperthermia as an adjuvant to chemotherapy in murine tumors. Cancer Treat Rep 63: 1311–1325

Rotin D, Wan P, Grinstein S, Tannock I (1987) Cytotoxicity of compounds that interfere with the regulation of intracellular pH: A potential new class of anticancer drugs. Cancer Res 47: 1497–1504

Smith PJ, Michera J, Bleehen NM (1986) Interaction of bleomycin, hyperthermia and a calmodulin inhibitor (trifluoperazine) in mouse tumour cells: II. DNA damage, repair and chromatin changes. Br J Cancer 53: 105–114

Song CW, Kang MS, Rhee JG, Levitt SH (1980) The effect of hyperthermia on vascular function, pH, and cell survival. Radiology 137: 795–803

Teicher BA, Kowal CD, Kennedy KA, Sartorelli AC (1981) Enhancement by hyperthermia of the *in vitro* cytotoxicity of mitomycin C toward hypoxic tumor cells. Cancer Res 41: 1096–1099

Terasima T, Yasukawa M, Umezawa, H (1970) Breaks and rejoining of DNA in cultured mammalian cells treated with bleomycin. Gann 61: 513–516

Tofilon PJ, Da Silva V, Gutin PH, Deen DF (1985) Effect of hyperthermia on DNA interstrand crosslinkings after treatment with BCNU in 9L rat brain tumor cells. Radiat Res 103: 373–382

Urano M (1986) The kinetics of thermotolerance in normal and tumor tissues. A review. Cancer Res 46: 474–482

Urano M (1988) Tumor response to hyperthermia. In: Urano M, Douple E (eds) Hyperthermia and Oncology, vol 1. VSP, Utrecht, Netherlands, pp 161–200

Urano M, Kahn J (1989) The effect of bleomycin administered in combination with hyperthermia on a C3H mouse fibrosarcoma. Int J Hyperthermia 5: 377–382

Urano M, Kahn J, Kenton L (1988a) Effect of bleomycin on murine tumor cells at elevated temperatures and two different pH values. Cancer Res 48: 615–619

Urano M, Kahn J, Kenton L (1988b) Thermochemotherapy-induced resistance to cyclophosphamide. Br J Cancer 57: 295–297

Urano M, Kahn J, Kenton LA (1990a) The effect of cis-diamminedichloroplatinum (II) treatment at elevated temperatures on murine fibrosarcoma, FSa-II. Int J Hyperthermia 6: 563–570

Urano M, Kahn J, Majima H, Gerweck LE (1990b) The cytotoxic effect of cis-diamminedichloroplatinum (II) on cultured Chinese hamster cells at elevated temperatures. Int J Hyperthermia 6: 581–590

Urano M, Kim MS (1983) The effect of hyperglycemia on thermochemotherapy of a spontaneous murine fibrosarcoma. Cancer Res 43: 3041–3044

Urano M, Kim MS, Kahn J, Kenton LA, Li ML (1985) Effect of thermochemotherapy (combined cyclophosphamide and hyperthermia) given at various temperatures with or without glucose administration on a murine fibrosarcoma. Cancer Res 45: 4162–4166

Von Arden M, Reitnauer PG (1980) Selective occlusion of cancer tissue capillaries as the central mechanism of the cancer multistep therapy. Jpn J Clin Oncol 10 (1): 31–48

Wallner KE, Banda M, Li GC (1987) Hyperthermic enhancement of cell killing by mitomycin C in mitomycin C-resistant Chinese hamster ovary cells. Cancer Res 47: 1308–1312

Wallner KE, Li GC (1987) Effect of drug exposure duration and sequencing on hyperthermic potentiation of mitomycin-C and cisplatin. Cancer Res 47: 493–495

Ward KA, Jain RK (1988) Response of tumours to hyperglycaemia: Characterization, significance and role in hyperthermia. Int J Hyperthermia 4: 223–250

Weinkan RJ, Deen DF (1982) Quantitative dose-response relations for the cytotoxic activity of chloroethylnitrosourea in cell culture. Cancer Res 42: 1008–1014

Wike-Hooley JL, Haveman J, Reinhold HS (1984) The relevance of tumour pH to the treatment of malignant disease. Radiother Oncol 2: 343–366

Woodhall B, Pickbell KL, Georgiade NG, Mahaley MS, Dukes HT (1960) Effect of hyperthermia upon cancer chemotherapy: Application to external cancer of head and face structures. Ann Surg 151: 750–759

Yatvin MB, Muhlensiepen, Porschen W, Weinstein JN, Feinendegen LE (1981) Selective delivery of liposome-associated cis-dichlorodiammineplatinum (II) by heat and its influence on tumor drug uptake and growth. Cancer Res 41: 1602–1607

4

Physical Aspects of Interstitial Hyperthermia

J. W. Hand

Medical Research Council Cyclotron Unit, Hammersmith Hospital, London, England

Introduction

Recent years have seen a developing interest in the use of hyperthermia, usually combined with radiotherapy or chemotherapy, in the treatment of some cancer patients. Experience has shown that induction of hyperthermia in patients in a predictable and sufficiently uniform manner is, in general, a major technical problem. One approach which has been investigated is to implant the sources of heat within the tumour and some surrounding normal tissue in ways analogous to techniques used in brachytherapy. This approach circumvents some of the problems encountered with most non-invasive methods such as limited penetration and excessive heating of intervening normal tissues (Gautherie, 1990). Interstitial methods are aften applicable to deep seated as well as superficial tumours. These advantages must be weighed against some drawbacks. For example, the invasive nature of the techniques may be impractical for many patients and, since the sources of energy are much more localized than in most non-invasive methods, the resulting temperature distribution is highly sensitive to both blood flow and the geometry of the implant. Nevertheless, considerable interest in the use of interstitial hyperthermia exists, as described elsewhere in this book. From a physical point of view, three major classes of technique for interstitial hyperthermia have been developed, namely radiofrequency (RF) techniques, microwave techniques and hot source techniques. The purpose of this chapter is to review some physical aspects of these methods.

Physical bases of electromagnetic interstitial hyperthermia

The presence of an electric field in the tissue can produce a drift, superimposed on their random thermal motion, of the free conduction charges within the tissue and polarization effects. The latter can arise because positive and negative charges of molecules may be displaced slightly from their equilibrium positions by the presence of the field. There may also be partial alignment with the applied field of those molecules possessing permanent electric dipoles. The degree of alignment is dependent upon the strength of the field and is opposed by random thermal motion and mutual interactions between molecules.

These interactions between electric field and tissue can be described by a parameter ε known as the complex permittivity of the tissue and which is defined by:

$$\varepsilon = \varepsilon_0(1 + \chi + \sigma/j\omega\varepsilon_0) = \varepsilon_0(\varepsilon' - j\varepsilon'') \quad [1]$$

where ε_0 ($= 8.8542 \times 10^{-12}$ F m^{-1}) is the permittivity of free space, χ is the electric susceptibility, ω (radian s^{-1}) is the angular frequency of the field and σ (S m^{-1}) is the electrical conductivity of the tissue. The effect of the free or conduction charges is described by ε'' whilst the polarization arising from bound charges is accounted for by ε'.

The values of both ε' and ε'' are dependent upon tissue type and the frequency f ($=\omega/2\pi$) of the field E. In tissues with high water content such as muscle, $\varepsilon''/\varepsilon' \approx 1$ at a frequency near 400 MHz; at higher frequencies, dielectric losses dominate whilst at lower frequencies losses due to conduction currents dominate. Values of ε' and ε'' in tissues with low water content (fat, bone) are about an order of magnitude smaller than those for tissues with high water content. Details of dielectric properties of tissues can be found in the reviews and tabulations of SCHWAN (1957; 1963), GEDDES and BAKER (1967), TINGA and NELSON (1973) and STUCHLY and STUCHLY (1980).

Time-varying electric and magnetic fields, **E** and **B**, are related to each other and to charge density ρ and current density **J** by the set of equations known as Maxwell's equations. If we assume a sinusoidal time dependence of **E**, **B**, **J** and ρ, we can separate the temporal and spatial dependencies and write, for example $\mathbf{E}(x,y,z,t) = \mathrm{Re}\,\{\mathbf{E}(x,y,z)e^{j\omega t}\}$ and define $\bar{\mathbf{B}}$, $\bar{\mathbf{J}}$ and $\bar{\rho}$ in a similar way. The differential forms of Maxwell's equations for an unbounded region of tissue may then be written (DURNEY, 1987):

$$\nabla \cdot (\varepsilon\bar{\mathbf{E}}) = \bar{\rho} \quad [2]$$

$$\nabla \times \bar{\mathbf{E}} = -j\omega\mu_0\bar{\mathbf{H}} \quad [3]$$

$$\nabla \cdot (\mu_0\bar{\mathbf{H}}) = 0 \quad [4]$$

$$\nabla \times \bar{\mathbf{H}} = \bar{\mathbf{J}} + j\omega\varepsilon\bar{\mathbf{E}} \quad [5]$$

where $\mathbf{H} (= \mu_0/\mathbf{B})$ is the magnetic field intensity (A m^{-1}) and $\mu_0 = 4\pi \times 10^{-7}$ H m^{-1} is the permeability of free space. Equations [3] and [5] show that when $\omega = 0$ (i.e. in the case of dc) electric and magnetic effects are distinct phenomena. Even when $\omega > 0$ the approximation of treating electric and magnetic effects separately remains good so long as the wavelength associated with the field is large with respect to the dimensions characterising the problem. This condition is satisfied at the frequencies used for rf interstitial hyperthermia (typically 0.5 to 27 MHz) and for the magnetic induction fields (typically 0.1 to 0.5 MHz) used for heating implanted ferromagnetic materials. However, electric and magnetic fields must be considered to be interdependent at the higher frequencies (300 to 2450 MHz) used in the microwave techniques.

RF techniques

In RF interstitial hyperthermia a voltage is applied between needle-like electrodes inserted into and around the tumour with the intention of elevating temperature by Ohmic heating due to conduction currents within the tissues. The first description of a radiofrequency (RF) interstitial hyperthermia technique was probably that by Doss (1975) although a similar idea had been proposed in 1970 by

ROBINSON (cited by DEWEY, 1989). Early studies of electric field distributions associated with this technique were reported by HUTSON (1975) and a more detailed account of "localized current fields" (LCF), a description coined by Doss, was given in Doss and MCCABE (1976).

If conduction currents are to be much greater than displacement currents, σ must be much greater than $\omega\varepsilon'\varepsilon_0$. This condition is satisfied in tissues with high water content at frequencies up to a few tens of MHz and in tissues with low water content such as fat at frequencies up to a few MHz; it sets an upper limit to the frequency which can be used in this technique. Furthermore, MILLIGAN and PANJEHPOUR (1983) found that the use of higher frequencies resulted in less uniform temperature distributions and created problems if thermocouple thermometry was used. The lower limit to the operating frequency should be sufficiently high to avoid direct electrical stimulation of nerve and muscle fibres. Although the premise that rf signals at frequencies above a few tens of kHz will not excite nerve or muscle has been long held, it has been reported that there is a monotonically increasing threshold excitation current for frequencies below 1 MHz above which excitation may be elicited (LACOURSE et al, 1985). At frequencies near 1 MHz however, tissue dessication occurred at current densities similar to the stimulus threshold. In practice, a frequency in the range 500 kHz to 1 MHz is usually selected for radiofrequency interstitial hyperthermia although some groups have used a frequency as high as 27 MHz. In this range of frequencies, the E-field can be assumed to be distributed in space as a static field. In the LCF technique the electric field arises predominantly from the potential differences which are imposed on the implanted electrodes; effects due to the H-field are negligible.

For many applications of RF interstitial hyperthermia, the basic element of the technique can be taken to be a pair of electrodes. In Fig. 1 the electrodes are represented in two dimensions by two parallel perfect conductors of circular cross-section (A and B) and a current I amp m^{-1} is passed between them resulting in line charges $q = \pm I/j\omega$ coulombs m^{-1}. Since equipotential surfaces for two line charges of opposite sign are circular cylinders, the potential in the region around the electrodes can be found by considering two lines of charge located at a distance $d = (b - \sqrt{\{b^2 - 4a^2\}})/2$ from the centres of the two electrodes. The potential at P(x,y) is:

$$\Phi(x,y) = \frac{q}{2\pi\varepsilon} \ln\left[\frac{r_B}{r_A}\right] \quad [6]$$

where r_A, r_B are the distances between P and the two line sources. The electric field $\mathbf{E}(x,y)$ is:

$$\mathbf{E} = -\nabla\Phi = -\left[\frac{\partial\Phi}{\partial x}\mathbf{i} + \frac{\partial\Phi}{\partial y}\mathbf{j}\right] \quad [7]$$

and the specific absorption rate (SAR) is:

$$\mathrm{SAR} = \frac{\sigma}{2\rho_m}|E|^2 \ \mathrm{W\,kg^{-1}} \quad [8]$$

where ρ_m kg m^{-3} is the density of the tissue.

Fig. 2 shows the SAR distribution associated with a pair of electrodes in a homogeneous medium and separated by a distance equal to 15 times their radius. Clearly, there is a rapid fall-off in SAR with increasing distance from each electrode. Indeed, the peak value of SAR along the line equidistant from the electrodes is only approximately 8% of that at the surface of the electrodes. In such regions, heat transport mechanisms

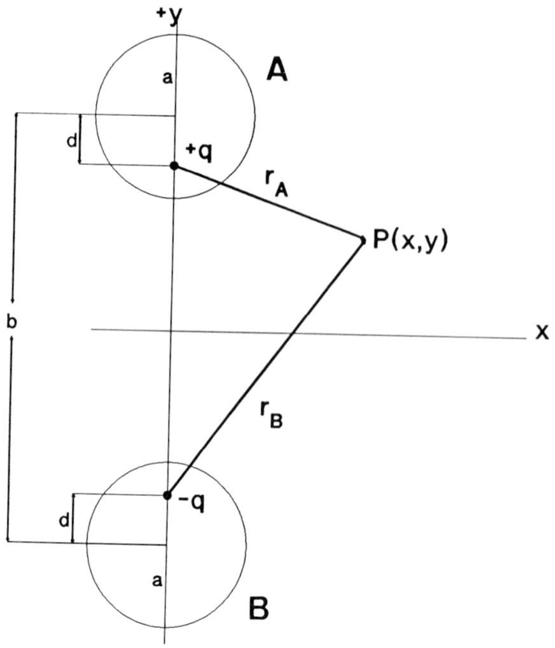

Fig. 1. The model used for calculating the potential and electric field associated with a pair of electrodes

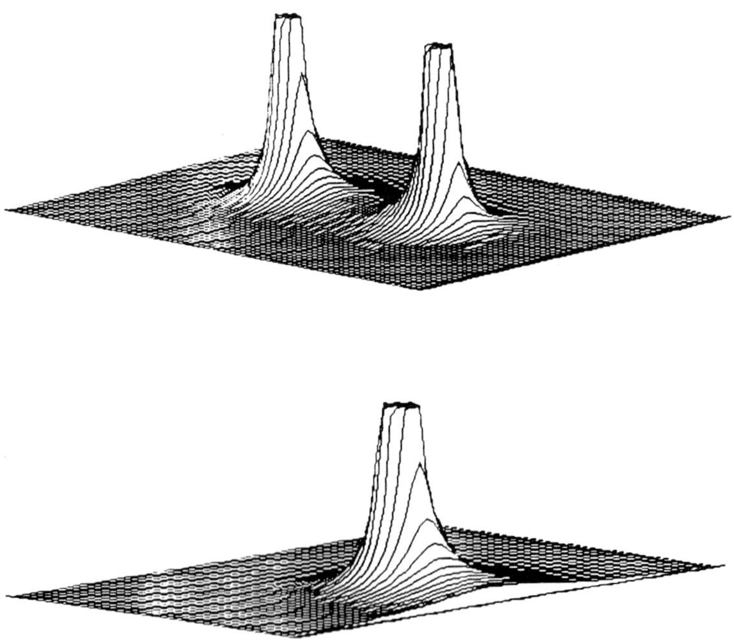

Fig. 2. SAR distribution for a pair of electrodes in a homogeneous medium. Each electrode has radius a and the separation is 15a. The lower figure shows a cut through the distribution in the plane midway between the electrodes

within the tissues, rather than direct absorption of electromagnetic energy, must be dominant factors in accounting for increase in temperature within the implanted region.

Such theoretical calculations suggest that inter-electrode spacing should be no more than about ten times the diameter of the electrodes. Clinical experience suggests that inter-electrode spacing should be limited to about 15 mm (COSSET et al, 1985). Typically, the diameter of interstitial electrodes is in the range 1 to 1.6 mm; the use of thinner electrodes would result in very high temperatures in the regions close to the electrodes whilst significantly larger electrodes would be unacceptable for the patient. Rigid metallic needles were often used in early applications of the LCF technique (GERNER et al, 1975; STERNHAGEN et al, 1977; ASTRAHAN and GEORGE, 1980) but problems such as patient discomfort due to the rigidity of the implant and the fact that normal tissue as well as tumour was heated because of the direct electrical contact between tissue and the electrode along its entire length (with the exception of short insulated sections at the entrance and exit points at the skin) called for new designs. COSSET et al (1985) used tubes which consisted of a central metallic section attached at each end to flexible plastic sections. The length of the metallic section was determined by the tumour dimensions. RF power was delivered via a metallic probe which was inserted through the lumen of one of the plastic sections to make electrical contact with the central section. The electrodes described by KAPP et al (1988) consisted of a coaxial arrangement of a flexible plastic tube, a fine-wire metal braid and an outer thin walled insulating layer. They were customised for individual treatments by removing an appropriate length of the outer insulating layer.

One method of implementing the LCF technique is to apply a rf voltage between two or more planes of electrodes as shown in Fig. 3(i); this was often used in early applications of rf interstitial hyperthermia. A 2-dimensional model of the method was described by STROHBEHN (1983) who showed that the potential Φ_k at each electrode k ($k = 1, \ldots N$) within an N-fold array could be found from equations of the form

$$\Phi_k = \frac{j}{2\pi\omega\varepsilon} \sum_{i=1}^{N} I_i \ln(r_{ik}) \qquad [9]$$

where r_{ik} is the distance from electrode i to surface of electrode k; $r_{ii} = a$, the radius of the electrodes. If the magnitudes of the voltages at each electrode are assumed to be equal, these N equations permit the unknown current I_i ($i = 1,N$) impressed on each electrode to be determined. The electric field in the region around the electrodes may be found from $-\nabla\Phi$. The imposition of equal magnitudes for the electrode voltages results in a dependence of I_i, and hence in SAR close to the electrode, on the position of the electrode within the array. In practice therefore, a means of adjusting the relative voltages at the electrodes should be provided (STROHBEHN, 1983).

An alternative technique which offers improved control was used by COSSET et al (1985). Predetermined pairs of electrodes are each driven by a generator (as shown schematically in Fig. 3(ii)) and the feedback signal for power control of each pair is derived from a thermistor within one of the electrodes. A system which has up to eight 20 W generators working either coherently (at 570 kHz) or incoherently at frequencies spaced at 20 kHz within the range 500–610 kHz was developed. However, a disadvantage with this approach is the small number of indi-

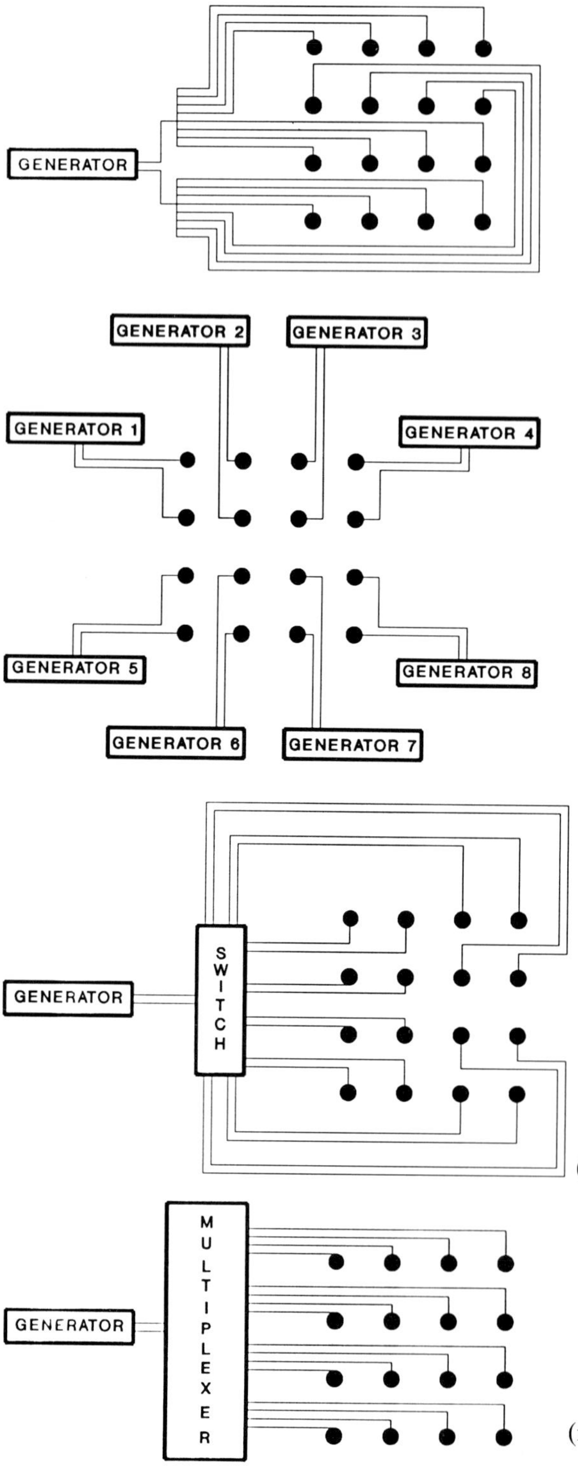

(i)

(ii)

(iii)

(iv)

Fig. 3. Methods of driving an array of electrodes;
(i) single generator and alternate rows of electrodes connected together;
(ii) several generators, each dedicated to a predetermined pair of electrodes;
(iii) single generator time sharing several pairs of predetermined electrodes;
(iv) single generator connected to any pair of electrodes via a multiplexer

vidually controlled electrode pairs available.

Another approach is to time-share the power from a single generator between predetermined pairs of electrodes (see Fig. 3(iii)). A commercial system was developed using this technique which is capable of switching up to 200 W of power at 500 kHz between up to 20 pairs of electrodes. The pattern of sequencing and its overall cycle time, the time power is applied to each pair of electrodes and the power level are adjustable. A feedback signal for control can be derived from the temperature at any of the locations of up to 32 thermocouple sensors provided in the system.

A fourth technique which provides an even greater degree of control has been described by KAPP et al (1988). In this case power from the generator can be delivered to any two electrodes within an array via a multiplexer (see Fig. 3(iv)). The technique results in a relatively uniform temperature distribution but requires at least one temperature sensor per electrode. One criterion which is used to control such a system is that power should be delivered to the pair of electrodes which is coolest at the time when temperatures are sampled. The power level and dwell times can also be controlled. Further improvement in the control of temperature distributions should be achieved by using segmented electrodes (PRIONAS et al, 1989). Each short segment of such electrodes is electrically insulated from its neighbours and connected to the multiplexer, allowing the power delivered to individual segments of an electrode to be controlled. In this way, some of the problems associated with simpler techniques which arise from a lack of parallelism of electrodes and/or the heterogeneity in the electrical and thermal properties of the tissues may be reduced. Another method which may improve temperature distributions within electrically heterogeneous tissue is to pass temperature regulated water through the electrodes, creating essentially constant temperature sources (PRIOR, 1991).

In a variation on the LCF technique, MARCHAL et al (1989) and VISSER et al (1989) used a frequency as high as 27.12 MHz to achieve capacitive coupling between the tissue and flexible electrodes inserted into flexible plastic catheters. In the system described by VISSER et al,

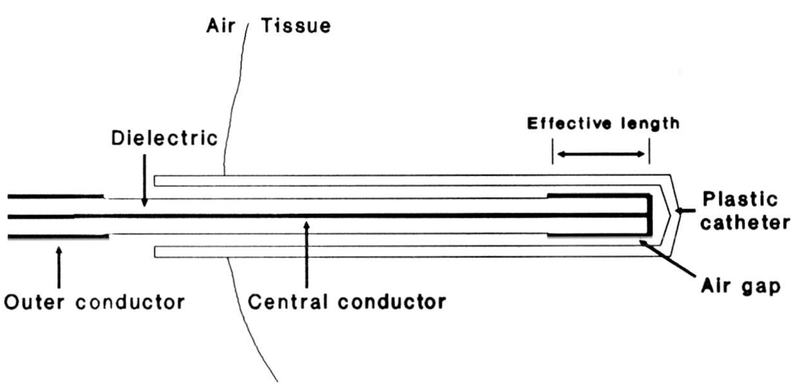

Fig. 4. 27 MHz electrode in plastic catheter (after VISSER et al, 1989)

heating is restricted to the desired section of the electrode by significantly reducing the capacitive coupling in other parts of the electrode/catheter assembly. This is achieved by constructing the electrode from a miniature coaxial cable with its shield removed except for a section of the desired length at the distal end of the cable where the remaining shield is connected to the central conductor (Fig. 4). Each electrode is connected to an impedance matching network and an amplifier; the return electrodes form a segmented external ground plane spaced from the skin by a bolus. This technique can be used with curved catheters having a small radius of curvature such as those used in some treatments in the head and neck regions.

Microwave techniques

In microwave techniques, needle-like antennas, designed to operate at a frequency which is usually within the range 300 to 2450 MHz, are implanted into the tissues. An early description of an interstitial microwave antenna was given by TAYLOR (1978). His device was formed from subminiature semi-rigid coaxial cable which was terminated by removing the outer conductor for a distance of about a quarter of a wavelength, leaving the exposed central conductor to act as the radiating element. The results of a study of several types of monopole antenna (DE SIEYES et al, 1981) showed that the fully insulated antenna had the best performance.

In contrast with the ohmic heating associated with RF electrodes, microwave antennas radiate electromagnetic waves and energy is transferred to the tissues increasingly through dielectric losses as the operating frequency is increased. In clinical practice, plastic catheters are usually implanted into the tissues and used to carry radioactive seeds during brachytherapy or antennas during hyperthermia. Indeed, inserting the antennas into suitable catheters can improve their charactersistics (KING et al, 1983; JONES et al, 1989). Typically, the heating pattern for a single microwave antenna is an elongated ellipsoid of revolution with a radial penetration of about 10 mm. Dipole-type antennas are often driven at resonance (which provides the best impedance match) and so in principle the length of the heating pattern can be selected by choosing the antenna length and the corresponding operating frequency. Although larger tumours can be heated using longer antennas, a correspondingly larger volume of tissue near the tip of the antenna will receive inadequate power since the power deposition for a dipole antenna is maximum at the junction and falls to zero at the tip of the dipole (JONES et al, 1989). Since the volume heated by a single antenna is small, an array of implanted antennas is usually used.

When using an array of antennas a choice must be made between incoherent and coherent operation. For incoherent operation, power from a single generator may be switched sequentially from one antenna to another over a period which is short compared with the thermal time constant of the tissue (Fig. 5). In practice, a complete cycle should be made within a few seconds. Alternatively, each antenna could be powered by its own signal source and amplifier. In both cases, the resulting SAR distribution is obtained by super-

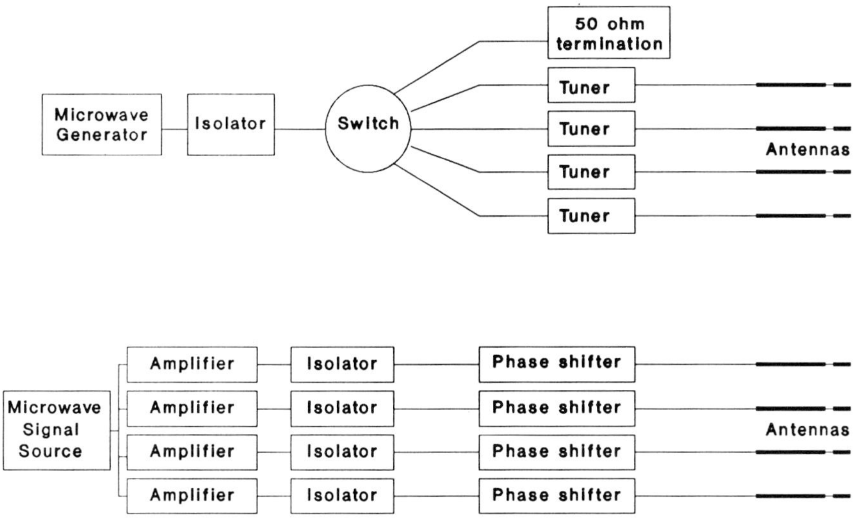

Fig. 5. Schematic diagrams of microwave systems. The upper diagram shows an incoherent system in which microwave power is switched sequentially between 4 antennas. Power may also be diverted away from the antennas into the 50-ohm termination. The lower diagram shows a coherent system. In this case, the power delivered to individual antennas may be adjusted at their respective amplifiers

imposing the SAR distributions associated with individual antennas. In a coherent system, power from a single amplifier (or from a common signal source and individual amplifiers) is fed simultaneously to all the antennas in the array. In this case the electric fields from each antenna are added vectorially and the SAR is determined in terms of (total electric field)^2. Coherent arrays can produce enhanced SAR compared with incoherent types in regions where the fields from individual antennas interfere constructively. On the other hand, if distances within the array are greater than half a wavelength, there will be corresponding areas of destructive interference leading to lower levels of SAR. The relative phases between antennas are also critical in determining the SAR distribution; we can take advantage of this by using phase shifters to change the relative phase angles intentionally. The relative phases may also be changed unintentionally be using tuners (Wong et al, 1986) and attenuators and, if each antenna has its own amplifier, by adjusting the output of the amplifier. Under carefully monitored conditions, coherent systems using dipole antennas can lead to better SAR distributions than similar incoherent systems (Trembly et al, 1986; Turner, 1986a; Wong et al, 1986). This may not be true for other types of antenna (e.g. helical antennas).

Dipole antennas

A common form of antenna consists of flexible miniature coaxial cable (outer diameter approximately 1 to 1.5 mm) with an extension of the inner conductor at the distal end. This extension can be formed by soldering a section of outer conductor to the inner one, leaving about 1 mm of the central conductor exposed at

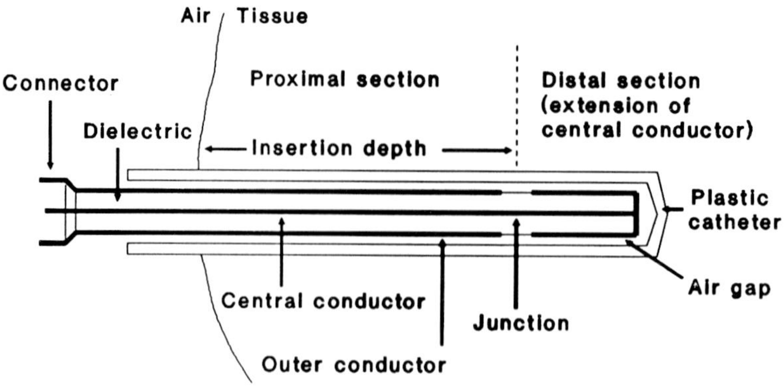

Fig. 6. Typical microwave dipole antenna inserted into a plastic catheter (after Strohbehn and Mechling, 1986)

the junction. The antenna is inserted into a plastic catheter as shown in Fig. 6. When power is applied to the antenna, a voltage is impressed at the junction and this produces currents which flow along the outside of the two sections of the antenna. These currents, in turn, give rise to an electromagnetic wave which propagates into the tissue. Characteristic dimensions of this type of antenna are the distance from the junction to the tip of the extended inner conductor, that from the junction to the tissue-air interface and the radii of the antenna and catheter.

King et al (1983) and Trembly (1985) considered the arrangement of the antenna (a symmetrical dipole) within its catheter to be an insulated antenna embedded in an electrically dense medium of infinite extent. Assuming that the diameter of the antenna was small compared to the wavelength in the tissue and that the permittivity of the catheter was much less than that of tissue, they treated the problem as a generalised coaxial transmission line formed by the antenna (taken to be the central conductor) and the tissue (taken to be an extensive outer conductor). Using a known approximation for the current distribution on the antenna – that for a transmission line of known wavenumber with an open circuit termination – (King and Smith, 1981), the electric field around the antenna could be determined. The value of the wavenumber used in determining the current distribution lies between that in the catheter material and that in the tissue.

Trembly (1985) reported the effects of driving frequency (300–915 MHz) and antenna length on the SAR distribution for an array of four antennas placed at the corners of a 3 cm × 3 cm square and driven coherently and in phase. For each frequency, the dipole halflength was chosen to be 3 cm, 6 cm or resonant ($\lambda_L/4$ where λ_L is the wavelength related to the wavenumber used for determining the current distribution on the antenna – see above). In the plane of the junctions, the 300 MHz antennas produced the smoothest SAR distribution although the length of a resonant antenna at this frequency was impractically large (>18 cm). At the higher frequencies, for example 915 MHz (a frequency commonly provided by commercial hyperthermia systems), the phase variations across the inter-antenna spacing considered in this study produced significant interference effects. In later studies discussed below, the spacing between antennas in an array operating at 915 MHz is usually reduced to 2 cm. When the length of the antenna was significantly shorter or longer than $\lambda_L/4$, relatively little power was deposited at the centre of the array compared with that in regions close to the antennas. However, in practice, cooling the surface of the antennas might improve this situation. A method which may reduce problems caused by the non-uniform SAR distribution in the central transverse plane of an array of 915 MHz antennas is to introduce time-dependent phase differences between the antennas (TREMBLY et al, 1986). The resulting time-averaged SAR distribution can be much smoother than those for arrays with static phase relationships.

Insertion depth

In practical use, the depth to which antennas are inserted into the tissues is an important variable. DENMAN et al (1988) and CHAN et al (1989) investigated the effects of changes in insertion depth on SAR distributions associated with arrays of 915 MHz antennas implanted in phantoms and (in the case of DENMAN et al) in canine thigh models. Both groups found that the maximum SAR shifted with respect to the junction plane in a complex manner over a range of insertion depths. The SAR distribution distal to the junction was relatively insensitive to insertion depth. JAMES et al (1989) carried out a theoretical study of the effect of insertion depth on the SAR distributions for 2×2 arrays of antennas which were either resonant (length of tip section $= \lambda_L/4$) or which simulated the antenna/catheter parameters of one of the commercially available microwave interstitial systems (length of tip section $\approx 1.13\,\lambda_L/4$). They explained the changes observed in SAR distributions in terms of the charge and current distributions on the antenna. The SAR near the surface of the antenna is associated with maxima in the charge distribution and that at the centre of the array is associated with maxima in the current distribution. The current is zero at the tip of an antenna and is approximately so at the point of insertion into the tissue.

JONES et al (1988) investigated the impedance of single insulated asymmetrical 915 MHz antennas implanted in a muscle-like medium. The input impedances and current and charge distributions associated with the two sections of the antenna are dependent upon the lengths of the respective sections and the two input impedances determine the distribution of power between the two sections. If the proximal section is significantly shorter than $\lambda_L/4$, it receives relatively little power. On the other hand, if it is much longer than $\lambda_L/4$, its impedance is relatively independent of the length and so the power radiated in this region is relatively constant. The SAR distribution in the vicinity of the distal section should be independent of changes in insertion depth since the impedance of that section is independent of the length of the proximal section of the antenna. The length of the distal section should be approximately $\lambda_L/4$ to optimise both coupling and the radial and longitudinal extents of the SAR distribution. ZHANG et al (1988) also modelled an asymmetrically driven insulated dipole implanted in a tissue-like medium. They found that the return loss for three 915 MHz antennas with tip lengths ranging from 1.5 to 3.5 cm was reasonably constant for insertion depths greater than 10 cm and that the length of the heating pattern depended upon the the properties of the antenna and the attenuation in the surrounding medium. For short-tipped antennas there was a secondary peak in the longitudinal distribution of SAR proximal from the junction.

Other antenna designs

A disadvantage of dipole antennas of the type discussed above is that power deposition falls off towards the tip of the antenna. This leads to inadequate heating in that area and requires that the tip of the antenna is inserted into normal tissue beyond the target volume if the tumour is to be heated effectively. Several antenna designs which have improved heating in the region of the tip have been reported. A modified dipole antenna in which two metal collars are added to the central conductor whilst a third collar is placed over the outer conductor proximal to the junction is described by TURNER (1986a). Since the diameter of the distal section increases towards the tip, the capacitance to the tissue through the catheter is increased and results in an increased current towards the tip compared with the conventional design. This type of antenna has also been designed with an integral thermistor which can provide continuous monitoring of temperature (TURNER, 1986b). However, care is needed in interpreting temperatures monitored in this way (ASTRAHAN et al, 1988). Another antenna designed to produce enhanced heating at the tip is that of ROOS and HUGANDER (1988). In this case the distal section of the dipole is replaced by a cone and a sleeve $\lambda_c/4$ long (λ_c = wavelength of the current on the sleeve) is placed proximal to the junction. A different approach to the problem is described by LIN and WANG (1987). These authors used a sleeved coaxial slot antenna consisting of two radiating slots seperated by $\lambda/8$ over a ground plane together an additional outer conductor and a short tip section ($\approx \lambda/8$). Antennas with two or three nodes and designed to produce longer heating patterns than those associated with single node antennas are discussed by LEE et al (1986).

Helical antennas have also been investigated as alternatives to dipole types with the aim of improving heating patterns in the longitudinal direction. In these antennas a helical coil is wound over a distal section of semi-rigid coaxial cable in which the dielectric and central conductor are exposed. WU et al (1987) describe an antenna in which the helical coil is connected to the central conductor at the tip and to the outer conductor at the proximal end of the exposed section. SATOH and STAUFFER (1988) and SATOH et al (1988) investigated the performance of antennas designed for 2450 MHz or 915 MHz operation. Several variations of the basic geometry were tested. At 2540 MHz the optimum antenna was found to be one for which the coil, 10 mm long with 1 turn per mm, was connected to the central conductor at the tip and separated from the outer conductor by a gap of 1 mm. At 915 MHz, the coil was 35 mm long and had 35 turns. Compared with that of a dipole, the heating pattern for this type of antenna was found to be more uniform in the longitudinal direction and extended to the tip. It was also less dependent upon insertion depth.

Hot source techniques

'Hot source' techniques differ markedly from the RF and microwave ones described in the previous sections in that energy transfer from these sources is dependent entirely upon heat transfer mechanisms present within the tissues. Since there is no (or, in the case of inductively heated ferromagnetic material, very little) direct energy deposition in the tissues, heterogeneity in the electrical properties of the tissues does not effect the resultant temperature distribution. This is dependent upon the geometry of the implant, the temperatures of the sources and the blood flow within the tissue. Examples of hot sources are tubes carrying hot water, electrically heated resistance elements and ferromagnetic seeds.

Hot water tube techniques

The simplest of these techniques is that in which hot water is passed with unidirectional flow through an array of stainless steel tubes or plastic catheters. The velocity and temperature profiles within a tube of circular cross section and diameter d are fully developed only beyond certain distances upstream from the tube entrance. These distances, known as the hydrodynamic and thermal entry lengths, x_{hd} and x_{th}, are given by:

$$x_{hd} = 0.05\, R_e d \text{ and } x_{th} - 0.05\, R_e P_r d \quad [10]$$

where

$$R_e = \frac{\rho_w u_m d}{\eta_w} \quad [11]$$

is the Reynolds number (the ratio of inertial forces (which tend to be destabilising) to viscous forces (which tend to be stabilising)) and

$$P_r = \frac{c_w \eta_w}{k_w} \quad [12]$$

is the Prandtl number (the ratio of momentum diffusivity to thermal diffusivity). ρ_w, η_w, c_w and k_w are respectively the density, dynamic viscosity, specific heat and thermal conductivity of water and u_m is the mean velocity of the water in the tube.

For water at 50°C, $P_r = 3.67$ and so it follows from equation [10] that in this case the velocity profile develops faster than the temperature profile. Assuming that there is a smooth inflow of water at the tube entrance, laminar flow will result when $R_e \leqslant 2300$ (Prandtl, 1963).

The radial heat flux may be considered to pass through a series of thermal resistances, namely those of the fluid boundary layer within the tube, the tube wall and the tissue. It can be shown that the thermal resistance of the tissue is an order of magnitude greater than the other two (Hand et al, 1991) and so Q, the radial heat flux through the wall of the tube, is approximately:

$$Q \approx h\pi dL(T_m - T_s) = N_u k_w \pi l(T_m - T_s) \quad [13]$$

where T_s is the temperature at the tube wall/tissue interface, T_m is the mean temperature in a given cross-section of the tube, L is the length of the tube and $N_u = hd/k_w$ is a non-dimensional heat flux known as the Nusselt number.

Assuming d = 1.6 mm, a typical value for tubes used for interstitial hyperthermia, and a flow rate of 1.5 ml s^{-1}, the normalised radial heat flux Q′ (i.e. heat flux per unit length and per °C temperature difference) is approximately 14 W m^{-1} °C^{-1} (Schreier et al, 1990). At somewhat higher flow rates (e.g. 2.5 ml s^{-1}) the flow becomes turbulent and the heat flux increases several fold. Brezovich (1988) has argued that hot sources (ferromagnetic seeds) should be capable of producing between 20 and 50 W m^{-1} to be useful in most clinical situations. Sufficient heating power should be available therefore from hot water tubes when the temperature difference between the water and tissue is

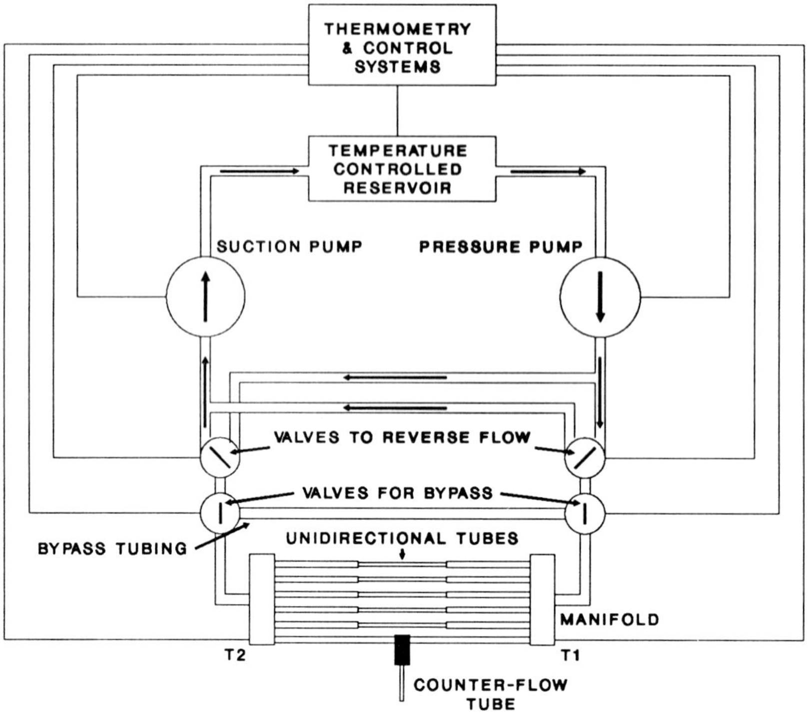

Fig. 7. Schematic diagram of a hot water interstitial hyperthermia system

a few °C. In practice water temperatures in the range of approximately 46–48°C have proved useful (SCHREIER et al, 1990; BREZOVICH et al, 1989). HAND et al (1991) studied the effects small changes in tube radius, tube spacing and blood flow had on the water temperature necessary to maintain an acceptable temperature distribution. Of these three parameters, blood flow has the greatest effect. The effect of tube radius is approximately three times that of tube spacing. If a smaller tube spacing is chosen, not only is a lower water temperature required but the time-constant governing the heat-up time of tissue is also reduced (STROHBEHN et al, 1982).

A practical hot water interstitial hyperthermia system (Fig. 7) consists of a temperature controlled reservoir of water, manifolds to distribute the water to the implanted tubes and one or more pumps to circulate the water. It is desirable to include valves which enable the direction of water flow to be reversed periodically. If provision for a secondary preheated circuit is made, the temperature of the implanted tubes can reach the desired level rapidly at the beginning of treatment.

The simplest technique is to use unidirectional flow through open ended tubes which may be of either stainless steel or plastic. As noted previously, the rigid metallic tubes may be less acceptable to the patient than the more flexible plastic ones. However, if the latter are used, a slightly higher water temperature is required to take account of the lower thermal conductivity of plastic compared with that of stainless steel. Where the use of open-ended tubes is inappropriate, tubes supporting counter-flow can be used (SCHREIER et al, 1990). These have greater normalised power and produce a smaller temperature gradient along the tubes than is the case for tubes in which there is unidirectional flow. Protection of normal tissue adjacent to proximal regions of implanted tubes is also possible by using tubes with two heating zones (HANDL et al, 1989).

Electrically heated resistance elements

An alternative 'hot source' source technique uses needles containing a resistance element and heated by ohmic losses (YOKOYAMA et al, 1985; MARCHOSKY et al, 1988). A DC or low frequency current I is passed through the element of resistance R ohm which results in a heating power $P = I^2R$. If the resistance is evenly distributed along the length of the needle, the power per unit length will be uniform along the needle. Where there is non-uniform heat loss from the needle, this will result in temperature variations along it. Some control over the longitudinal temperature distribution would be possible if the heating elements were segmented with individual power control to each segment. The integrity of the electrical isolation of the heating elements from the tissue is essential for the safety of the patient.

Ferromagnetic seeds

In this technique, implanted ferromagnetic material in the form of thin cylindrical 'seeds' is subjected to a radiofrequency magnetic field. Of the two mechanisms of heating – hysteresis losses and resistive heating by induced eddy currents – the latter is predominant in heating the seeds at the frequencies used (typically 100–200 kHz). Early reports of its use include those by MEDAL et al (1959), BURTON et al (1971), MERRY et al (1973) and MOIDEL et al (1976). More recently, ATKINSON et al (1984) and STAUFFER et al (1984a,b) applied the technique to interstitial hyperthermia.

ATKINSON et al (1984) considered the heating power per unit length of long cylindrical ferromagnetic implants. When the implants are orientated parallel to the magnetic field:

$$P_{//} = \pi H_0^2 a \sqrt{\frac{\omega\mu}{2\sigma}} f(x) \qquad [14]$$

where $x = a\sqrt{\omega\mu\sigma}$. a, σ and μ are the radius, conductivity and permeability of the implanted seed and ω and H_0 are the angular frequency and strength of the magnetic field. f(x) is a function of ber(x) and bei(x) and their derivatives (SIMPSON, 1960). When the implants are perpendicular to the field, the heating power is:

$$P_{perp} = 8\pi H_0^2 a \sqrt{\frac{\omega\mu}{2\sigma}} g(x,\mu_r) \qquad [15]$$

where $g(x,\mu_r)$ is a function of ber(x), bei(x) and their derivatives and μ_r, the relative permeability of the implanted material (SMYTHE, 1950). ATKINSON et al (1984) calculated that at frequencies below about 200 kHz, ferromagnetic seeds 1 mm in diameter and implanted parallel with the magnetic field should achieve adequate heating power (20 to 50 W m^{-1}) for a range of materials ($\mu_r \geq 8$) using magnetic field strengths which should not lead to excessive heating in tissues away from the implanted region. Perpendicular orientation of the seeds with respect to the magnetic field is best avoided since larger diameter seeds would be needed and there would be significant dependence of the heating power on misalignment of the implant from true orthogonality with the field. As the operating frequency is increased, the heating power associated with both orientations tends to decrease although this could be offset by increasing the diameter of the seed, choosing a material with higher permeability or increasing H_0. As the frequency is decreased, larger values of H_0 are required and eventually magnetic saturation of the seed will occur leading to a reduction in its permeability and consequently to a reduction in its heating power. The lower limit to the frequency which can be used is about 50 kHz (BREZOVICH, 1988).

The rf magnetic field also induces eddy currents to flow in the tissues and the direct heating which results from these must not cause a problem for the patient, either in terms of local hot spots or as excessive systemic heating. BREZOVICH (1988) discusses this point for solenoidal rf induction coils. The local absorbed power density in cylindrical loads associated with such magnetic induction systems is proportional to $\sigma_t (\mu_t H_0 f r)^2$ where σ_t, μ_t are the conductivity and permeability of the tissue ($\mu_t \approx \mu_0$, the permeability of free space) and r is the radial distance from the central axis to the point in question. BREZOVICH suggests that the operating parameters of a system designed for treating regions within the torso should be such that the product ($H_0 f$) has an upper limit of about 4.3×10^8 amp m^{-1} s^{-1}. This limit could be increased in the case of a system which was dedicated to treatments in the head and neck region or in limbs. STAUFFER et al (1984a) suggested that the power absorption per unit volume by an implanted array should be an order of magnitude greater than that induced directly in the tissues. This would give a slightly lower value to the upper limit for ($H_0 f$) than that suggested by BREZOVICH. STAUFFER and his colleagues also pointed out that solenoidal coils which require the target volume to be placed within their boundaries are restrictive since seed alignment should be paralel with the longitudinal axis of the body or limb. They suggested that the use of coaxially aligned pairs of coils may be less restrictive in clinical use.

The spontaneous magnetization of ferromagnetic materials vanishes above a temperature T_c known as the Curie temperature or Curie point. The Curie temperature of nickel is 358°C. Clearly, this is much too high for hyperthermia but nickel alloys have lower values of T_c. BURTON et al (1971) took advantage of self-regulating ‘thermo-seeds’ of nickel and palladium which had a Curie point of about 95°C, consistent with tissue coagulation. More recently materials which are suited to hyperthermia have been investigated. These include alloys of nickel-silicon (DESHMUKH et al, 1984; DEMER et al, 1986; CHEN et al, 1988), nickel-copper (BREZOVICH et al, 1984; BABA et al, 1987), nickel-palladium (BREZOVICH et al, 1984; KOBAYASHI and AMEMIYA, 1985; KOBAYASHI et al, 1985), iron-platinum and iron-platinum-silicon (MATSUI et al, 1987).

Ferromagnetic seed techniques can be classified into two general groups. On one hand there are ‘constant power seeds’ which are made from material with a T_c much higher than the desired operating temperature. Stainless steel seeds are an example of this type. In this case the heating power for a given seed depends upon ($H_0 f$) and is essentially independent of its temperature. The equilibrium temperature attained by each seed is dependent upon the environmental conditions around it and temperature regulation must be achieved through external control of the power delivered to

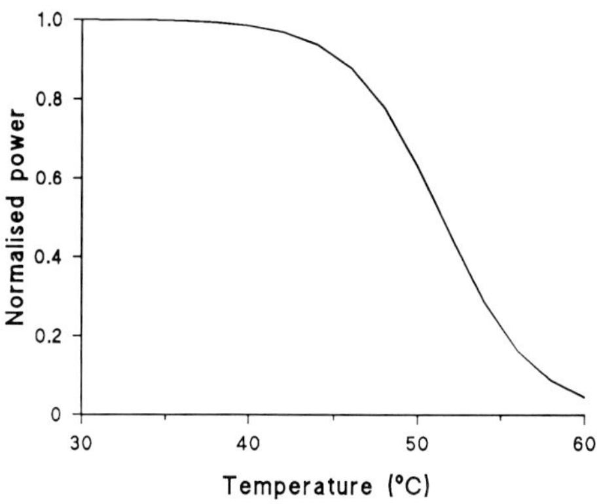

Fig. 8. The temperature dependence of the normalised power of a self regulating ferromagnetic seed, $P = (1 + a \exp[bT])^{-1}$. In this case, the Curie point is approximately 56°C and the normalised power falls from 0.9 to 0.1 over a temperature range of approximately 13°C

the seeds. On the other hand there are 'constant temperature seeds' which are produced from material with T_c close to the desired operating temperature. For seeds in this group, the dependence of heating power on temperature can be approximated by an expression of the type

$$P = \frac{1}{1 + a \exp(bT)} \qquad [16]$$

where P is the normalised power absorption and a and b are constants describing a particular type of implant (HAIDER et al, 1987). Since the heating power is strongly dependent upon temperature in the region of the Curie point and decreases as the seed temperature approaches T_c, the implants are thermally self-regulating if sufficient power is supplied. For seeds investigated to date, the transition from ferromagnetic to non-ferromagnetic state occurs over a temperature range of about 10°C. This range is minimised by choosing the lowest frequency and seeds with the smallest diameter compatible with a sufficiently large heating power (BREZOVICH, 1988). In practice a frequency near to 100 kHz and seeds of about 1 mm in diameter have been used (MEREDITH et al, 1989; SHIMM et al, 1989).

When temporary implants are used in the interstitial therapy, problems related to the biocompatiblity of ferromagnetic seeds are circumvented since the seeds are inserted into plastic catheters and do not come into direct contact with the tissues. The problem of biocompatibility remains to be solved for applications in which permanent implants are envisaged. There have been investigations into using inert coatings for the seeds (CHEN et al, 1988; BREZOVICH et al, 1990) but practical and effective solutions have yet to be determined.

Comparison of techniques

Several theoretical and experimental studies of the performance of the various interstitial techniques have been reported. Most theoretical studies concerned with prediction of temperature distributions have used models based on 2-dimensional solutions to the bioheat transfer equation, although some 3-dimensional models have been reported recently. The 3-dimensional models

(Furse and Iskander, 1989; James et al, 1989; Uzonoglu and Nikita, 1988; Zhu and Gandhi, 1988) show that the predictions of 2-dimensional models are over-optimistic in the region of the tip of an implant. The limitations of the bioheat transfer equation have been discussed at length in the literature (Chen and Holmes, 1980; Weinbaum and Jiji, 1985; Lagendijk, 1987; Sekins, 1989) and the predictions of the models should be interpreted accordingly. Lim (1988) showed that the bioheat transfer equation tended to predict lower temperatures than a convective heat transfer model in simulations of heating by ferromagnetic implants in a phantom with directional perfusion. Crezee and Lagendijk (1990) compared predictions of the temperature distributions around a single vessel within vascularized tissue using the bioheat transfer equation and a model based on an effective thermal conductivity. Experimental measurement agreed with the predictions of the effective thermal conductivity model but were at variance with those of the bioheat transfer equation. In some cases SAR distributions alone have been studied, particularly for microwave antennas. Whilst SAR distributions are very useful as an aid to our understanding of the behaviour of microwave systems, it must be stressed that temperature distributions achieved during the clinical use of interstitial techniques are very dependent upon heat transport mechanisms within the tissue (Strohbehn and Mechling, 1986). The use of SAR alone is of little help in predicting performance in patients.

Effects of spacing of implants and blood flow

Strohbehn and Mechling (1986) compared the performance of an array of 4 implants consisting of RF electrodes, microwave antennas or constant temperature ferromagnetic seeds as functions of spacing and blood flow. This study showed that in the absence of blood flow, all three techniques could be expected to produce excellent temperature distributions (temperatures above 43°C throughout the target region) for spacings of 1, 2 and 3 cm. When blood flow was present and the spacing was 1 cm, the temperature distributions were excellent for blood flows up to 100 ml 100 g^{-1} min^{-1} in the case of microwave antennas and up to 20 ml 100 g^{-1} min^{-1} for the other techniques. When the spacing was 2 cm, microwave antennas still produced excellent temperature distributions for blood flows up to 20 ml 100 g^{-1} min^{-1}. RF electrodes performed marginally better than seeds at this spacing but the performance of both techniques was compromised by blood flows of 5 ml 100 g^{-1} min^{-1}. None of the techniques performed well when the implants were spaced at 3 cm. These findings are somewhat at variance with the results of a comparison in vivo of RF LCF electrodes and microwave antennas (Stauffer et al, 1989). Although confirming that the optimal spacing of implants was 10 – 20 mm, Stauffer et al found that temperature distributions produced by the RF LCF technique were more uniform than those for the array of microwave antennas. It must be remembered that Strohbehn and Mechling's predictions are from a 2-dimensional model which does not address the problem of decreased power deposition around the tips of the microwave antennas. Another reason for the discrepancy may have been deviation from idealised phase relationships between antennas in the experimental study. Clinical experience with RF LCF electrodes is that their spacing should be no more than approximately 15 mm (Cosset et al, 1985). Studies with various hot source techniques suggest that an array of implants spaced at approximately 10 mm should produce acceptable temperature distributions over a large range of perfusion rates (Stea et al, 1990; Brezovich et al, 1990; Schreier et al, 1990).

Summary

RF LCF techniques appear to be useful when tumours can be implanted with an array of parallel electrodes of approximately equal length. Flexible custom built electrodes are advantageous compared to rigid tubes. Inter-electrode spacing should be no more than 15 mm. Careful pretreatment selection of electrode pairs is necessary with most techniques. Current research is aimed at improving temperature distributions along electrodes and making the technique more tolerant of deviations from perfect geometry.

Microwave antennas are compatible with plastic catheters used in brachytherapy. The method requires the lowest density of sources (typically 1 per 4 cm^2) and is the most robust in regions of high blood flow. Improvements in antenna design to overcome low power deposition near the tip and to improve the longitudinal uniformity in temperature distributions are underway as is work on arrays aimed at optimum power deposition and control.

Hot water tube techniques offer a simple and low cost approach to interstitial hyperthermia. When the flow through tubes is turbulent, a temperature differential between the tissue and the water of a few °C is sufficient to achieve acceptable temperature distributions. Both open- (unidirectional flow) and closed- (counter flow) ended tubes may be used. As is the case for all hot source techniques, tubes should have the largest possible diameter and minimum spacing, subject to practical restrictions, to make the method more insensitive to increased blood flow. An implant density of 1 per cm^2 is typical. By using tubes with two heating zones, normal tissue adjacent to the proximal section of a tube may be protected from the hyperthermal treatment.

Self regulating ferromagnetic seeds have been developed in several institions. Since this is a hot source technique, a relatively high implant density (typically 1 per cm^2) is required. However, because of thermal regulation in the seeds, the technique is less demanding of perfect implant geometry. There is also less sensitivity to variable perfusion than is the case with methods which employ sources of constant power. Permanent implants may be possible when biocompatible seeds become available. Access to a supply of seeds with a range of Curie temperatures is likely to be necessary to implement the requirements of pretreatment planning.

Improvements in three dimensional modelling and in our understanding of the distribution of perfusion are required for all interstitial techniques.

A list of some advantages and disadvantages of various techniques for interstitial hyperthermia is given in Table 1. A similar format has been used by Stauffer (1990).

Table 1

LCF electrodes

Advantages	Disadvantages
* simplest EM technique	* flexible electrodes must be custom made
* commercial systems available	* parallelism of electrodes important
* relatively inexpensive	* set-up can be tedious
* longitudinal control of heating pattern possible using segmented electrodes	
* thermometry is relatively simple	

Microwave antennas

Advantages	Disadvantages
* commercial systems available	* longitudinal control of heating pattern difficult
* compatible with plastic catheters used in brachytherapy	* heating pattern depends on insertion depth
* offers greatest spacing between implants	* optical or other nonperturbing thermometry preferable
* most robust performance in regions with high blood flow	* relatively expensive
* control of SAR by amplitude and phase adjustments to individual antennas (coherent arrays)	

Hot source techniques

General features

Advantages	Disadvantages
* heating patterns independent of electrical heterogeneities in tissue	* closer spacing between implants required
* simple thermometry	* least robust robust performance in regions with high blood flow
* no restrictions on length of implants	

Specific features

Hot water tubes

Advantages	Disadvantages
* simple and low cost	* set up may be awkward
* commercially available	
* no problems with EMI or potential EM hazards	
* maximum temperature known	
* essentially constant temperature sources	

Specific features

Self-regulating ferromagnetic seeds

Advantages	Disadvantages
* implants heated remotely	* treatment planning critical
* thermally self-regulating	* difficult to change temperature of implants during treatment
* long term of permanent implants possible	* high cost
* tolerant of imperfect geometry	
* simple thermometry	

References

Astrahan MA, George FW (1980) A temperature regulating circuit for experimental localized current field hyperthermia systems. Med Phys 7: 362–364

Astrahan MA, Luxton G, Sapozink MD, Petrovich Z (1988) The accuracy of temperature measurement from within an interstitial microwave antenna. Int J Hyperthermia 4: 593–607

Atkinson WJ, Brezovich IA, Chakraborty DP (1984) Usable frequencies in hyperthermia with thermal seeds. IEEE Trans Biomed Engng BME-31: 70–75

Baba M, Itani K, Naito H, Suzuki A, Minamitani H (1987) An estimation of the ferromagnetic seeds for hyperthermia. In: Onoyama Y (ed) Hyperthermic Oncology '86 in Japan. Mag Bros Inc, Tokyo, pp 135–136

Brezovich IA (1988) Low frequency hyperthermia: Capacitive and ferromagnetic seed methods. In: Paliwal B, Hetzel FW, Dewhirst MW (eds) Biological, Physical and Clinical Aspects of Hyperthermia. American Institute of Physics, New York, pp 82–110

Brezovich IA, Atkinson WJ, Chakraborty DP (1984) Temperature distributions in tumor models heated by self-regulating nickel-copper alloy thermoseeds. Med Phys 11: 145–152

Brezovich IA, Lilly MB, Meredith RF, Weppelmann B, Henderson RA, Brawner Jr W, Salter MM (1990) Hyperthermia of pet animal tumours with self-regulating ferromagnetic thermoseeds. Int J Hyperthermia 6: 117–130

Brezovich IA, Meredith RF, Henderson RA, Brawne WR, Weppelmann B, Salter MM (1989) Hyperthermia with water-perfused catheters. In: Sugahara T, Saito M (eds) Hyperthermic Oncology 1988, vol 1. Taylor & Francis, London, New York, Philadelphia, pp 809–810

Burton C, Hill M, Walker AE (1971) The RF thermoseed – a thermally self regulating implant for the production of brain lesions. IEEE Trans Biomed Engng BME-18: 104–109

Chan KW, Chou CK, McDougall JA, Luk KH, Vora NL, Forell BW (1989) Changes in heating patterns of interstitial microwave antenna arrays at different insertion depths. Int J Hyperthermia 5: 499–507

Chen JS, Poirier DR, Damento MA, Demer LJ, Biencaniello F, Cetas TC (1988) Development of Ni-4 wt. % Si thermoseeds for hyperthermia cancer treatment. J Biomaterials Res 22: 303–319

Chen MM, Holmes KR (1980) Micro-vascular contributions in tissue heat transfer. Ann NY Acad Sci 335: 137–151

Cosset JM, Dutreix J, Haie C, Gerbaulet A, Janoray P, Dewar JA (1985) Interstitial thermoradiotherapy: A technical and clinical study of 29 implantations performed at the Institut Gustave-Roussy. Int J Hyperthermia 1: 3–13

Crezee J, Lagendijk JJW (1990) Experimental verification of bioheat transfer theories: Measurement of temperature profiles around large artifical vessels in perfused tissue. Phys Med Biol 35: 905 – 923

Demer LJ, Chen JS, Buechler D, Damento MA, Poirier DS, Cetas TC (1986) Ferromagnetic thermoseed materials for tumor hyperthermia. Proc. IEEE 8th Annual Conference of the Engineering in Medicine and Biology Society (vol 3). IEEE, New York, pp 1448–1453

Denman DL, Foster AE, Cooper Lewis G, Redmond KP, Elson HR, Breneman JC, Kereiakes JG, Aron BS (1988) The distribution of power and heat produced by interstitial microwave antenna arrays: II. The role of antenna spacing and insertion depth. Int J Radiat Oncol Biol Phys 14: 537–545

Deshmukh R, Damento M, Demer L, Forsyth K, DeYoung D, Dewhirst M, Cetas TC (1984) Ferromagnetic alloys with curie temperatures near 50°C for use in hyperthermic therapy. In: Overgaard J (ed) Hyperthermic Oncology 1984, vol 1. Taylor & Francis, London, New York, Philadelphia, pp 571–574

de Sieyes DC, Douple EB, Strohbehn JW, Trembly BS (1981) Some aspects of optimization of an invasive microwave antenna for local hyperthermia treatment of cancer. Med Phys 8: 174–183

Dewey WC (1989) Dr. Eugene Robinson (1925–1983). Int J Radiat Oncol Biol Phys 16: 531–532

Doss JD (1975) Use of RF fields to produce hyperthermia in animal tumors. In: Wizenberg MJ, Robinson JE (eds) Proceedings of International Symposium on Cancer Therapy and Radiation, Washington, DC, April 28–30, 1975. American College of Radiology, Bethesda, MD, pp 226–227

Doss JD, McCabe CW (1976) A technique for localized heating in tissue: An adjunct to tumor therapy. Med Instrum 10: 16–21

Durney CH (1987) Electromagnetic field generation and propagation. In: Field SB, Franconi C (eds) Physics and Technology of Hyperthermia. Martinus Nijhoff, Dordrecht, The Netherlands, pp 123–151

Furse CM, Iskander MF (1989) Three-dimensional electromagnetic power deposition in tumors using interstitial antenna arrays. IEEE Trans Biomed Engng BME-36: 977–986

Gautherie M (ed) (1990) Methods of External Hyperthermic Heating. Springer, Berlin, Heidelberg, New York, Tokyo

Geddes LA, Baker LE (1967) The specific resistance of biological material – a compendium of data for the biomedical engineer and physiologist. Med & Biol Engng 5: 271–293

Gerner EW, Connor WG, Boone MLM, Doss JD, Mayer EG, Miller RC (1975) The potential of localized heating as an adjunct to radiation therapy. Radiology 116: 433–439

Haider SA, Chen ZP, Cetas TC, Roemer RB (1987) Interstitial ferrmomagnetic implant heating: Practical guidelines for use. Proceedings of 9th Annual Conference of IEEE Engineering in Medicine and Biology Society (vol 3). IEEE, New York, pp 1626–1628

Hand JW, Trembly BS, Prior MV (1991) Physics of interstitial hyperthermia: Radiofrequency and hot water tube techniques. In: Urano M, Douple E (eds) Hyperthermia and Oncology, vol 3: Interstitial Hyperthermia. VSP, Zeist (in press)

Handl O, Handl-Zeller L, Schreier K, Lesnicar H, Budihna M (1989) Interstitial hyperthermia with microheat exchangers – system KHS-9/W18. In: Sugahara T, Saito M (eds) Hyperthermic Oncology 1988, vol 1. Taylor & Francis, London, New York, Philadelphia, pp 811–812

Hutson RL (1975) Modeling electric fields from implanted electrodes. In: Wizenberg MJ, Robinson JE (eds) Proceedings of International Symposium on Cancer Therapy and Radiation, Washington, DC, April 28–30, 1975. American College of Radiology, Bethesda, MD, pp 229–230

James BJ, Strohbehn JW, Mechling JA, Trembly BS (1989) The effect of insertion depth on the theoretical SAR patterns of 915 MHz dipole antenna arrays for hyperthermia. Int J Hyperthermia 5: 733–747

Jones KM, Mechling JA, Trembly BS, Strohbehn JW (1988) SAR distributions for 915 MHz interstitial microwave antennas used in hyperthermia for cancer therapy. IEEE Trans Biomed Engng BME-35: 851–857

Jones KM, Mechling JA, Trembly BS, Strohbehn JW (1989) Theoretical and experimental SAR distributions for interstitial dipole antenna arrays used in hyperthermia. IEEE Trans Microwave Theory & Tech MTT-37: 1200–1209

Kapp DS, Fessenden P, Samulski TV, Bagshaw MA, Cox RS, Lee ER, Lohrbach AW, Meyer JL, Prionas SD (1988) Stanford University institutional report. Phase 1 evaluation of equipment for hyperthermic treatment of cancer. Int J Hyperthermia 4: 75–115

King RWP, Smith GS (1981) Antennas in Matter. MIT Press, Cambridge, MA, pp 489–526

King RWP, Trembly BS, Strohbehn JW (1983) Electromagnetic field of an insulated antenna in a conducting or dielectric medium. IEEE Trans Microwave Theory & Tech MTT-31: 574–583

Kobayashi H, Amemiya Y (1985) Combined effect of implant heating and whole-body heating. In: Abe M, Takahashi M, Sugahara T (eds) Hyperthermia in Cancer

Therapy. Mag Bros Inc, Tokyo, pp 178–179

Kobayashi T, Kida Y, Ohta M, Kageyama N, Amamiya Y, Kobayashi H (1985) Experimental study on magnetic induction hyperthermia for brain tumor. In: Abe M, Takahashi M, Sugahara T (eds) Hyperthermia in Cancer Therapy. Mag Bros Inc, Tokyo, pp 158–159

Lacourse JR, Miller III WT, Vogt M, Selikowitz SM (1985) Effect of high-frequency current on nerve and muscle tissue. IEEE Trans Biomed Engng BME-32: 82–86

Lagendijk JJW (1987) Heat transfer in tissues. In: Field SB, Franconi C (eds) Physics and Technology of Hyperthermia. Martinus Nijhoff, Dordrecht, Netherlands, pp 517–552

Lee DJ, O'Neill MJ, Lam KS, Rostock R, Lam WC (1986) A new design of microwave interstitial applicators for hyperthermia with improved treatment volume. Int J Radiat Oncol Biol Phys 12: 2003–2008

Lim J (1988) Evaluation of temperature fields in two dynamic phantoms heated by the ferromagnetic implant hyperthermia. MS Thesis. Dept Aerospace and Mechanical Engineering, University of Arizona, Tucson.

Lin JC, Wang YJ (1987) Interstitial microwave antennas for thermal therapy. Int J Hyperthermia 3: 37–47

Marchal C, Nadi M, Hoffstetter S, Bey P, Pernot M, Prieur G (1989) Practical interstitial method of heating operating at 27.12 MHz. Int J Hyperthermia 5: 451–466

Marchosky JA, Moran C, Fearnot N (1988) A system for volumetric interstitial hyperthermia. Abtracts 36th Annual Meeting of Radiation Research Society, RRS, Philadelphia, p 32, abstract Ce-8

Matsui M, Shimizu T, Kobayashi T (1987) Research on hyperthermia implant materials from a point of view of material science. In: Onoyama Y (ed) Hyperthermic Oncology '86 in Japan. Mag Bros Inc, Tokyo, pp 63–64

Medal R, Shorey W, Gilchrist RK, Barker W, Hanselman R (1959) Controlled radiofrequency generator for production of localized heat in intact animal. Am Med Assoc Arch Surg 79: 427–431

Meredith RF, Brezovich IA, Weppelmann B, Henderson RA, Brawner WR, Kwapien RP, Bartolucci AA, Salter MM (1989) Ferromagnetic thermoseeds: Suitable for an afterloading interstitial implant. Int J Radiat Oncol Biol Phys 17: 1341–1346

Merry GA, Hale R, Zervas NT (1973) Induction thermocoagulation – a power seed study. IEEE Trans Biomed Engng BME-20: 302–303

Milligan AJ, Panjehpour M (1983) The relationship of temperature profiles to frequency during interstitial hyperthermia. Med Instrum 17: 303–306

Moidal RA, Wolfson SK, Selker RG, Weine SB (1976) Materials for selective heating in a radiofrequency electromagnetic field for the combined chemothermal treatment of brain tumours. J Biomed Mater Res 10: 327–334

Prandtl L (1963) Essentials of Fluid Dynamics. Blackie & Sons, Glasgow, pp 98–114

Prionas SD, Fessenden P, Kapp DS, Goffinet DR, Hahn GM (1989) Interstitial electrodes allowing longitudinal control of SAR distributions. In: Sugahara T, Saito M (eds) Hyperthermic Oncology 1988, vol 2. Taylor & Francis, London, New York, Philadelphia, pp 707–710

Prior MV (1991) A comparative study of RF-LCF and hot source interstitial hyperthermia techniques. Int J Hyperthermia 7: 131–140

Roos D, Hugander A (1988) Microwave interstitial applicators with improved longitudinal heating patterns. Int J Hyperthermia 4: 609–615

Satoh T, Stauffer PR (1988) Implantable helical coil microwave antenna for interstitial hyperthermia. Int J Hyperthermia 4: 497–512

Satoh T, Stauffer PR, Fike JR (1988) Thermal distribution studies of helical coil microwave antennas for interstitial hyperthermia. Int J Radiat Oncol Biol Phys 15: 1209–1218

Schreier K, Budihna M, Lesnicar H, Handl-Zeller L, Hand JW, Prior MV, Clegg ST, Brezovich IA (1990) Preliminary studies of

interstitial hyperthermia using hot water. Int J Hyperthermia 6: 431 – 444
Schwan HP (1957) Electrical properties of tissues and cell suspensions. Adv Biol Med Phys 5: 147–209
Schwan HP (1963) Electric characteristics of tissues – a survey. Biophysik 1: 198–208
Sekins KM (1989) Microvascular bioheat transfer equations. In: Sugahara T, Saito, M (eds) Hyperthermic Oncology, vol 2. Taylor & Francis, London, New York, Philadelphia, pp 758–760
Shimm D, Cetas T, Buechler D, Chen J, Dean S, Fletcher A, Haider S, Lutz W, Sinno R, Stauffer P, Cassady J (1989) Inductively heated, thermoregulating ferromagnetic seeds for interstitial thermoradiotherapy. In: Sugahara T, Saito M (eds) Hyperthermic Oncology, vol 1. Taylor & Francis, London, New York, Philadelphia, pp 594–595
Simpson PG (1960) Induction Heating. McGraw-Hill, New York
Smythe WR (1950) Static and Dynamic Electricity. McGraw-Hill, New York
Stauffer PR (1990) Techniques for interstitial hyperthermia. In: Field SB, Hand JW (eds) An Introduction to the Practical Aspects of Clinical Hyperthermia. Taylor & Francis, London, New York, Philadelphia, pp 344–370
Stauffer PR, Cetas TC, Fletcher AM, DeYoung DW, Dewhirst MW, Oleson JR, Roemer RB (1984a) Observations on the use of ferromagnetic implants for inducing hyperthermia. IEEE Trans Biomed Engng BME-31: 76–90
Stauffer PR, Cetas TC, Jones RC (1984b) Magnetic induction heating of ferromagnetic implants for inducing localized hyperthermia in deep seated tumours. IEEE Trans Biomed Engng BME-31: 235–251
Stauffer PR, Sneed PK, Suen SA, Satoh T, Matsumoto K, Fike JR, Phillips TL (1989) Comparative thermal dosimetry of interstitial microwave and radiofrequency-LCF hyperthermia. Int J Hyperthermia 5: 307–318
Stea B, Cetas TC, Cassady JR, Guthkelch AW, Iacono R, Lulu B, Lutz W, Obbens E, Rossman K, Seeger J, Shetter A, Shimm DS (1990) Interstitial thermoradiotherapy of brain tumors: Preliminary results of a phase I clinical trial. Int J Radiat Oncol Biol Phys 19: 1463 – 1471
Sternhagen CJ, Doss JD, Day PW, Edwards WS, Dobernek RC, Herzon FS, Powell TD, O'Brien GF, Larkin JM (1977) Clinical use of radiofrequency current in oral cavity carcinomas and metastatic malignancies with continuous temperature control and monitoring. In: Streffer C, et al (eds) Cancer Therapy by Hyperthermia and Radiation. Urban & Schwarzenberg, Munich, pp 331–334
Strohbehn JW (1983) Temperature distributions from interstitial rf electrode hyperthermia systems: Theoretical predictions. Int J Radiat Oncol Biol Phys 9: 1655–1667
Strohbehn JW, Mechling JA (1986) Interstitial techniques for clincial hyperthermia. In: Hand JW, James JR (eds) Physical Techniques in Clinical Hyperthermia. Research Studies Press, Letchworth, pp 210–287
Strohbehn JW, Trembly BS, Douple EB (1982) Blood flow effects on the temperature distributions from an invasive microwave antenna array used in cancer therapy. IEEE Trans Biomed Engng BME-29: 649–661
Stuchly MA, Stuchly SS (1980) Dielectric properties of biological substances – tabulated. J Microwave Power 15: 19–26
Taylor (1978) Electromagnetic syringe. IEEE Trans Biomed Engng BME-25: 303–304
Tinga WR, Nelson SO (1973) Dielectric properties of materials for microwave processing – tabulated. J Microwave Power 8: 23–65
Trembly BS (1985) The effects of driving frequency and antenna length on power deposition within a microwave antenna array used for hyperthermia. IEEE Trans Microwave Theory & Tech MTT-32: 152–157
Trembly BS, Wilson AH, Sullivan MJ, Stein AD, Wong TZ, Strohbehn JW (1986) Control of the SAR pattern within an interstitial microwave array through variation of antenna driving phase. IEEE Trans Micro-

wave Theory & Tech MTT-34: 568–571

Turner PF (1986a) Interstitial equal-phased arrays for EM hyperthermia. IEEE Trans Microwave Theory & Tech MTT-34: 572–578

Turner PF (1986b) Interstitial em applicator/temperature probes. In: Proceedings of 8th Annual Conference IEEE Engineering in Medicine and Biology Society, vol 3. IEEE, New York, pp 1454–1457

Uzonoglu NK, Nikita KS (1988) Estimation of temperature distribution inside tissues heated by interstitial RF electrode systems. IEEE Trans Biomed Engng BME-35: 250–255

Visser AG, Deurloo IKK, Levendag PC, Ruifrok ACC, Cornet B, van Rhoon GC (1989) An interstitial hyperthermia system at 27 MHz. Int J Hyperthermia 5: 265–276

Weinbaum S, Jiji LM (1985) A new simplified bioheat equation for the effect of blood flow on local average tissue temperature. J Biomech Eng 107: 131–139

Wong TZ, Strohbehn JW, Jones KM, Mechling JA, Trembly BS (1986) SAR patterns from an interstitial microwave antenna-array hyperthermia system. IEEE Trans Microwave Theory & Tech MTT-34: 560–567

Wu A, Watson ML, Sternick ES, Bielawa RJ, Carr KL (1987) Performance characteristics of a helical coil microwave interstitial antenna for local hyperthermia. Med Phys 14: 235–237

Yokoyama M, Wada J, Nagara H, Kasagi Y, Itaoka T (1985) Insertion of electric heater into the tumor tissue. In: Abe M, Takahashi M, Sugahara T (eds) Hyperthermia in Cancer Therapy. Mag Bros Inc, Tokyo, pp 94–95

Zhang Y, Dubal NV, Takemoto-Hambleton R, Joines WT (1988) The determination of the electromagnetic field and SAR pattern of an interstitial applicator in a dissipative medium. IEEE Trans Microwave Theory & Tech MTT-36: 1438–1443

Zhu XL, Gandhi OP (1988) Design of RF needle applicators for optimum SAR distributions in irregularly shaped tumors. IEEE Trans Biomed Engng BME-35: 382–388

5

Quality Assurance for Interstitial Radiofrequency-Induced Hyperthermia

S. D. Prionas and *D. S. Kapp*

Department of Radiation Oncology, Stanford University School of Medicine, Stanford, California, U.S.A.

Introduction

During the last decade, various interstitial techniques have been developed to induce and maintain hyperthermia (HT) in implantable solid deep-seated tumors. These techniques can be classified into two broad categories; those which utilize externally generated electromagnetic (EM) energy and a form of conversion of EM energy into heat [radiofrequency (RF) electrodes, capacitively-coupled RF implants, microwave (MW) antennas, and Curie point ferromagnetic seeds], and those which deliver energy in the form of heat with no need for an intermediate conversion (hot water tubes, low frequency resistive wire elements, and other hot source techniques). The principles of operation and detailed descriptions of the technical aspects of each heating delivery technique have been published elsewhere (Stauffer, 1989; Hand, 1990a; Hand, 1990b; International Consensus Report, 1990).

Although the nature of the heating technique, and the intricate details of the technology differ for each interstitial heating modality, they all share a common objective: to selectively induce elevated temperatures in the tumor, compared to normal surrounding tissues. The extent to which this objective is achieved depends on numerous parameters including the physical/physiological properties of the tumor and the normal surrounding tissues, the technique of implantation, the choice of the interstitial heating modality, details of the implementation which are specific to the heating device, as well as the ability of the heating device to adapt to dynamic changes occurring during the HT treatment. In order to assure optimum heating, control over the quality of each component of the HT treatment is essential Therefore, the various aspects of quality assurance (QA) for interstitial HT, to a certain extent, should address each of these issues.

There are at least three important areas where QA should be directed. The first relates to the safety of the patient undergoing an interstitial HT treatment: this includes the electrical safety of the heating device, the potential toxicities of the implantable materials (their biocompatibility), the safety of the implant technique (e.g. sterile conditions; avoidance of major blood vessels), and attention to ensure that non-tumor bearing tissues and vital organs of the patient are not exposed to the potentially cytotoxic effects of elevated temperatures. The second area for QA relates to the safety of the operator(s) of the heating device (clinician, radiation technologist, physicist, engineer, or nurse). These issues include the electrical safety of the heating device, power generator, and potential side-effects associated with exposure to stray fields. The third area for QA relates to the quality of the HT treatment delivered to the patient, the effectiveness of the treatment, the meticulous documentation of treatment-related parameters such as the adequacy of coverage of the tumor volume, the site of implantation, results of pre-treatment dosimetry, concurrent radiation dosimetry, post-treatment evaluation and data analysis. This area for QA should include issues involved with the standardization of the HT such as the number, location, and spacing of the interstitial inserts (e.g. RF electrodes, MW antennas, ferromagnetic seeds), the number, location, and orientation of thermometry catheters, temperature probe calibration, documentation of treatment set-up, the data acquisition of temperature-time profiles, frequency of temperature mapping, spatial increment of temperature maps, recording of the power (forward and reflected), and format of data recording/storage.

At Stanford University, the clinical utility of interstitial HT induced by means of RF electrodes has been under investigation for the past ten years (Kapp et al, 1988; Goffinet et al, 1990; Kapp and Prionas, 1991). In this chapter we will highlight areas where QA is essential; present some important aspects of our pre-treatment planning; describe the salient features of our heating and thermometry systems; and summarize the step-by-step procedure of the various items of QA that are implemented at the Stanford HT clinic in preparation for, during, and following an interstitial RF (IRF) HT treatment. Although we will concentrate on the QA for IRF HT systems, most of these QA issues are similarly applicable to other interstitial heating modalities (e.g. microwaves – Seegenschmiedt et al, 1989).

Areas for quality assurance

Patient safety

Our primary concern is the safety of the patient. This includes the issues of electrical safety, the biocompatibility of the implantable devices, and concerns about the implant technique. To ensure electrical safety of the patient a set of very stringent criteria of electrical safety should be implemented in the clinic (Bassen and Coakley, 1982; AAMI, 1988). The main electrical power should be filtered prior to its distribution within the shielded room. Each electrical device should be thoroughly checked for adherence to good grounding techniques. A test to evaluate the magnitude of leakage current should be performed on an annual basis. With respect to our specific device: main electrical power is provided to the IRF instrument through an ultra-isolation transformer, and the output of the high power RF amplifier is coupled to the implanted electrodes by means of a 1:1 isolation transformer (single-ended to balanced operation), so that the RF output signals are floating with respect to chassis ground. The safety of the implantable devices (e.g. RF electrodes and thermometry catheters) is assured by sterilizing all implantable devices prior to their use; employing coating or sheathing materials known to be non-toxic; and testing the mechanical durability and resistance to stress of the various coatings for loosening, breaks or chips prior to use.

Issues of patient safety which relate to the implant technique are clearly of major importance. Prior to the interstitial implant, laboratory tests should be conducted to determine that the patient's blood clotting time, differential blood counts and platelet counts are within normal limits. During the operation there should be strict adherence to sterile technique and extreme caution should be exercised to avoid puncturing major blood vessels, or vital organs. Pretreatment CAT scans or MRI studies should be obtained to help delineate the tumor volume and adjacent normal tissues. Patients should not be treated while under general anaesthesia, and should be fully responsive to pain at the time of HT. The time-temperature exposure to sensitive normal tissues should be considered. Special care need be directed to tissues with poor blood flow, since these areas can overheat with resultant complications. Normal tissue denervation resulting from prior surgery can also lead to excessive heating since the patient's pain sensation has been compromised and hot spots in unmonitored areas may develop. Electrical excitation of nerve fibers can potentially lead to involuntary contraction of skeletal muscle or possibly "referred pain".

Although no adverse effects have been reported following incidental exposure to EM energy at 500 KHz, certain organs (e.g. lens, testicles) can be at risk for thermal damage. The magnitudes of stray electric and magnetic components of the EM field in the proximity of the implant (5 cm from the electrodes) should be measured (ANSI, 1982; ANSI, 1990; Chou, 1990). Various exposure limits are being considered in different countries, and different safety guidelines have been established (Table 1). For example, the exposure limit that has been proposed by the American National Standard Institute (ANSI, 1990) in the USA is frequency-dependent: at 500 KHz, the proposed maximum values of the electric and magnetic field components, spatially averaged over a volume equivalent to the human body, are 614 V/m and 32.6 A/m, respectively; the maximum power density

Table 1. RF safety guidelines for operating personel

Source	Frequency Range (MHz)	Electric Field (V/m)	Magnetic Field (A/m)	Averaging Time (min)
United States of America – 1990 (proposed by ANSI)	0.1 – 3.0	614	16.3/f*	6
United Kingdom – 1986	0.3 – 10	600/f	5.0/f	N/A⁺
Federal Republic of Germany – 1984	0.03 – 2	1500	7.5/f	N/A

Modified from Tables 18.1A, 18.2 and 18.3, Chou, 1990.
*f = frequency (MHz).
⁺N/A = Not available.

of RF exposure, averaged over periods greater than 6 min, is 100 mW/cm^2.

The presence of metallic implants (e.g. large metal clips, prosthetic devices) located in close proximity to an interstitial implant may perturb the EM field and may lead to local hot spots. Contact of adjacent electrodes to a metallic clip may result in an electrical short. Caution should be exercised with such implants. Cardiac pacemakers worn by patients may present additional problems during IRF HT. Although present designs of cardiac pacemakers are significantly more immune to EM interference compared with older designs, such devices should be carefully evaluated prior to the treatment. The fetus in pregnant patients may be at high risk to exposure to EM energy during an interstitial HT treatment. Careful assessment of the risk to benefit ratio should be considered prior to such treatments.

Safety of operator

Each IRF HT treatment is delivered within a shielded room located in our HT clinic, to ensure that EM energy generated by the IRF system is effectively contained within the treatment room. Patient and operator safety is ensured by following well established safety procedures (AAMI, 1988). Main power is supplied through ultra-isolation power supplies, and grounding and good shielding techniques are implemented to minimize stray EM fields and ensure adherence to established exposure standards (Shrivastava et al, 1989; Chou, 1990; ANSI, 1982; ANSI, 1990).

In order to minimize RF exposure to personnel, it is recommended that a screen window in the shielded room be used to observe the patient during the treatment and that control of the power generator be performed in this separate adjoining room. The magnitude of stray EM fields at several key locations inside the shielded room (e.g. in close proximity of high RF power generators, coaxial cables, and at 5 cm from the interstitial implant) should be measured and documented during the treatment. Operators of RF units should be aware of the potentially detrimental side effects from exposure to stray EM fields and attempt to minimize their exposure.

Quality of treatment: Pre-treatment planning

Perhaps the most important steps in preparation for an interstitial HT treatment are related to the evaluation of the patient, documentation of the extent of the disease, estimation of the tumor volume, and planning the implant. This preplanning needs to take into consideration the nature of the surrounding normal tissues and the proximity of the tumor to neighboring vital organs and structures. Careful physical examination of the patient, a series of consecutive CAT scans through the treatment area taken every 0.5–1.0 cm, and/or MRI studies are essential in this evaluation. Since the size of the tumor may be influenced by therapy given prior to the implant it is important that reexamination and repeat scans be obtained close to the time of the implant. In addition, since the location and orientation of the tumor relative to the surrounding tissues can change depending on the position of the patient, it is important to scan the patient in a position as similar to the treatment position as possible. Based on these studies, parameters including the total number of electrodes (partially insulated stainless steel catheters or flexible RF electrodes), the active length of each electrode, the length of the electrode traversing normal tissues, the relative configuration of the implant, and the overall geometry are determined. This information is then used to prepare a set of electrodes of appropriate length and with the desired insulation. These are then sterilized prior to the implant. Also, a computer algorithm can be utilized, which through an iterative process, can optimize the three-dimensional (3-D) pattern of power deposition. Eventually we hope to be able to generate a family of 3-D temperature distributions assuming a set of "realistic" values for blood flow rate, thermal conductivity, and other parameters involved in the bioheat transfer equation.

An important QA issue relates to the spacing between electrodes in a given implant. The power depositon depends, among other things, on the electrical properties of the tumor and normal surrounding tissues. The 3-D isothermal contours depend on the blood flow rate, as well as on the thermal conductivity of the tissues. The former may change dramatically during HT and may differ in normal tissues compared with tumor. Therefore, it is expected that the "ideal" spacing is tissue- as well as site-dependent. From a practical standpoint, perhaps the best spacing is the one used to optimize the dose distribution of X-irradiation delivered during the brachytherapy procedure. Spacings of the order of 0.8 to 1.5 cm have been utilized in most implants. In our experience, the closer spacings lead to more uniform temperature distributions. As a result, most of our recent implants utilized a template-guided approach, employing a transparent template (plexiglas) which had pre-drilled holes in a rectangular grid pattern to maintain a spacing of 0.8 cm between columns and rows of the needles used for electrodes.

Although a significant amount of theoretical and experimental work has been devoted to thermal dosimetry, there is no consensus with respect to the choice of the "appropriate" formulation of the bioheat transfer equation (International Consensus Report, 1990). At the present time, we feel that temperature distributions predicted by computer simulations are not accurate enough to substitute for measured temperature profiles obtained during treatment. We consider it essential to plan the number, location, and orientation of thermometry catheters to be used for thermal dosimetry. The number of catheters placed for temperature monitoring should be proportional to the total number of electrodes implanted in a given tumor (and therefore proportional to the tumor volume), while their locations should be selected to yield the maximum amount of thermal information. Multipoint or mechanically mapped thermometry systems are essential.

Currently we are following the RTOG QA guidelines for interstitial HT (Emami et al, 1991). Table 2 summarizes the recommended distribution of thermometry catheters as a function of the number of implanted heating sources (RF electrodes). As an example, Fig. 1 illustrates a typical small implant consisting of 2 rows of 4 electrodes per row. Each electrode (solid rings) can be identified by a pair of coordinates (letter/numeral combination). In addition each electrode can be identified by a sequential number (1–8). The locations of additional pre-drilled holes which could be potentially used for thermometry have also been identified (dotted rings). In general, it is suggested that at least one thermometry catheter be placed close to the "center" of the tumor, and a second catheter be placed close to the tumor–normal tissue interface. Additional thermometry catheters should be

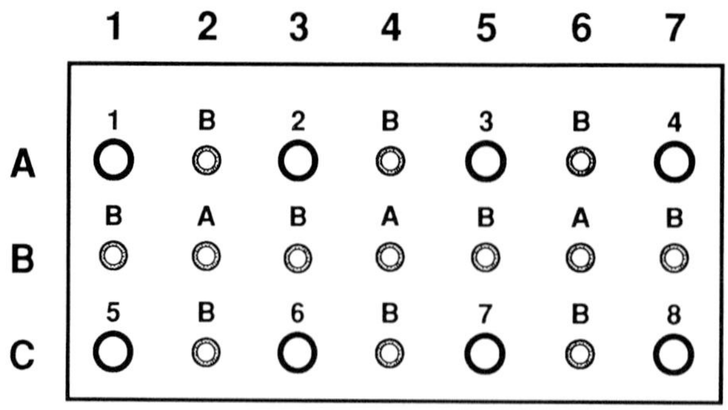

Fig. 1. Cross section of a hypothetical interstitial RF implant of two planes with four RF electrodes per plane. Electrodes (solid black rings) are numbered sequentially (*1–8*). The positions available for the insertion of thermometry catheters are also shown (dotted rings). The actual position of each insert is referenced in the Cartesian coordinate system by means of its column number (*1–7*) and row letter (*A–C*). Thermometry catheters located at the center of the square created by the four closest neighboring electrodes are termed (*A*). Thermometry catheters located between two neighboring electrodes are termed (*B*)

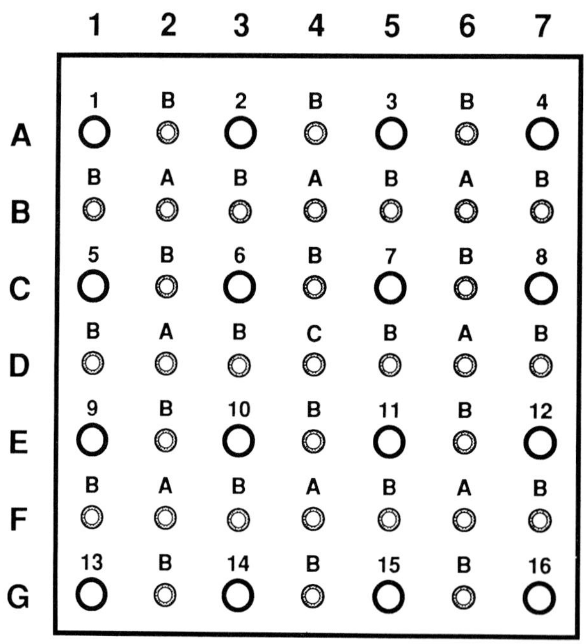

Fig. 2. Cross section of a hypothetical interstitial RF implant of four planes with four RF electrodes per plane. Electrodes (solid black rings) are numbered sequentially (*1–16*). The positions available for the insertion of thermometry catheters are also shown (dotted rings). The actual position of each insert is referenced in the Cartesian coordinate system by means of its column number (*1–7*) and row letter (*A–G*). Thermometry catheters located at the center of the square created by the four closest neighboring electrodes are termed (*A*). Thermometry catheters located between two neighboring electrodes are termed (*B*). One thermometry catheter is located at the center of the implant (*C*)

placed either at the center of a group of four electrodes (e.g. location A at the center of the square formed by electrodes #1, #2, #5, and #6) or between two neighboring electrodes (e.g. location B between electrodes #3 and #7). When clinically safe, one catheter should be placed outside the periphery of the tumor, to provide a record of the temperature distribution induced in the normal surrounding tissues. Also, if possible, catheters for thermometry should be placed perpendicular to the long axis of the implant. Furthermore, temperatures should be monitored in any tumor or adjacent normal tissue area of particular concern (e.g. scars; necrotic areas). Thus, a total of at least 2 catheters for thermometry should be used in this implant (e.g. one at location A and one at location B) and possibly one in neighboring normal tissues. Fig. 2 illustrates an implant consisting of 4 × 4 electrodes. A total of at least 3 catheters for thermometry should be used in this implant (e.g. one at location A, one at location B, and one at location C).

Quality of treatment: Verification of implant geometry

It is advisable to obtain X-ray placement films (AP and lateral) prior to removing the patient from the operating room. Strings of dummy seeds inserted into thermometry catheters should be used to help document their locations. These films can help as a guide for determining the quality of the implant, and to ensure that the implanted stainless steel trocars and the thermometry catheters are as parallel as possible. Repositioning and re-orientation might be possible at this time. When the patient has recovered from the implantation, a CAT scan should be obtained to document the precise geometry of the implant. At our facility, we have developed a CAT scan protocol which minimizes the "streaking" artifact caused by stainless steel needles. Based on these scans we can establish the 3-D orientation of the thermometry catheter(s) relative to the trocars, the boundaries of the implant volume, and can identify the part of the thermometry catheter(s) traversing normal surrounding tissues. Additional orthogonal X-rays are obtained, when appropriate, with contrast in adjacent normal organs (e.g. in the bladder and rectum for pelvic implants), to aid in dosimetry for brachytherapy and HT.

Quality of treatment: Standardization of HT treatment

The actual lengths of the catheters for thermometry should be chosen such that the temperature maps cover the maximum longitudinal dimension of the implanted tumor with an additional margin (0.5–1.0 cm) whenever possible. Temperature maps should be taken using non-perturbing probes, by manual or mechanical scanning, using a spatial increment of 0.5–1.0 cm. These temperature probes should meet the QA specifications previously established including: an accuracy of at least ±0.2 °C over the range of 30–50°C; a precision of ±0.1 °C or better; a stability of ±0.1 °C for the duration of treatment; and a response time of < 10 sec (SHRIVASTAVA et al, 1989). The temperature maps should be taken as often as possible during treatment. At least two maps should be obtained; the first soon after steady-state conditions have been achieved (early map), and the second later into the treatment (late map). The lateral extent of the heating element (active element) should be identified on these maps. Additionally, the part of the map in tumor versus normal surrounding tissue (proximal and distal to the tumor) should be delineated. Ideally, HT treatment goals should be standardized and should include a prescription as to the desired tumor temperature, duration of treatment, the temperature uniformity, the maximum intratumoral temperature and maximum normal tissue temperature permitted. At the present time, there is no consensous with respect to whether or not a tumor treated at a given iso-SAR level will indeed lead to an acceptable 3-D temperature distribution throughout the tumor volume. Tumor volume coverage based on the use of the 50%, 70%, or 80% iso-SAR contour lines has been suggested (Hand, 1990c). Considering the multitude of physical/physiological parameters that can affect the 3-D temperature distribution in a given tumor, we believe that our effort at the present time should be devoted to inducing, maintaining, and especially *documenting* the actual temperatures achieved. Perhaps in the future, one might be able to establish a relationship between the physiology of a given tumor, and the temperature distribution as a function of the iso-SAR level.

Quality of treatment: QA of our specific equipment

A block diagram of the interstitial RF heating system developed at Stanford University and a brief description of its operation have been provided in the previous chapter (Kapp and Prionas, 1991). In this section several elements of QA critical to the operation of this instrument are reviewed. The RF component of this instrument consists of a power amplifier cascade operating at 0.5 MHz. In order to ensure reliable and reproducible operation, a frequency counter is used to provide a continuous display of the operating frequency. The amplitude of the sinusoidal waveform generated by the signal generator is modulated by means of the voltage generated by a computer-controlled digital to analog converter. A portable oscilloscope is employed to verify that the output level and the quality of the waveform are reproducible from treatment to treatment. The gain of the high power amplifier is adjustable to provide for some additional flexibility in control. This is important during the early phase of HT induction in a given tumor, when there is the most uncertainty concerning the patient's thermal/electrical parameters (e.g. blood flow rate, thermal conductivity, electrical properties of the tumor). The instantaneous values of the RF voltage appearing across the output of the power amplifier and the RF current which flows through the complex load are monitored continuously by means of a voltage probe and a current probe. Visualization of the phase angle difference between the voltage and current provides the necessary feedback needed for adjusting the impedance matching network so as to minimize the power standing wave ratio (PSWR), as well as a convenient means for detecting the occurrence of a shorted or an opened circuit. The instantaneous levels of RF power generated by the amplifier in the "forward" direction, and the RF power "reflected" by the load are digitized and displayed by the computer, to augment the process of interpreting the temperature measurements taken during the HT treatment.

During a HT treatment, and for the purpose of thermal dosimetry, two separate groups of temperature probes are used. The first group of temperature probes, the so-called control sensors, is comprised of all those probes which are used to control the operation of the interstitial RF system. Each probe is essentially a teflon-coated twisted pair of copper/constantan wires forming a thermocouple junction (Physitherm, Corp., model IT-18) which is introduced at the center of the active element of a given electrode. The second group of temperature probes is used for temperature mapping. For this purpose, non-perturbing fiberoptic probes (Luxtron, Inc., model MPM) are utilized. These are mechanically scanned inside plastic thermometry catheters (Deseret, Inc.) which have been implanted for this purpose.

In general, established guidelines for thermometry developed by the Hyperthermia Physics Center (HPC) in the USA should be followed (SHRIVASTAVA et al, 1989). On a daily basis, the operation of each group of temperature probes is verified against an NBS-traceable mercury-in-glass thermometer prior to the HT treatment. If the temperature readings from any sensor deviate by more than ±0.1 °C, then the probes are recalibrated. For fiberoptic probes, a daily record of the deviations from true temperature is maintained for each probe. For thermocouple probes a two-point calibration procedure is utilized, and a permanent record of the calibration coefficients is maintained.

Traditionally, bare stainless steel trocars have been used for IRF HT induction. The need to protect normal surrounding tissues led to the development of partially insulated electrodes (GOFFINET et al, 1990). The need to improve the temperature distributions induced along the longitudinal axis of the implant has led to the development of segmented electrodes allowing control of the power deposition along their longitudinal axis (PRIONAS

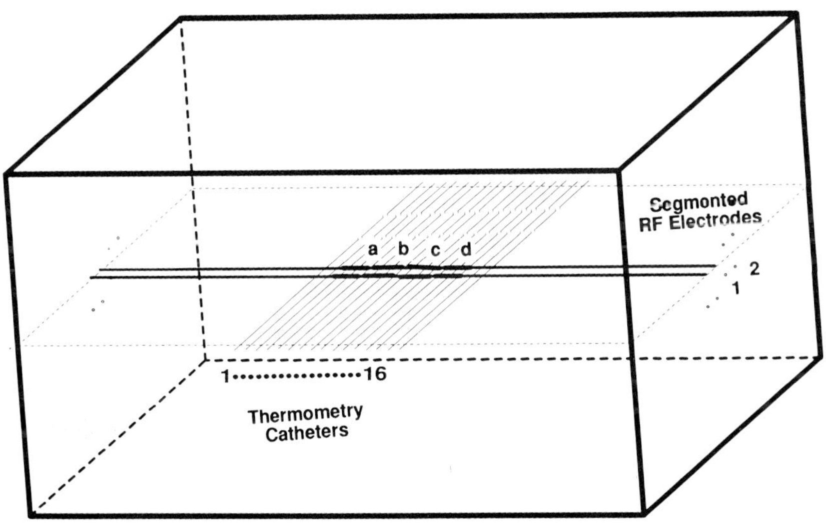

Fig. 3. Schematic drawing of experimental set-up illustrating the relative positions of interstitial RF electrodes and thermometry catheters used to measure the two-dimensional pattern of power deposition induced by interstitial RF electrodes in a static tissue equivalent phantom. Two segmented electrodes, #1 and #2, with four segments per electrode, labeled a, b, c, and d, are shown. A set of sixteen copper/constantan thermocouples inserted in plastic catheters (labeled 1 ··· 16) is used for temperature measurement

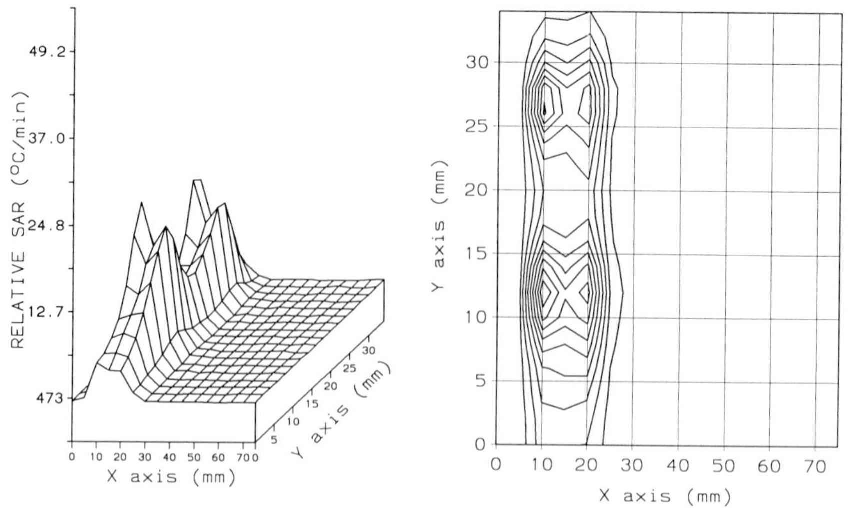

Fig. 4. Two-dimensional distribution of power deposition (relative SAR) generated by a pair of segmented interstitial RF electrodes. Electrode diameter was 2.1mm. The distance between the two segmented electrodes was 15 mm. Each segmented RF electrode had four electrically independent elements. The length of each electrode element was 13 mm. The separation between electrode elements was 2 mm. These data were generated from the initial positive slope of the temperature-time profiles acquired during sequential activations of electrode pair 1a & 2a (see Fig. 3). Net electrical power was 5 Watts. Activation time interval was 15 sec. Left panel: Axonometric plot. Right panel: Iso-SAR contour plot. Contour level increment was 10% of SAR_{max}

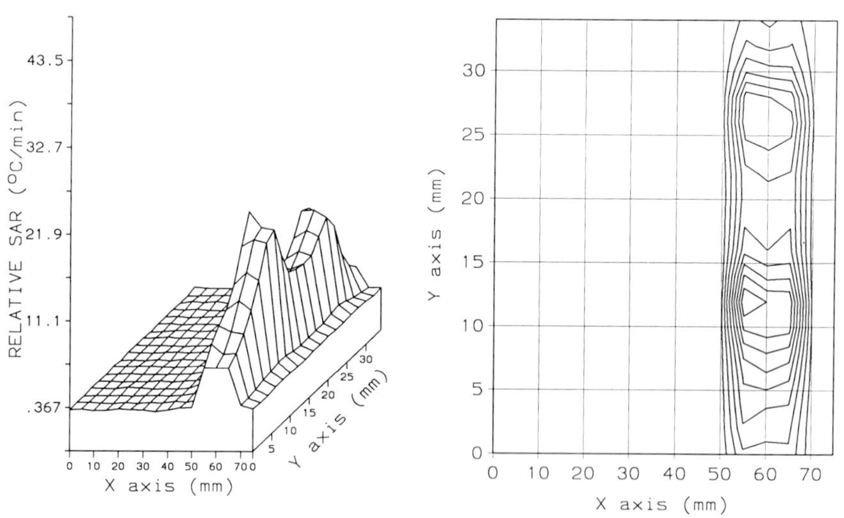

Fig. 5. Two-dimensional distribution of power deposition (relative SAR) generated by a pair of segmented interstitial RF electrodes as configured in Fig. 4. These data were generated from the initial positive slope of the temperature-time profiles acquired during sequential activations of electrode pair 1d & 2d (see Fig. 3). Net electrical power was 5 Watts. Activation time interval was 15 sec. Left panel: Axonometric plot. Right panel: Iso-SAR contour plot. Contour level increment was 10% of SAR_{max}

et al, 1989; KAPP and PRIONAS, 1991). Assurance of proper function and specific QA procedures must be developed for these recent developments. At our institution we have developed a technique to characterize the two-dimensional (2-D) distribution of specific absorption rate (SAR) generated by single and multiple-aperture (segmented) RF electrodes. These SAR distributions are determined in a static tissue equivalent phantom, suitable for IRF heating systems. Fig. 3 illustrates a schematic drawing of the device. A set of sixteen copper/constantan thermocouple sensors are utilized for temperature measurement. An example of the 2-D SAR generated by activating a pair of electrode elements (pair 1a & 2a, located at one end of the segmented electrodes) is shown on Fig. 4. A similar 2-D SAR distribution is generated when the pair of elements located at the opposite end of the electrodes (pair 1d & 2d) is activated (Fig. 5). Fig. 6 illustrates a 2-D distribution of SAR generated when all eight electrode elements are active.

The conversion efficiency of a given hyperthermia applicator is a characteristic parameter that describes the ability of the applicator to convert electrical energy into heat. Calorimetric techniques have been developed to allow rapid and accurate evaluation of this parameter. We feel that a similar technique should be developed to evaluate the functional status and perform routine QA for interstitial RF electrodes.

Quality of treatment: Data analysis

At the conclusion of an IRF treatment, the data collected during the treatment are analyzed so as to ensure the integrity of the data, and to identify problematic areas in need for improvement on subsequent treatments. The data consist of a time series of temperature measurements recorded by each sensor, as well as power measurements. Each temperature-time profile and power-time record is plotted and analyzed to compute several measures of thermal distribution (e.g. mean temperature during the steady-state condition, standard deviation, and minimum and maximum temperatures detected during this phase as previously described (KAPP et al, 1988). Temperature maps are treated similarly. These processed data are then transferred to a host computer (VAX; Digital Equipment Corporation) to be appended to our clinical data base for later processing. It should be realized that one needs to implement some means of data reduction, to ensure a meaningful interpretation of these data. A simple approach that allows us to accomplish this objective is to calculate the percentage of temperature data points measured in a linear temperature map with a value greater than or equal to a given temperature (index temperature).

Electrode multiplexing can aid in steering and modification of the 3-D pattern of

Table 2. Minimum number of thermometry catheters recommended for implantation to map temperature distributions induced by interstitial heating modalities. (Modified from Emami et al, 1991)

	Number of thermometry catheters		
Number of heating sources	A	B	C
3–8	0	1	1
9–16	1	1	1
17–32	2	1	1
>32	3	2	1

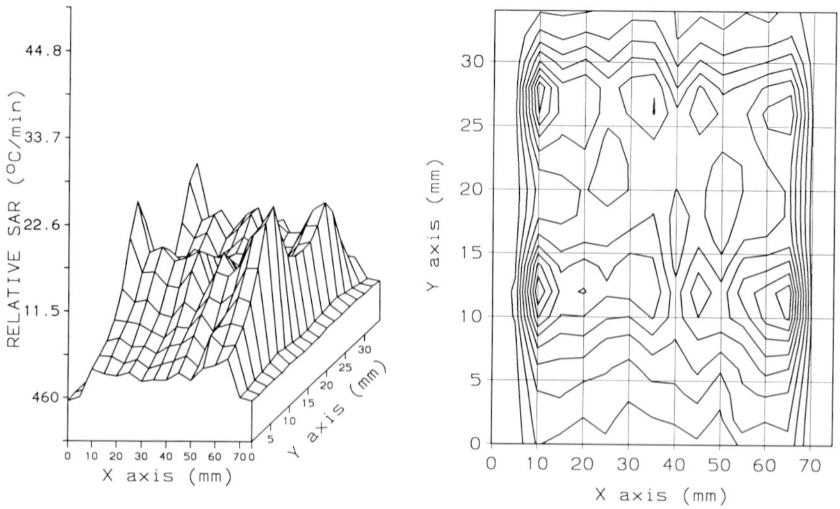

Fig. 6. Two-dimensional distribution of power deposition (relative SAR) generated by a pair of segmented interstitial RF electrodes as configured in Fig. 4. These data were generated from the initial position slope of the temperature-time profiles acquired during sequential activations of segmented electrode #1 (by electrically connecting all four elements, 1a/1b/1c/1d, to one terminal) with segmented electrode #2 (by electrically connecting all four elements, 2a/2b/2c/2d, to one terminal). Net electrical power level was 20 Watts. Activation time interval was 15 sec. Left panel: Axonometric plot. Right panel: Iso-SAR contour plot. Contour level increment was 10% of SAR_{max}

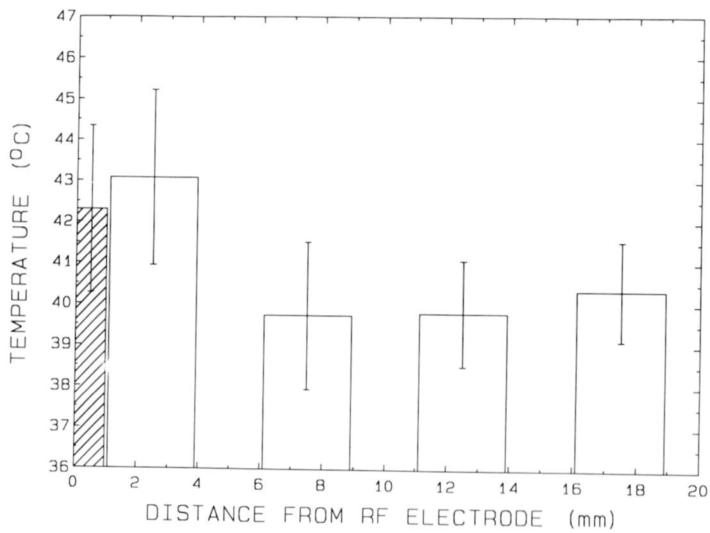

Fig. 7. Summary of steady-state temperatures measured during the 20 HT treatments of tumors located in the head & neck (5 patients) and the pelvic region (5 patients). The bar graph was generated by combining the temperature values measured either at the center of the active element of an active interstitial RF electrode (shaded bar) or within a thermometry catheter (open bars), at a point located at the shortest distance away from the center of the neighboring active RF electrode. Temperature distribution is plotted as a function of distance away from the closest interstitial RF electrode. Error bar is ± S.D.

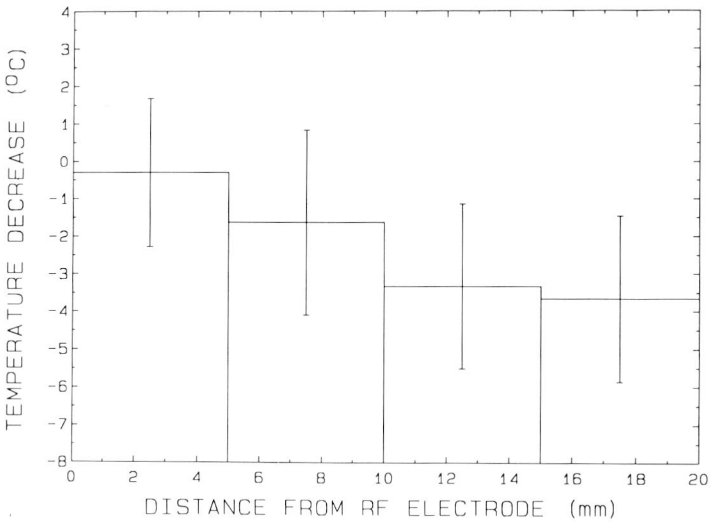

Fig. 8. Summary of temperature differences measured between interstitial RF electrodes and thermometry catheters in the steady-state condition during 20 treatments of ten tumors as in Fig. 7. Each temperature difference was calculated by subtracting the temperature value measured within a thermometry catheter, at a point located proximal to center of the active element of the closest neighboring RF electrode, from the steady-state temperature measured at the center of the active element of the closest interstitial RF electrode. Temperature differences are plotted as a function of distance away from the closest interstitial RF electrode. Error bar is ± S.D.

energy deposition during the treatment. A measure of this ability can be developed from evaluation of the temperature distributions induced along the axis perpendicular to the RF electrodes. Fig. 7 illustrates the results of our attempts to derive this distribution based on the temperature measurements recorded at the centers of the active elements of RF electrodes surrounding a thermometry catheter (control points) and at a point inside the thermometry catheter located proximal to these control points. These thermometry data were obtained during twenty treatments delivered to patients with head and neck (5 patients), and pelvic tumors (5 patients) (see Goffinet et al, 1990). Temperature differences between mapped probes and closest control probes are shown on Fig. 8. The same data plotted in the form of temperature distribution functions are shown on Fig. 9. This mode of data analysis has the potential for deriving information useful in evaluating the dynamic performance of the heating device, and as a means of ensuring the quality of the software and it's potential to adapt to changes occurring during heating.

Step-by-step procedure for QA of IRF HT treatment

To aid others in the establishment of their own in-house QA procedure the QA procedure for our IRF system is presented in outline form.

Before the IRF treatment

Verify that each copper/constantan thermocouple probe, to be used during the IRF treatment, is operational.

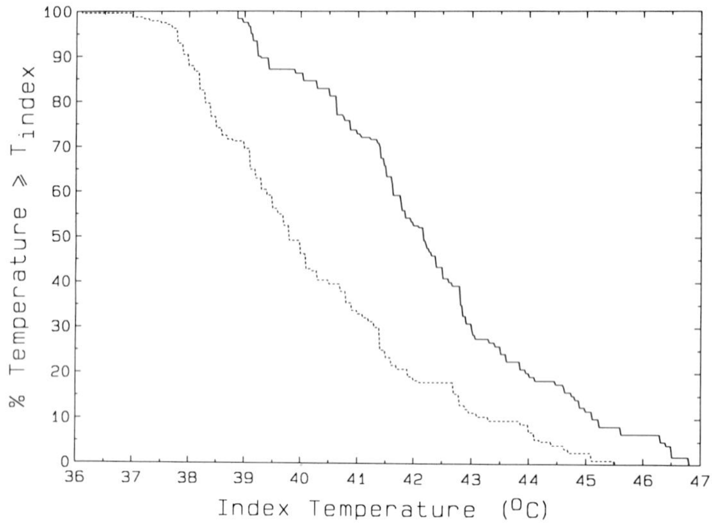

Fig. 9. Temperature distributions measured during 20 treatments delivered to ten patients with tumors as in Fig. 7. The percentage of temperature points with a value greater than or equal to a given temperature (index temperature) is plotted as a function of index temperature. Curve #1 (solid line): steady-state temperatures measured at the center of active element (control point) located proximal to the thermometry catheter. Curve #2 (dashed line): steady-state temperature measured inside the thermometry catheter at a point located the shortest distance away from the control point

a. Measure the resistance of each sensor – check for continuity.
b. Use a calibration water bath equipped with an NBS-traceable mercury-in-glass thermometer to check for long- or short-term drift of the calibration constants.

Verify that each thermocouple extension cable is operational (contacts are free from surface oxides, electrical connections are of good quality, wires are not loose, number-coding is correct).

Prior to sterilization, verify that each electrode is prepared correctly and working correctly.

a. With partially insulated stainless steel trocars, verify that the electrical insulation is intact, the length of the active zone is correct, the insulation is fixed and does not slide, the area of electrical contact is clear (free from electrically insulating materials such as heat-shrinking tubing, varnish, or paint).
b. With flexible electrodes (single or multiple element), verify the integrity of the complete assembly, make sure that each element is electrically insulated from each other, and that each electrode is electrically connected to the corresponding pin on the miniature connector (continuity test). If these electrodes have temperature sensors embedded in the plastic wall, verify that each temperature sensor is operational.

Ensure that the correct number of interconnecting (extension) wires is available. Verify that each is properly color- and number-coded. Verify that each is functioning properly (continuity test).

Verify that the power cable (for 110 Volts

AC) is safe to use (check resistance between ground pin to chassis, check to make sure that each power plug is firmly seated). Ensure that the ultra-isolation transformer is functioning properly.

Verify that each hardware device is operating properly.

a. Computer, display, printer.
b. Signal generator and frequency counter.
c. Data acquisition and control unit.
d. Power amplifier, impedance matching network.
e. Oscilloscope, voltage/current probes, 50 Ohm dummy load.
f. Switching matrix (electrode multiplexer).
g. Thermocouple "distribution" box (check for corroded copper or constantan contacts, bent, twisted, or broken shielded cable).
h. RF isolation transformer.

Turn the computer "ON". Display the contents of the root directory on the hard disc. Make sure that the hard disc is functioning correctly. Park the read/write head before moving the instrument rack to the HT suite.

Check the date and time; correct if necessary.

Use the portable, pseudo-dynamic phantom, and simulate the actual configuration of RF electrodes. This is a simple phantom which allows for a quick but extensive test of the functional performance of the IRF system (setup time is of the order of 10–15 min).

Connect the RF output to the built-in 50 Ohm dummy load. Remove the control signal from the AM input of the signal generator (by disconnecting the BNC cable which connects the output from the DAC to the external AM modulation input of the signal generator). Manually adjust the level of the input signal and/or the gain of the power amplifier, to maintain a constant output power level (e.g. 10 Watts). Verify that the RF voltage and RF power readings displayed on the front panel of the power amplifier, the D.C. voltage being output from the power meter(s), and oscilloscope readings (peak-to-peak voltage, peak-to-peak current, and phase angle difference) are in agreement. Reconnect the control signal.

Execute the diagnostic routine(s) to verify that each hardware component operates normally (static tests).

Verify that the temperature readings are correct. Recalibrate the thermocouple sensors if necessary.

Execute the IRF program to ensure that each component of the closed loop is functioning correctly (dynamic test). Generate a sample data file, store it on the hard disc, and then TYPE it out on the CRT, to verify that the data are stored correctly.

Park the read/write head of the hard disc (in preparation for transport).

During the IRF treatment

Oversee the operation of the clinical IRF instrument. Switch to semi-automatic control if necessary.

Observe temperature readings, watch out for temperature outlyers indicative of RF interference, a poor electrical connection, or an intermittent electrical contact.

Observe readings of RF power (forward & reflected), RF voltage, RF current, and changes in their phase angle difference. Adjust settings of impedance matching network as necessary.

Make sure that patient and operator(s) are safe (electrically) by ensuring that each electrical device is properly grounded and electrically insulated (provide filtered AC power through ultra-isolation transformer).

Use the electric and magnetic field probes (Holaday Industries, Inc., model HI-3003) to measure the intensity of the stray EM fields in the proximity of the implant as well as other key locations inside the shielded room.
Make sure that the temperature data, power levels, date, and time are properly recorded on the hard disc for later processing.
Document with diagram and photograph patient and implant position.
Document the occurence and nature of any treatment limiting events (e.g. patient pain, excessive normal tissue temperatures, excessive tumor temperatures) and what corrective measures were undertaken.

After the IRF treatment

Thoroughly clean and safely package each thermocouple sensor.
Disconnect, and save all BNC coaxial cables.
Rename data file (to be appended in archive file).
Ready all equipment for safe transport back to the laboratory.
Plot temperature data, power data, print patient notes, etc.
Analyze data to derive useful results.
Archive the raw data file in patient's archive file (on floppy diskette and magnetic tape cartridge).

Discussion

The need for QA to assure optimum quality of HT results has been well illustrated by initial clinical experience (Perez et al, 1989). An extensive set of general guidelines resultant from clinical investigations has been published for RTOG cooperative HT trials in the USA (Dewhirst et al, 1990). A list of specific guidelines for interstitial HT in general has also been compiled (Emami et al, 1991).
We believe that it is imperative for each institution clinically utilizing HT (either alone or in conjunction with XRT or chemotherapy), to establish their own in-house general QA measures for HT, as well as equipment specific QA measures. This is especially relevant for interstitial HT techniques which invasively position applicators or heating sources directly into the patient.
Care must be taken to ensure patient and operator safety, optimization of treatment, and documentation of HT treatment. As experience with IRF is accumulated and equipment development continues, QA measures may need to be modified both in terms of the frequency of QA checks and the type of studies needed. For example, temperature measurements from actual treatments, we well as computer assisted thermal modeling have demonstrated the need for power control along the longitudinal axis of the implant, related both to heterogeneity in blood flow, thermal conductivity, and electrical properties of the tumor model, and to the geometry of the needle placement. This will necessitate additional thermometry to permit better power regulation during treatment. In the future 3-D modeling of SAR and temperature distributions will permit better pretreatment planning. QA procedures to ensure optimum functioning of this more complex system – including the computer based models – should accompany these future developments. Further

improvements in the clinical results already obtained by IRF (KAPP and PRIONAS, 1991) are anticipated.

Acknowledgments: We gratefully acknowledge the technical assistance of John L. Sokol in preparing the illustrations. This work was supported by NCI Grant CA-44665.

References

AAMI (1988) American national standard, safe current limits for electromedical apparatus (ES1 – 1985). In: Essential Standards for Biomedical Equipment Safety and Performance. Association for the Advancement of Medical Instrumentation, Arlington, Virginia, pp 1–20

ANSI (1982) American National Standard Safety Levels with Respect to Human Exposure to Radiofrequency Electromagnetic Fields, 300 KHz to 100 GHz. IEEE, New York, pp 1–24

ANSI (1990) American National Standard Proposed Safety Levels with Respect to Human Exposure to Radiofrequency Electromagnetic Fields, 3 KHz to 300 GHz (proposed)

Bassen HI, Coakley RF Jr (1982) United States radiation safety and regulatory considerations for radiofrequency hyperthermia systems. In: Nussbaum GH (ed) Physical Aspects of Hyperthermia. American Association of Physicists in Medicine, Medical Physics Monograph No. 8. American Institute of Physics, Inc., New York, pp 372–392

Chou CK (1990) Safety considerations for clinical hyperthermia. In: Field SB, Hand JW (eds) An Introduction to the Practical Aspects of Clinical Hyperthermia. Taylor & Francis, London, New York, Philadelphia, pp 533–564

Dewhirst MW, Phillips TL, Samulski TV, Stauffer P, Shrivastava P, Paliwal B, Pajak T, Gillin M, Sapozink M, Myerson R, Waterman FM, Sapareto SA, Corry P, Cetas TC, Leeper DB, Fessenden P, Kapp DS, Oleson JR, Emami B (1990) RTOG quality assurance guidelines for clinical trials using hyperthermia. Int J Radiat Oncol Biol Phys 18: 1249–1259

Emami B, Stauffer P, Prionas SD, Ryan T, Corry P, Dewhirst M, Herman T, Kapp DS, Myerson R, Samulski TV, Sapareto S, Sapozink M, Shrivastava P, Waterman F (1991) Quality assurance guidelines for interstitial hyperthermia (an RTOG document). Int J Radiat Oncol Biol Phys 20: 1117–1124

Goffinet DR, Prionas SD, Kapp DS, Samulski TV, Fessenden P, Hahn GM, Lohrbach AW, Mariscal JM, Bagshaw MA (1990) Interstitial ^{192}Ir flexible catheter radiofrequency hyperthermia treatments of head and neck and recurrent pelvic carcinomas. Int J Radiat Oncol Biol Phys 18: 199–210

Hand JW (1991) Physical aspects of interstitial hyperthermia. Chapter 4 in this book, pp 51–75

Hand JW, Trembly BS, Prior MV (1990b) Physics of interstitial hyperthermia: Radiofrequency and hot water tube techniques. In: Urano M, Douple E (eds) Hyperthermia and Oncology, vol 3. Interstitial Hyperthermia. Vsp BV, Utrecht

Hand JW (1990c) Quality assurance in hyperthermia. In: Field SB, Hand JW (eds) An Introduction to the Practical Aspects of Clinical Hyperthermia. Taylor & Francis, London, New York, Philadelphia, pp 513–532

International consensus meeting on Hyperthermia: Final report (1990) Int J Hyperthermia 6: 837–877

Kapp DS, Prionas SD (1991) Experience with radiofrequency – local current field interstitial hyperthermia: biological rationale, equipment development, and clinical results. Chapter 6 in this book, pp 95–119

Kapp DS, Fessenden P, Samulski TV, Bagshaw MA, Cox RS, Lee ER, Lohrbach

AW, Meyer JL, Prionas SD (1988) Stanford University institutional report: Phase I evaluation of equipment for hyperthermia treatment of cancer. Int J Hyperthermia 4: 75–115

Perez CA, Gillespie B, Pajak T, Hornback NB, Emami B, Rubin P (1989) Quality assurance problems in clinical hyperthermia and their impact on therapeutic outcome: A report by the Radiation Therapy Oncology Group. Int J Radiat Oncol Biol Phys 16: 551–558

Prionas SD, Fessenden P, Kapp DS, Goffinet DR, Hahn GM (1989) Interstitial electrodes allowing longitudinal control of SAR distributions. In: Sugahara T, Saito M (eds) Proceedings of the 5th International Symposium on Hyperthermic Oncology 1988, vol 2. Taylor & Francis, London, New York, Philadelphia, pp 707–710

Seegenschmiedt MH, Sauer R, Herbst M, Thiel H-J, Fietkau LW, Karlsson U (1989) Interstitial hyperthermia for H & N tumors: Treatment planning and quality assurance (QA). In: Sugahara T, Saito M (eds) Proceedings of the 5th International Symposium on Hyperthermic Oncology 1988, vol 2. Taylor & Francis, London, New York, Philadelphia, pp 524–527

Shrivastava P, Luk K, Oleson J, Dewhirst M, Pajak T, Paliwal B, Perez C, Sapareto S, Saylor T, Steeves R (1989) Hyperthermia quality assurance guidelines. Int J Radiat Oncol Biol Phys 16: 571–587

Stauffer P (1990) Techniques for interstitial hyperthermia. In: Field SB, Hand JW (eds) An Introduction to the Practical Aspects of Clinical Hyperthermia. Taylor & Francis, London, New York, Philadelphia, pp 344–370

6

Experience with Radiofrequency-Local Current Field Interstitial Hyperthermia: Biological Rationale, Equipment Development, and Clinical Results

D. S. Kapp and *S. D. Prionas*

Department of Radiation Oncology, Stanford University, School of Medicine, Stanford, California, U.S.A.

Introduction

Considerable progress has been made in the clinical utilization of local hyperthermia (HT) as an adjunct to radiation therapy (XRT) in the treatment of superficially-located malignancies during the past 15 years (ANDERSON and KAPP, 1990). Evidence is accumulating demonstrating a correlation between the ability to heat tumors and the therapeutic outcome as measured by complete response rates or duration of local control (KAPP, 1988; VALDAGNI et al, 1988). While the parameters which best define our ability to heat tumors remain to be better elucidated, most studies show a relationship between some measure reflecting the average minimum or average intratumoral temperature distribution and outcome (KAPP, 1988). However, currently available non-invasive microwave or ultrasound heating techniques have limited field sizes and depths of penetration, making it difficult to obtain effective heating (goal ≥43°C for 30–60 minutes) at tumor depths of greater than 2–3 cm. Investigational systems employing radiative electromagnetic arrays or capacitive heating have some promise for deeper heating but, in general, result in regional rather than local heating of the tumors (HIRAOKA et al, 1984; PETROVICH et al, 1989).

One potential solution for providing improved and more homogeneous heating for accessible superficial or deep-seated tumors involves the implantation of the heating sources directly into the tumor in a manner analogous to that used in brachytherapy (BT). This permits minimizing the heating of the adjacent normal tissues. Furthermore, one can design the heating element such that simultaneous or closely sequenced HT and BT can be administered.

Several general methods have been developed for the induction of interstitial HT. Broadly grouped, these include: (1) radiofrequency (RF)-local current field techniques; (2) microwave antenna arrays; (3) hot source techniques – including ferromagnetic seeds, hot wires, circulating hot water systems, and laserthermia; and (4) hybrid techniques – including the 27 MHz capacitive coupled local current field heating technique (VISSER et al, 1989). This chapter will review the biological rationale, physics and engineering, clinical results and future plans for two RF systems developed and tested at our facility. The clinical results of RF-local current field techniques and interstitial heating with microwave antennas will be summarized. Other studies employing interstitial HT techniques are presented elsewhere in this volume and have been reviewed in recent publications (COUGHLIN and STROHBEHN, 1989; STAUFFER, 1989; PEREZ and EMAMI, 1989).

Biological rationale for low-dose rate brachytherapy and RF interstitial hyperthermia

The results of laboratory studies investigating the interaction of XRT and HT were considered in the initial design of the RF-interstitial systems developed and used in the clinical protocols employed at our facility. One major criterion was to design systems that could induce interstitial HT and accommodate 192-Ir seeds for the administration of low dose rate BT. Cell culture and murine tumor studies had suggested that the thermal enhancement ratio varied inversely with dose rate and was greater for a dose rate of one to several cGy per minute than for acute exposure at rates of approximately 100 cGy per minute (BEN-HUR et al, 1974; HARISIADIS et al, 1987; MOORTHY et al, 1984). Systems were, therefore, designed to employ BT at a dose rate of approximately one cGy per minute, our standard dose rate for interstitial BT for head and neck and pelvic tumors. Murine tumor studies (OVERGAARD, 1980) and clinical trials (ARCANGELI, 1984; OVERGAARD, 1984) had also demonstrated that the maximum enhancement of tumor cell killing occurred for simultaneous administration of HT and radiation. If the tumor could be selectively heated, the simultaneous administration of HT and XRT would produce the maximum therapeutic gain. Therefore, a second criterion was to develop interstitial systems that could selectively heat the tumors. Systems were designed to insulate the portions of the electrodes passing through the normal tissues adjacent to tumor such that only the portions of the electrode within the tumor were active. Electrodes were developed with hollow central cores so that standard ribbons of 192-I iridium seeds could be rapidly loaded, permitting minimum delay between the HT and XRT. Simultaneous HT and XRT was not employed in our studies because of the potential radiation exposure hazards to the personnel. Since it is unclear whether pre- or post-radiation HT was more advantageous, our trials elected to give HT both immediately prior to as well as immediately following the BT. Equipment development and clinical trials attempted to exploit both biological complementation between the HT and the BT as well as spatial complementation – limiting the heating to the tumor volume and, thereby, minimizing any potentiation of the radiation effects in the surrounding normal tissues.

Physics and engineering

The basic concept of local-current field interstitial heating was introduced by DOSS and MCCABE (1976). In principle, a source of alternating voltage connected between two metal catheters (electrodes) implanted in tissue, generates an alternating current which flows across the tissue between the two electrodes. The instantaneous value of this current is equal to the ratio between the applied voltage, and the impedance present between the electrodes (Ohm's law). In general, this impedance is a complex quantity with a real, or resistive component, and an imaginary, or reactive component. The magnitude of either component depends on the frequency of the alternating current, the distance between the two electrodes, the physical dimensions of each electrode, and the electrical properties of the tissue (i.e. electrical conductivity and permittivity or relative dielectric constant). The resulting current can be thought of as consisting of a real (or resistive) component and an imaginary (or reactive component). The resistive (or ionic) component generates heating (Joule's law), while the reactive component (displacement current) allows for the exchange of energy stored in the form of an electric or a magnetic field.

Interstitial RF hyperthermia systems operate in the frequency range between 100 KHz and 27 MHz. The low frequency limit is selected to avoid the effects of depolarization of nerve and muscle fibers. The high frequency end is limited by design constraints imposed on the impedance matching network and other practical considerations involving the nature and type of the temperature sensors used for thermometry. Typically, interstitial radiofrequency local current field (IRF/LCF) hyperthermia systems operate in the range of 0.5–1.0 MHz. At these low frequencies, the predominant carriers of electric charge include free electrons, small ions, and several species of charged macromolecules. At the cellular level, the presence of biological membranes composed of lipid bilayers, and the overabundance of polar molecules leads to an increase in relative dielectic constant, and a proportional decrease in the magnitude of the displacement current (Takashima and Fishman, 1977).

Mathematical models

The mathematical formulation describing LCF heating has been reported in detail previously (Strohbehn and Mechling, 1987) for the two-dimensional case. However, for most of the clinical uses of RF interstitial HT, volume implants are utilized and a three-dimensional model is necessary. Uzunoglu and Nikita fulfilled this need with their elegant analytical formulation of an idealized 3-D volume implant (Uzunoglu and Nikita, 1988). This model is applicable to a homogeneous tissue (e.g. the liver) and for a perfect geometrical configuration of the implanted electrodes. Fig. 1 illustrates the distribution of relative specific absorption rate (SAR) generated by a single pair of IRF electrodes. In this simulation, the two electrodes have been placed precisely parallel to each other. Unfortunately, in many clinical situations, various anatomical constraints preclude the placement of the heating electrodes along a predefined lattice or 2-D grid, and it is quite common to see electrodes converging as much as 5°–10°. We have developed an analytic solution which incorporates the angle of convergence between two convergent IRF electrodes. Fig. 2 illustrates the results of a 3-D calculation of the relative SAR generated by a pair of convergent electrodes. In this simulation, the angle of convergence was taken as 20° (i.e. each electrode is rotated by 10° about the midpoint of its long axis). The results are illustrated for the same plane

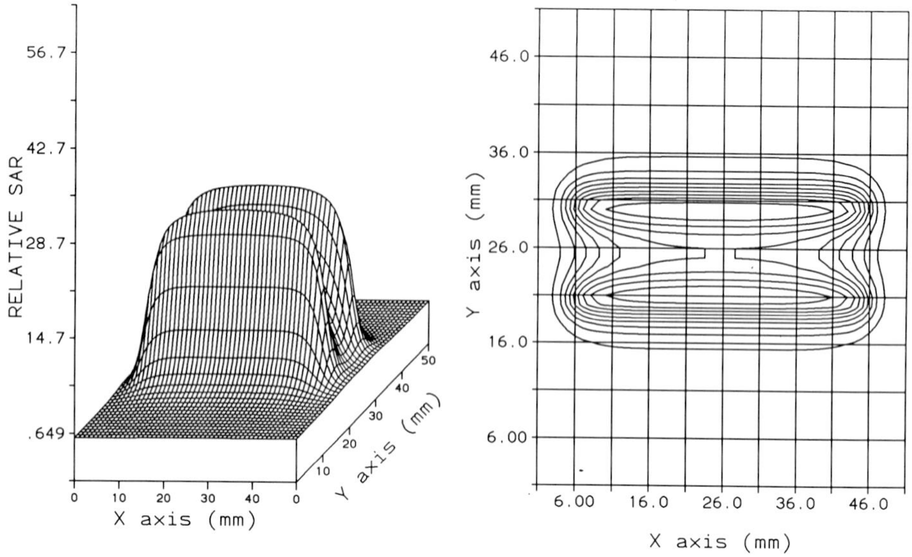

Fig. 1. Two-dimensional distribution of relative SAR generated by a pair of parallel IRF electrodes. The measurement plane was parallel to the plane defined by the two electrodes. The separation between planes was 1.1 cm. Electrode diameter was 2.1 mm. Length of active element was 4.0 cm. The separation between electrodes was 1.5 cm. Grid size was 51 × 51 points. Spatial resolution was 1 mm. Left panel: relative SAR plotted in the form of a pseudo 3-D (axonometric) plot. Right panel: relative SAR plotted in the form of closed contour lines. Contour interval was 10% of SAR_{MAX}

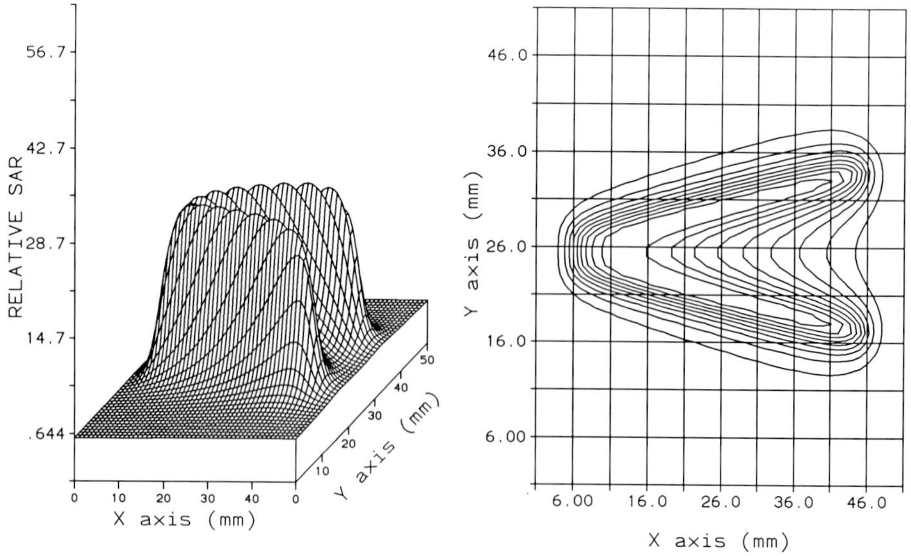

Fig. 2. Two-dimensional SAR distribution generated by a pair of convergent IRF electrodes. Angle of convergence was 20°. For additional details see legend for Fig. 1.

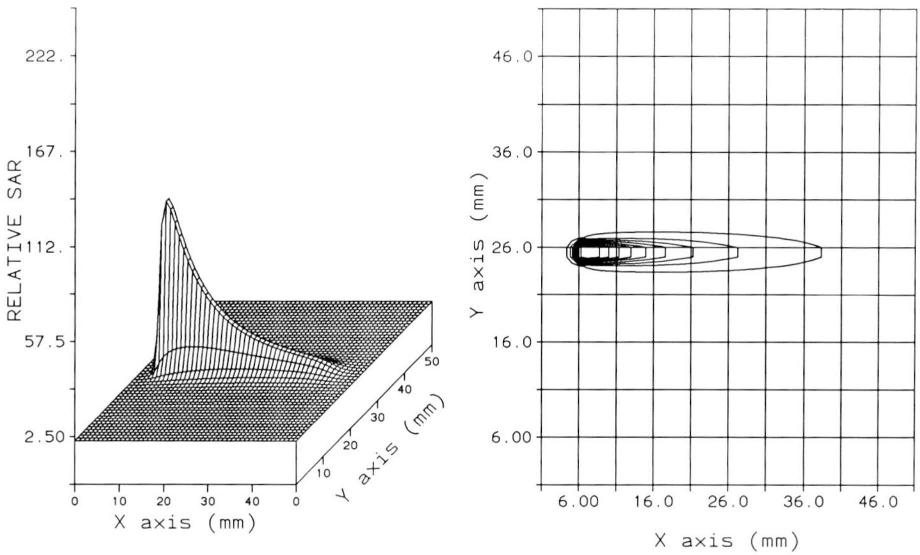

Fig. 3. Two-dimensional SAR distribution generated by a pair of convergent IRF electrodes across a plane (measurement plane) which was perpendicular to the plane defined by the two electrodes. Measurement plane was equidistant from both electrodes. Angle of convergence was 20°. For additional details see legend for Fig. 1.

as that in Fig. 1. Notice the considerable increase in power deposition (relative SAR) occurring near the tips of the two electrodes (X = 10 mm, Y = 25 mm on the contour map). A better visualization of this effect is shown in Fig. 3, which shows the distribution of relative SAR generated across the central plane. Notice the tremendous variation of SAR along the longitudinal axis (X axis) and the considerably narrow width of the distribution along the Y axis. The temperature distribution induced in a homogeneous tissue will of course be related to the pattern of the SAR distribution. However, in the clinical situation, tissue heterogeneity, variations in blood flow, and tissue thermal conductivity will tend to modulate these temperature distributions and smooth out the sharp discontinuities.

IRF equipment

Clearly, any interstitial hyperthermia system should be equipped with the necessary hardware, software and components to provide a sufficient amount of flexibility in control to compensate for any of the limitations discussed in the previous section. At Stanford University, we have developed an interstitial RF-based hyperthermia instrument, which is adaptable to a number of possible configurations. A schematic diagram of this system is shown in Fig. 4. The instrument has been described elsewhere (KAPP et al, 1988; GOFFINET et al, 1990). Briefly, a signal generator operating at 500 KHz provides a low level, computer controlled RF signal, which is amplified, and subsequently applied between a pair of IRF electrodes. The pair of these electrodes is selected from the total number of implanted elec-

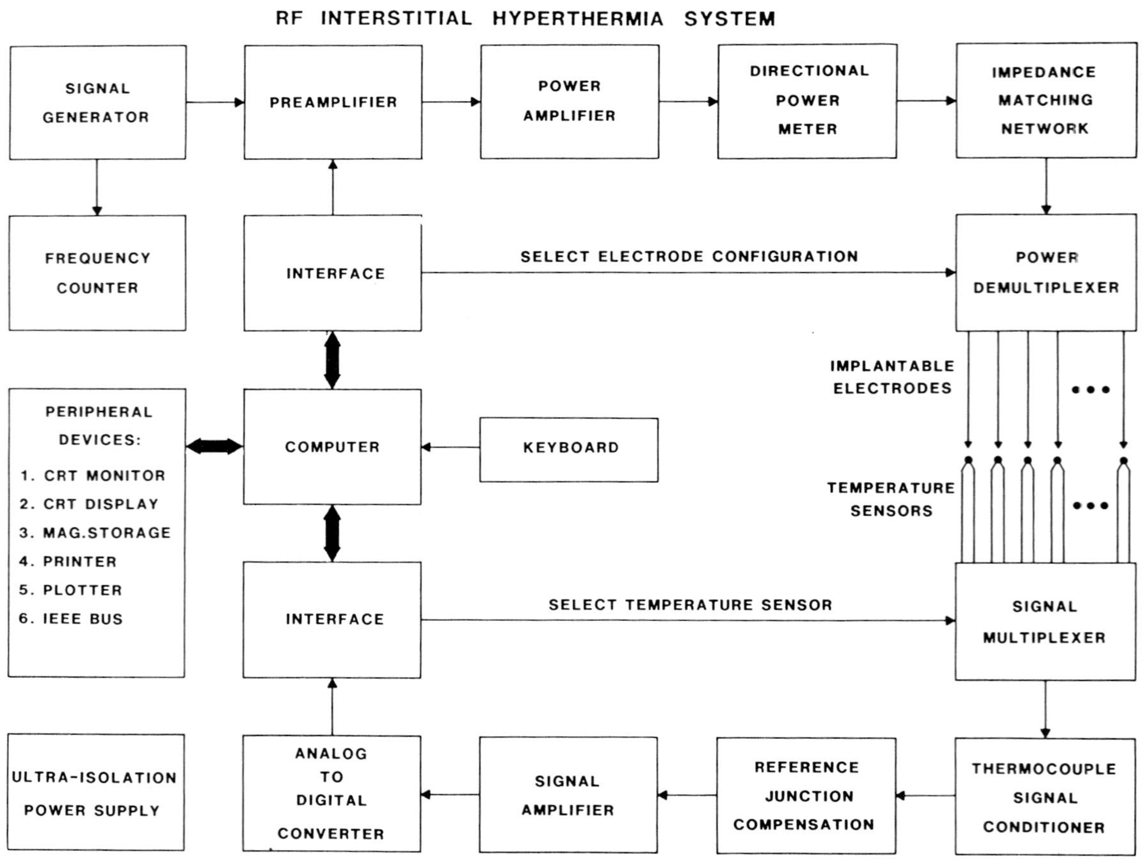

Fig. 4. Schematic diagram of RF-based interstitial hyperthermia system developed at Stanford University. See text for details. (Reproduced with permission from Kapp DS, et al, 1988.)

trodes using an M × N switching matrix (M = 2, N = total number of electrodes or electrode elements, in the range of 2 to 32). Measurement of the instantaneous net electrical power is provided by means of a four-quadrant analog multiplier. Temperature measurements are taken from the center of each electrically active electrode element using electrically shielded and insulated copper/constantan thermocouple sensors.

The temperature from each sensor is sampled by a high speed dual-slope integrating digital voltmeter, at a rate of 1–3 samples/sec. The system controller, an IBM-PC/AT microcomputer, operates the data acquisition and control unit, the electrode multiplexer, and supporting peripheral devices. The software has been written to utilize the fullest extent of the flexibility offered with this hardware configuration. During each iteration, the software, based on the values of the temperatures measured in each electrode, determines the next pair of electrodes to be activated. Usually, this pair is the one at the lowest average temperature, unless this criterion is overridden by other considerations having higher priority (for example, the rate of sequential activation of a given pair, pain threshold, and choice of target temperature). We have elected to implement a simplistic algorithm which allows us to set and control the power level and the average temperature of *each* electrode individually. During normal operation, this feature allows us to increase or decrease the target temperature in the range of 37°C to 49°C being recorded by a given control sensor. This provides a convenient means to compensate for temperature inhomogeneities attributable to the effects of thermally significant blood vessels, and in addition, it provides a simple means of minimizing or eliminating the pain occasionally caused by a localized hot spot.

IRF electrodes

Rigid electrodes

Early designs of IRF electrodes were based on the use of a section of bare stainless steel tubing (trocar). In an attempt to eliminate or at least minimize the detrimental effects of inadvertently exposed normal tissue to the cytotoxic effects of elevated temperatures, we elected to use a thin layer of electrical insulation to coat the parts of each electrode traversing the normal tissue neighboring a deep-seated tumor. Prototypes of partially insulated IRF stainless steel trocars were coated with a thin layer of modified polyvinylidene fluoride (KYNAR)[1] heat-shrinkable tubing (wall thickness = 0.25 mm). Currently, we are evaluating the utility of a thin coating of polyimide (thickness = 5–10 μm) applied by a process of sequential and repetitive dipping and baking at 325°C.

Flexible IRF electrodes

Hollow, stainless steel-based electrodes offer some unique advantages. For instance, a template-guided trocar with a closed and sharpened tip has a tendency to be inserted straight when it is applied through the skin and subcutaneous soft tissues. This leads to a more parallel implant, which in tumors, results in a more uniform radiation dose distribution and power deposition. However, in several anatomically difficult to access sites, it is more convenient and less traumatic to use flexible IRF electrodes. The basic design and the performance of these electrodes has been reported elsewhere (Kapp et al, 1988; Goffinet et al, 1990). The flexible insert is composed of a hollow, electrically insulated tubing coated with a thin braid of electrical conductor (nickel). The sections of the electrical conductor which traverse the normal surrounding tissue are electrically insulated with a thin layer of vinyl.

Segmented electrodes

We are presently developing rigid – and flexible – substrate based segmented (multiple element) IRF electrodes (PRIONAS et al, 1989). The electrodes provide the additional capability of control over the SAR distribution along the longitudinal axis of the electrode. Clinical use of segmented electrodes should help to improve the 3-D distribution of power deposition in a volumetric implant.

Advantages and disadvantages of IRF systems

The key advantages of an RF-based interstitial hyperthermia system compared to other interstitial systems relate to its simplistic design and concomitant lower cost. The use of low RF frequencies leads to greater depths of penetration and more uniform energy deposition (compared to MW antennas). Compared with hot water systems, which do not have the ability to dissipate any energy in tissue away from the source of heating other than by conduction, the IRF systems should be expected to generate more uniform temperature distributions.

The most important disadvantage of IRF systems is related to the fact that a large number of individual electrodes are required to cover an average-sized tumor. Although the dependency of tissue type and tumor site on electrode spacing has not been rigorously evaluated, it is expected that electrode spacings ranging from 0.7 cm to 1.6 cm will be required in most clinical situations.

Clinical results

RF/LCF hyperthermia using flexible electrodes

A series of ten patients with locally recurrent or advanced primary tumors of the head and neck or pelvic regions were treated at Stanford University Medical Center using individually constructed flexible catheters for interstitial BT and RF-interstitial HT. The patient and implant details have been presented previously and will be summarized here (GOFFINET et al, 1990). Five patients had advanced primary head and neck tumors (three, base of tongue; two, floor of mouth). They all had received 3000–6000 cGy external beam irradiation, followed by interstitial hyperthermic implant (Table 1). HT was given immediately prior to and immediately after BT (2000 cGy–4270 cGy). The goals of the HT were to obtain intratumoral temperatures of 43–44°C for 45 minutes duration without exceeding intratumoral temperatures of 50°C or normal tissue temperatures of 43°C. One patient (#3) had received prior XRT to the treatment

Table 1. Interstitial hyperthermia using an Ir-192 flexible catheter RF system for head and neck tumors

Pt. No.	Age (Yrs)	Site	Stage
1	40	Base of Tongue	T_4N_0
2	76	Base of Tongue	T_4N_1
3	35	Base of Tongue	T_4N_0
4	60	Floor of Mouth	T_4N_0
5	67	Floor of Mouth	T_4N_3

Modified from GOFFINET et al, 1990.

Table 2. Treatment and results with interstitial hyperthermia using an Ir-192 flexible catheter RF system for head and neck tumors

Pt. No.	Ext. Beam Dose (cGy)	Implant Dose (cGy)	Implant Volume (cm^3)	Response	Outcome (Time-Months)
1	6000	2000	125	CR	LF-24
2	6000	2534	70	CR	DID-15
3	3000	4270	80	CR	DF-8
4	5000	2420	86	CR	LF-8
5	5940	2013	66	CR	NED-60

LF, Local failure; DID, Died other causes, no evidence of recurrence; NED, no evidence of disease; DF, recurrence outside of implant volume.
Modified from GOFFINET et al, 1990.

Table 3. Interstitial hyperthermia with an Ir-192 flexible catheter RF system for recurrent pelvic tumors

Pt. No.	Age	Site of Recurrence	Primary Site	Prior Treatment
6	73	Persacral	Colorectal	Surgery
7	54	Presacral	Colon	Surgery, then EBRT
8	51	Pelvic Wall	Rectal	Multiple Surgeries, EBRT
9	62	Perineum	Rectal	Surgery, EBRT & Superficial HT
10	56	Presacral	Sigmoid Colon	Surgery, I-125 implant, EBRT

EBRT, External Beam Radiation Therapy; HT, Hyperthermia.
Modified from GOFFINET et al, 1990.

field for the management of Hodgkin's disease 12 years earlier. Therefore, his external beam dose at the time of retreatment was limited to 3000 cGy and his BT dose was increased (4270 cGy). All patients tolerated the treatment without significant complications and complete responses were obtained in all five tumors. One patient remains free of disease at five years; two have had local failures at eight and 24 months; one died of other causes at 15 months; and one died following distant metastases at eight months (Table 2).

Five additional patients were treated with this RF interstitial HT system for pelvic recurrences of colorectal cancers (Table 3). They all had failed prior treatment with surgery alone (one patient) or surgery and XRT (four patients). Retreatment was with external beam XRT (one patient) as well as BT with RF interstitial HT (five patients: dose 1900–4348 cGy) with the dose utilized based on the extent of prior XRT. HT treatment goals were identical to those employed in the head and neck tumors and all treatments were accomplished without

Table 4. Treatment and results with interstitial hyperthermia using an Ir-192 flexible catheter RF system for recurrent pelvic tumors

Pt. No.	Ext. Beam Dose (cGy)	Implant Dose (cGy)	Implant Volume (cm^3)	Response	Outcome (Time-Months)
6	5400	4000	44	Stable	LF-12
7	none	4000	24	CR	LF-3
8	none	3407	29	NR	LF
9	none	1900	62	CR	LF-3
10	none	4348	20	CR	DF-4

LF, Local failure; DF, recurrence outside of implant volume.
Modified from GOFFINET et al, 1990.

complications. Three patients obtained complete responses; one had stable disease for one year; and one failed to respond. Two of the complete responders failed locally at three months while one patient died following distant metastases at four months (Table 4).

Thermometry in patients heated with flexible electrodes

Temperatures were measured and thermal distributions calculated using techniques and formulations as previously described (KAPP et al, 1988; GOFFINET et al, 1990). At the time of implantation, two to four additional closed-end 16 gauge catheters[2] were inserted into the tumor and adjacent normal tissues. High impedance thermistors (Bowman probes) and/or fiberoptic temperature sensors[3] were inserted into these catheters and mechanically or manually moved at 0.5 cm or 1.0 cm intervals to monitor temperatures. Steady-state conditions or near steady-state conditions were obtained approximately five to ten minutes after power was turned on. Temperature maps were made at least twice during treatment – the first shortly after steady-state was obtained, and the second approximately 30 minutes later. In addition, single-point temperature measurements were recorded (during power off cycles) at the center of each implanted electrode using copper/constantan thermocouple sensors.[4]

An example of the temperature versus location (mapped measurements Fig. 5) illustrates the temperature variation both with time during treatment and with location within the tumor.

Table 5 summarizes the thermal placement data. The total number of RF electrodes utilized in these ten patients was 76 and an additional 136 control electrode temperatures were utilized during the first and second heat treatments. Ninety-three temperature maps were recorded. Temperature distributions were obtained as a function of: (a) time during treatment comparing temperature maps measured early in treatment (<27 minutes) with those obtained later in treatment (>27 minutes); (b) temperatures of the control probes within the RF electrodes versus intratumoral map temperatures; (c) normal tissue temperatures versus intratumoral temperatures; (d) tumor site (head and neck versus pelvis) and (e) control temperatures measured

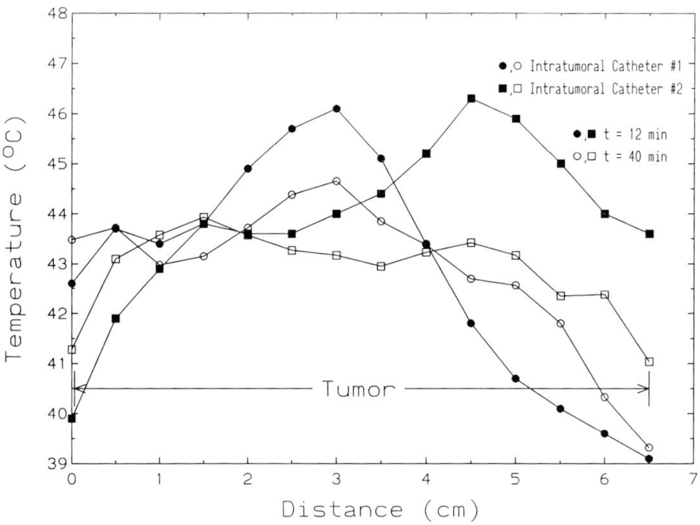

Fig. 5. Temperature maps measured along the length of two catheters oriented parallel to the longitudinal axis of the implanted electrodes during a hyperthermia treatment given to a patient with a presacral recurrence of colorectal cancer (Patient #6, Tables 3 and 4)

Table 5. Thermometry placement in flexible catheter Ir-192 RF hyperthermia

Tumor Location	No. Patients	No. RF Catheters		No. of Thermometry Catheters		No. of Temperature Maps	
		Average	Range	Average	Range	Average	Range
Head & Neck	5	10.8	8–15	3.6	2–5	12.4	8–16
Pelvic	5	4.4	3–5	2.2	2–3	6.2	4–8

Modified from GOFFINET et al, 1990.

during the first versus the second heat treatment.

No statistically significant differences were noted in temperature distributions between maps obtained early into treatment (<27 minutes) or later during the same treatment (>27 minutes) ($p = 0.09$). This suggests that there were no dramatic changes in blood flow or vascular collapse occurring as a result of the treatment. The control temperatures were statistically greater than the mapped temperatures ($p < 0.0001$) reflecting the expected fall-off of temperature in tissues distant to the electrodes. Only 56% of the temperature control sites were at temperatures ⩾42°C reflecting patient pain which limited our ability to maintain control temperatures set at the desired (43°C to 44°C) temperature levels. Mapped tumor temperatures were significantly higher than measured adjacent normal tissue temperatures ($p < 0.0001$). This confirmed our ability to selectively heat the tumor by tailormaking the active lengths of the electrodes to conform to the tumor dimensions. Less than 1% of the mapped temperatures in normal tissues were >42°C. Relatively high blood flow in the adjacent normal tissues probably also contributed to the rapid temperature fall-off at the normal tissue-tumor boundaries (SAMULSKI et al, 1987). Higher temperature distributions were obtained in tumors in the pelvic region than for head and neck tumors ($p < 0.0001$). This probably reflects the influence of higher blood flow rates in the head and neck area during HT. Only 7.1% of the mapped temperatures in tumors of the head and neck exceeded 42°C compared to 40.7% for the pelvic tumors.

Temperature maps measured for each patient during the first HT treatment compared with the second heat treatment revealed improved heating in the first heat treatment ($p = 0.04$). This probably reflects the residual influence of the anesthesia on pain control during the first HT treatment. A comparison of the temperature distributions for the control point temperatures (measured in the electrodes) for the first versus the second treatment (Fig. 6) also showed higher minimum temperatures as well as average temperatures measured during steady state conditions for the first treatment ($p = 0.0001$ and $p = 0.0027$, respectively).

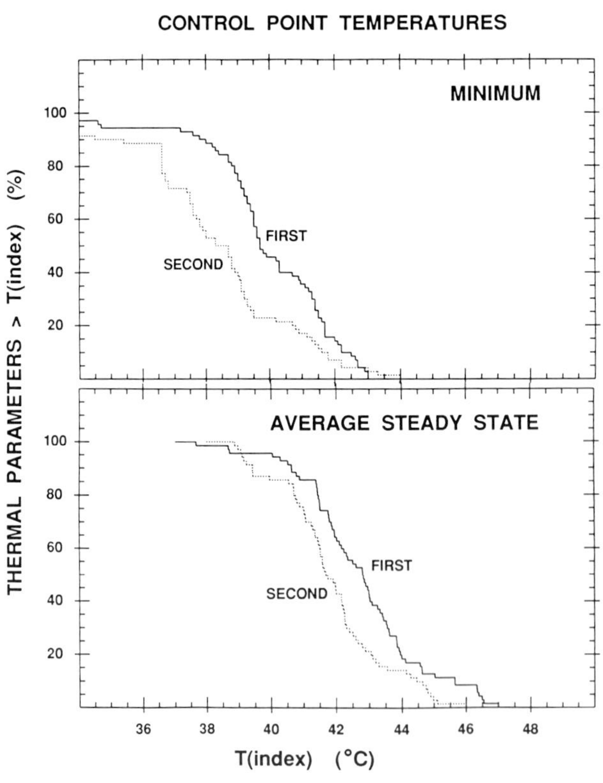

Fig. 6. Comparison of temperature distribution based on temperature measurements taken from within the flexible IRF electrodes (control point temperatures) for the first versus the second hyperthermia treatment. Top panel: Minimum control point temperatures ($p = 0.0001$). Bottom panel: Average control point temperatures during steady state ($p = 0.0027$)

RF/LCF hyperthermia with rigid electrodes

Clinically detectable local failure rates in Stages B_2 and C prostatic cancer following external beam XRT are high (SHIPLEY, 1988). Even higher rates of persistent microscopic disease have been noted in biopsies obtained after radiation therapy (KABLIN et al, 1989). This has led to the investigation of more intensive therapies for large localized prostatic cancers. One approach currently being studied at Stanford involves the utilization of 192-Ir implant boosts following external beam irradiation (BAGSHAW, 1990). A further extension of this approach utilizes interstitial HT implants in locally-advanced (Stages B_2, C) or recurrent prostatic cancers. We have employed the same treatment guidelines as for the flexible electrode RF implants described above. HT is administered for 45 minutes both prior to and after the BT. However, in place of the flexible catheters, hollow (O.D. = 1.45 mm) steel trochars[5] have been utilized. These steel trochanters can accommodate the ribbons of 192-Ir seeds as employed for our standard BT treatments of prostatic cancer. The steel needles also serve as electrodes for the interstitial HT treatments. The portions of the steel needles that remain in normal tissue can be insulated with heat shrink tubing (thickness = 0.25 mm) applied to the desired segment of the electrode based on an assessment of the tumor volume from pretreatment CT or MRI scans.

A steel needle electrode implant in a patient with Stage C prostatic cancer is illustrated in Fig. 7. The electrodes were implanted into the tumor and an extra catheter was placed in the tumor for temperature monitoring. One additional catheter was also placed in the adjacent normal tissue approximately 1 cm from the desired implant volume for normal tissue temperature monitoring. A rapid fall-off of temperatures was noted in this adjacent normal tissue, with tempera-

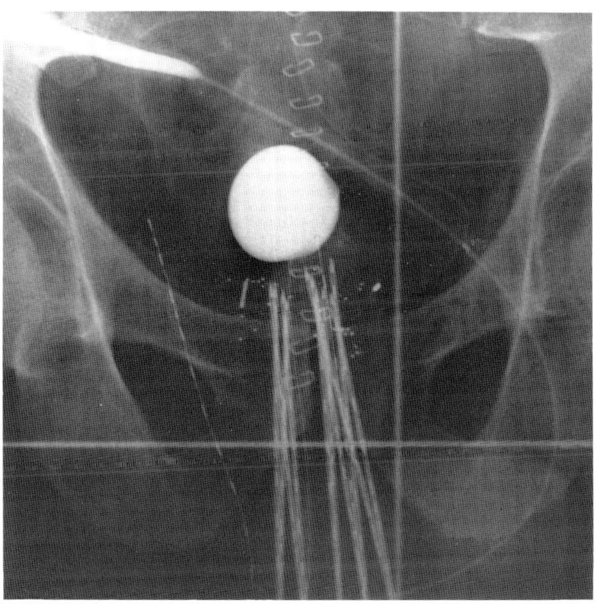

Fig. 7. Radiograph of implant in a patient with stage C prostatic cancer. The most lateral catheter on the patient's right was placed in the tissue adjacent to the prostate to permit monitoring of normal tissue temperatures

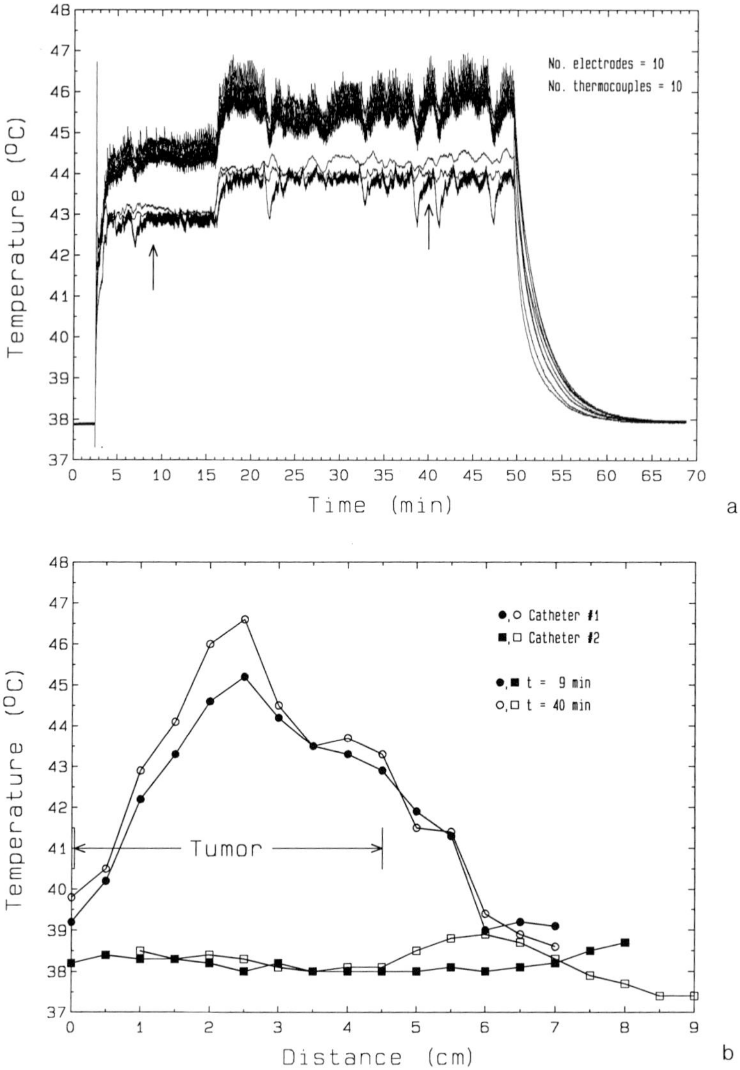

Fig. 8. Temperatures measured during interstitial hyperthermia treatment of a patient with Stage C carcinoma of the prostate. **a** Temperature-time profiles measured by copper/constantan thermocouples placed at the center of the active length of each of 10 implanted electrodes. Each electrode consisted of a partially insulated 16 gauge stainless steel trochar. The length of each active element was 6 mm. Arrows indicate times at which temperature maps were obtained. **b** Temperature maps measured along the length of two additional catheters. Catheter #1 transversed 4.5 cm of prostatic tumor and then extended through normal tissue to the surface of the perineum. Fiberoptic probes were mechanically mapped at 0.5 cm intervals early (9 minutes, closed circles) and late (40 minutes, open circles) during the treatment. Catheter #2 transversed normal tissues 1 to 2 cm lateral to the prostate gland. Fiberoptic probes were mapped at the same times during treatment as catheter #1 (closed and open squares)

tures remaining <40°C during the treatment of the tumor to 43–45°C (Fig. 8b, Catheter 2). A total of thirteen hyperthermic interstitial BT implants have been performed during the past year in patients with advanced stage (nine patients) or recurrent (4 patients) prostatic cancer. All treatments were well tolerated without complications. On initial follow-up assessment, all tumors appeared to regress. The rate of fall of PSA, the rate of tumor regression, and the local tumor control will be reported at a later date pending additional patient accrual and follow-up. At this time, the preliminary results appear encouraging (personal communication; GOFFINET, 1990).

Review of the literature for interstitial thermobrachytherapy

Clinical response and local-control rates have been recently reviewed for both microwave (MW) and RF interstitial HT techniques (PEREZ and EMAMI, 1989; COUGHLIN and STROHBEHN, 1989). Table 6 summarizes the clinical results obtained from studies employing RF electrode systems. Most studies employed one or two HT treatments, with HT administered immediately prior to or both prior to and immediately after the BT. Treatment goals ranged from 41°C for 30 minutes to 43.5°C for up to 60 minutes. High complete response (CR) and partial response (PR) rates were obtained.

Table 7 summarizes the clinical results obtained with interstitial HT and BT using MW antenna systems. Most studies employed MW at a frequency of 915 MHz with HT administered immediately prior to and immediately after BT with temperature goals in the same range as those utilized in the RF interstitial treatments. CR and PR rates similar to those reported for RF interstitial hyperthermia were obtained. Table 8 summarizes disease site-specific response rates for interstitial thermal BT for head and neck, pelvic, breast and chest wall sites. High CR rates were noted at all sites in most series.

Prognostic factors

Several of the larger series of patients treated with RF interstitial HT attempted to identify tumor or treatment factors which correlated with the rate of CR. ARISTIZABAL and OLESON (1984), in an evaluation of 64 patients, reported significant correlations between CR rate and: increasing radiation dose ($p = 0.008$), increasing time-averaged intratumoral temperatures ($p = 0.014$), and decreasing tumor volume ($p = 0.024$). Logistic regression models revealed the most significant parameters in predicting response to be tumor volume, radiation dose, and minimum intratumoral temperature. An analysis of the combined patient material from the University of Arizona, the City of Hope National Medical Center and the Institute Gustave-Roussy, revealed that high CR rates occurred in regimens employing radiation doses of greater than 6000 cGy or those obtaining a minimum tumor temperature of 44°C. Other studies (Table 9) have confirmed the prognostic importance of tumor volume (EMAMI et al, 1987; RAFLA et al, 1989; PETROVICH et al, 1989), radiation dose (RAFLA et al, 1989), and "satisfactory" HT treatment (EMAMI, 1987; PEREZ and EMAMI, 1989).

Complications

In general, interstitial hyperthermic BT treatments have been well-tolerated, considering the advanced nature of the tumors treated and their extensive prior treatment. However, serious toxicities

Table 6. Interstitial thermobrachytherapy: clinical results of studies which employed RF electrode systems

Study, Yr	No. Evaluable Pts (Sites)	Treatment Parameters			% CR	% PR
		HT (°C, min)	Sequence	No. Implants		
Vora et al, 1982	15 (16)	41°–43°, 30 min	HT-BT ± HT	1	69%	6%
Oleson et al, 1984	52	42°, 30 min	HT-BT	1	38%	42%
Cossett et al, 1985	(23)	44°, 45 min	HT-BT ± HT	1	83%	17%
Linares et al, 1986	11 (10)	43.5°, 45 min	HT-BT	1 or 2	36%	64%
Dunlop et al, 1986	9	20 min Eq. 43°	HT-BT-HT	1	0%	44%
Emami et al, 1987	9	42°, 60 min	HT-BT	1	56%	33%
Vora et al, 1988	19	42°–43°, 30 min	HT-BT	1 or 2	53%	5%
Gautherie et al, 1989	96	42°–43.5°, 45–60 min	HT-BT-HT	1	61%	15%
Goffinet et al, 1990	10	43°–44°, 45 min	HT-BT-HT	1	80%	0%

HT, interstitial hyperthermia; BT, brachytherapy; CR, complete response; PR, partial response.

Table 7. Interstitial thermobrachytherapy: clinical results of studies which employed microwave antenna systems

Study, Yr	No. Evaluable Pts (Sites)	Antenna Frequency (MHz)	Treatment Parameters			% CR	% PR
			HT (°C, min)	Sequence	No. Implants		
Strohbehn & Douple, 1984	6	915	42.5°, 60 min	HT-BT-HT	1	50%	33%
Puthawala et al, 1985	43	915	41.5°–43°, 60 min	HT-BT-HT	1 or 2	86%	14%
Emami et al, 1987	39	915	42°, 60 min	HT-BT-HT	1	54%	23%
Rafla et al, 1989	(35)	915/251	42.5°, 60 min	HT-BT-HT	1	54%	37%
Petrovich et al, 1989	39 (44)	915/630	42.5°, 45–60 min	HT-BT-HT*	1	64%	34%

HT, interstitial hyperthermia; BT, brachytherapy; CR, complete response; PR, partial response.

* 20% did not receive second heat treatment.

Table 8. Interstitial thermobrachytherapy: site specific results

Study, Yr	HT System (Type, Freq)	Site (No. CR/Total No. Pts; %)			
		Head & Neck	Pelvis	Breast & Chest Wall	Other
Surwit et al, 1983	RF, 0.5 MHz	—	7/21 (33%)	—	—
Puthawala et al, 1985*	MW, 915 MHz	15/20 (75%)	10/13 (77%)	5/8 (63%)	2/2 (100%)
Vora et al, 1988	RF, 0.5 MHz	—	10/19 (53%)	—	—
Gautherie et al, 1989	MW, 915 MHz	24/35 (69%)	23/39 (59%)	11/14 (79%)	3/8 (39%)
Rafla et al, 1989	MW, 915 MHz	8/15 (53%)	8/14 (57%)	3/6 (50%)	—
Petrovich et al, 1989	MW, 915,630 MHz	16/23 (70%)	3/4 (75%)	7/9 (78%)	2/8 (25%)
Goffinet et al, 1990	RF, 0.5 MHz	5/5 (100%)	3/5 (60%)	—	—

HT, hyperthermia; CR, complete response.

* Local control rates.

Table 9. Prognostic factors in treatment with interstitial thermobrachytherapy

Author, Yr	No. Evaluable Patients	Prognostic Factors	Relationship
Aristizabal & Oleson, 1984 University of Arizona	64	Radiation Dose: Tmin: Tumor Volume:	CR increases with dose CR increases with Tmin CR decreases with volume
Composite: 3 Series	97	Radiation Dose, Tmin	High CR with dose >6000 cGy or Tmin = 44°
Emami et al, 1987	48	Tumor Volume: No. Satisfactory HT Treatments:*	Smaller tumors do better At least one: CR = 70% None: CR = 0%
Rafla et al, 1989	35	Radiation Dose: Tumor Volume:	>6000 cGy: CR = 78% <6000 cGy: CR = 8% ≤30 cm³: CR = 100% >30 cm³: CR = 47%
Petrovich et al, 1989	44	Tumor Volume:	<150 cm³: CR = 75% >150 cm³: CR = 12%
Perez & Emami, 1989 Composite Series	110	No. Satisfactory HT Treatments:*	At least one: CR = 80% None: CR = 0%

Tmin, time-averaged minimum intratumoral temperature; CR, complete response rate.

* Temperature at some point in tumor >42°, entire volume included in hyperthermia implant.

Table 10. Complications of interstitial thermobrachytherapy

Author, Yr	No. Evaluable Pts	Complications
Oleson et al, 1984	52	Overall Rate: 25% "Serious" Toxicity: 14%
Puthawala et al, 1985	43	Burns: 5% Soft Tissue Necrosis: 14% (Including 7% Fistula) Brachial Neuropathy: 2%
Cosset et al, 1985	23	Necrosis: 52% (Including Large Areas of Necrosis – 17%)
Emami et al, 1987	48	Delayed Wound Healing: 4% Delayed Healing of Necrotic Crater: 13% Cutaneous Sinus: 4% Fistulas: 4%
Vora et al, 1988	19	Rectovaginal Fistula: 5%
Petrovich et al, 1989	44	Erythema: 14% Moist Desquamation: 16% Blister: 4% Aspiration Pneumonia: 2% Skin Necrosis: 4%

have been reported in approximately 14% of patients, with soft-tissue necrosis, burns, and fistulas most frequently noted (Table 10). The lack of uniform criteria for reporting complications or their severity makes intercomparison between the various studies and between the different interstitial techniques difficult.

Discussion and future directions

Equipment development

Interstitial RF-induced HT combined with interstitial BT has numerous potential theoretical advantages in the treatment of implantable locally advanced or recurrent malignancies. RF interstitial systems are relatively simple to operate (compared to the more complex multiple MW antenna systems or laserthermia systems); the length of the electrodes can be individualized to fit the tumor dimensions and insulation of the portions of the electrodes transversing normal tissues will limit normal tissue heating; there is no intrinsic limit to the length of the active elements (as is the case for frequency-dependent MW antennas); flexible electrodes can be utilized to permit better tumor access and localization in difficult-to-implant sites; pairs of electrodes can be individually activated to improve the uniformity of intratumoral heating during the actual HT treatments to help adjust for variations in tissue electrical and thermal properties as well as variations in blood flow; and the geometry requirements for the spacing of the electrodes are similar to those for BT (so that the same catheters can be used for both BT and HT providing the possibility of doing simultaneous HT-BT or closely sequenced treatments).

Radiofrequency-based interstitial hyperthermia systems have certain relative disadvantages. First, the heating is very sensitive to the spacing and orientation of the electrodes. This results in hot-spots in regions where the electrodes converge and cooler regions where the electrodes diverge. Second, the tumor-temperature distributions obtained are dependent on blood-flow. The current density (and, therefore, the temperature) is highest on the surface and adjacent to the electrodes with conduction playing a role in the heating of the tissues between the electrodes. Third, there is a lack of longitudinal control of power deposition with currently employed systems. The power to each electrode pair can be modulated, but the power (current density) applied along the length of the electrode is uniform. A fourth limitation of interstitial RF systems is that each electrode needs to be individually connected to the power supply. In a large implant with 32 or more electrodes, this is a tedious and time-consuming process.

Ongoing studies, at Stanford and elsewhere, are directed at improving the RF electrode systems to overcome these specific limitations. Segmented electrodes are being developed to permit power modulation along the longitudinal axis of each electrode. This will theoretically permit more uniform heating and a

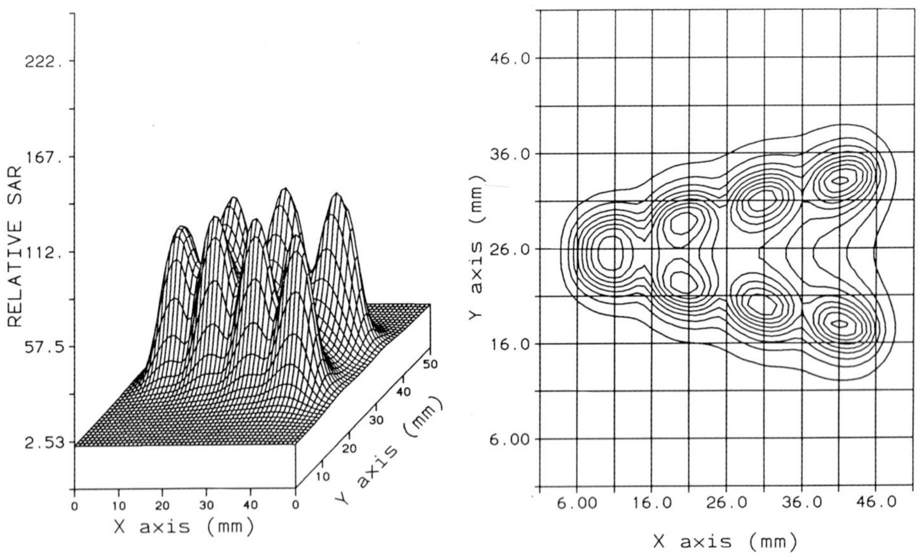

Fig. 9. Two dimensional SAR distribution generated by a pair of four-element segmented electrodes. The angle of convergence was 20°. The power level applied to each pair varied as a function of the distance between complementary pairs. Length of each electrically independent segment was 8 mm. Electrode diameter was 2.1 mm. Grid size was 51 × 51 points. Contour interval was 10% of SAR_{MAX}

diminution of the effect of non-parallel electrodes. For example, if a pair of electrodes converge, then the power can be proportionally applied to the various segments of the electrodes such that less power is applied to the portions of the electrode pair closest together and more power is supplied to those segments of the electrodes that are furthest apart (Fig. 9). The use of segmented electrodes should also permit better adjustment for variation in tissue properties and/or blood flow along the longitudinal axis of the implanted tumor. The use of water cooling of the RF electrode is also being explored in an attempt to adjust the surface temperature of the electrode to attain more uniform heating. A similar approach has been successfully developed for cooling of the interstitial MW antennas used in the treatment of brain tumors (Moriyama et al, 1988). Improved software systems are also under development to provide automatic multiplexing of power between selected electrode pairs based on real time temperature measurements within the tumor volumes located between the electrode pairs. In addition, an electrically controlled template system is being developed to permit multiplexing between all possible electrode pairs without the need for individual electrode connections (Corry, 1990). Finally, the use of pretreatment CT and/or MRI scans with the patient in the implant position is being explored to better evaluate the tumor dimensions and to permit more precise insulation of the portions of the electrodes that will be in normal tissues.

Biological considerations

Several thermal and radiobiological factors require further investigation to permit optimization of interstitial hyperthermic BT regimens. Although the initial studies employing cell culture systems suggested that the magnitude of the thermal potentiation of radiation-induced cell killing varied inversely with dose rate (Ben-Hur et al, 1974; Harisiadis et al, 1978), not all subsequent studies confirmed this dose rate effect. For example, Gerner et al (1983) utilizing a rat astrocytoma cell line and radiation dose rates from 0.6–300 cGy per minute, showed that the thermal enhancement ratios *did not* vary inversely with dose rate but were maximal at the two extremes tested. Additional studies employing cell lines from human tumors as well as in vivo studies are needed to help determine the optimum radiation dose rate to be utilized in combined interstitial HT-BT regimens.

The optimum sequencing of the HT and XRT also remains to be clarified. Most laboratory and clinical studies have utilized HT followed by XRT with or without a second HT treatment after the BT. Jones et al (1989) recently reported on sequencing HT and low-dose rate BT in a murine mammary adenocarcinoma. Using growth delay in tumor volume doubling as their endpoint, they compared: (a) single HT treatment before BT; (b) single HT after BT; (c) single HT given in the middle of BT; (d) one HT before and one HT after BT; (e) BT alone; and (f) HT alone. In terms of the duration of the growth delay and thermal enhancement ratio (TER) at 44°C, the sequence of a single HT given in the middle of the BT was most effective. However, studies on the effects of these treatments on normal tissues were not reported. Similar TER's at 44°C were obtained for HT-BT or HT-BT-HT suggesting that the second HT treatment contributed little to improving the TER. Additional clinical studies are, therefore, warranted to compare HT pre-

and post-BT, HT given only prior to the implant, and HT administered in the middle of the BT treatment. In addition, if remote afterloading systems are available, truly simultaneous HT and BT can be safely tested.

There exists little information on the optimum number of HT-BT implants necessary for the treatment of a given tumor. Studies on superficially-located tumors treated with externally administered HT and low-dose XRT suggested that as few as two HT treatments may be sufficient to obtain the maximum clinical response (DUNLOP, 1986; KAPP et al, 1989). Other questions including the optimum time and temperature duration of the HT treatment, and the utilization of pre-implant external beam XRT also warrant further study.

Clinical studies

The excellent results obtained by interstitial HT-BT suggest their potential value in the management of implantable tumors. However, several investigators including ARISTIZABAL and OLESON (1984) and KAPP (1986) have called attention to the high CR rates that have been reported in similar patient groups treated with interstitial BT without the addition of HT. The value of the interstitial HT therefore needs to be confirmed in randomized prospective clinical trials – carefully controlling for pretreatment prognostic factors and adequately documenting the thermal distributions obtained. One such trial is currently being carried out by the Radiation Therapy Oncology Group (RTOG #84-19) in which tumors are stratified by participating institute, size of lesion, extent of prior XRT exposure and type of lesion (recurrent versus persistent). The patients are then randomized to interstitial XRT with or without interstitial HT (43°C for one hour, one treatment before and one treatment immediately after the BT). Enrollment of appropriate patients in such trials is to be strongly encouraged. Additional randomized trials should be instituted attempting to establish the optimum treatment parameters for combined modality management as discussed above. Other clinical issues to be investigated include a determination of the possible limitations of tumor size for effective interstitial HT; the dose response curves for HT-BT for normal tissue toxicities; the optimal HT techniques for individual tumor sites; the optimum spacing of the RF electrodes (or MW antennas or ferromagnetic seeds); the risks and potential benefits of the use of analgesia during the HT treatments; and the use of whole-body HT in conjunction with interstitial HT for improving the temperature distributions and treatment outcome in patients with implantable tumors.

In summary, although technical problems currently exist limiting our ability to obtain optimum HT distributions in implantable tumors, many innovative approaches are being brought from the laboratory into the clinic to meet these challenges. Concurrently with these technical developments, our understanding of the fundamental biology of HT-induced cytotoxicity and radiation sensitization is increasing and the results of early clinical trials are shedding additional light not only on potential problem areas, but on important prognostic treatment parameters. It is, therefore, anticipated that the next decade should see considerable clinical advances in the interstitial HT-BT treatment of locally-advanced or recurrent human cancers.

Endnotes

1. Aerospace Materials Corporation, Placentia, CA 92670, U.S.A.
2. Deseret Medical, Inc., Sandy, UT 84070, U.S.A.
3. Luxtron, Inc., Mountain View, CA 94043, U.S.A.
4. Sensortek, Inc., Clifton, NJ 07013, U.S.A.
5. Superior Tube, Inc., Norristown, PA 19404, U.S.A.

Acknowledgments: We gratefully acknowledge the expertise and skill of D.R. Goffinet, M.D. in the performance of the interstitial hyperthermic implants and in patient care. The technical assistance of Joseph Mariscal, R.T.T. for brachytherapy dosimetry, of Allen W. Lohrbach, R.T.T. for aid in hyperthermia administration, John Sokol for assistance with the preparation of the illustrations, and of Sharon Clarke in the preparation of this manuscript are also to be acknowledged. This work was supported by NCI Grant CA-44665.

References

Anderson RL, Kapp DS (1990) Hyperthermia in cancer therapy: Current status. Med J Aust 152: 310–315

Arcangeli G, Nervi C, Cividalli A, Lovisolo GA, Mauro F (1984) The clinical use of experimental parameters to evaluate the response to combined heat (HT) and radiation (RT). In: Overgaard J (ed) Hyperthermic Oncology, vol 1, Summary Papers. Taylor & Francis, London, pp 363–366

Aristizabal SA, Oleson JR (1984) Combined interstitial irradiation and localized current field hyperthermia: Results and conclusions from clinical studies. Cancer Res (Suppl) 44: 4757s–4760s

Bagshaw MA (1990) The status of prostatic cancer as treated by irradiation at Stanford University. In: Proceedings of the Tenth Annual: Current Approaches to Radiation Oncology, Biology and Physics. University of California San Francisco School of Medicine, 28 Feb–2 March 1990, San Francisco, California, pp 113–128

Ben-Hur E, Elkind MM, Bronk BV (1974) Thermally enhanced radioresponse of cultured Chinese hamster cells. Radiat Res 58: 38–51

Corry PM (1990) A flexible multielectrode HF interstitial hyperthermia system. In: Abstracts of Papers for the Thirty-Eighth Annual Meeting of the Radiation Research Society, 7–10 April 1990, New Orleans, Louisiana, p 33

Cosset JM, Dutreix J, Haie C, Gerbaulet A, Janoray P, Dewar JA (1985) Interstitial thermoradiotherapy: A technical and clinical study of 29 implantations performed at the Institut Gustave-Roussy. Int J Hyperthermia 1: 3–13

Coughlin CT, Strohbehn JW (1989) Interstitial thermoradiotherapy. Radiol Clin N Am 27: 577–588

Doss JD, McCabe CW (1976) A technique for localized heating in tissue: An adjunct to tumor therapy. Med Instrum 10: 16–21

Dunlop PRC, Dickinson RJ, Hand JW, Munro AJ, Vallis KA (1986) Early experience with combined interstitial hyperthermia and brachytherapy. Br J Radiol 59: 525–527

Dunlop PRC, Hand JW, Dickinson RJ, Field SB (1986) An assessment of local hyperthermia in clinical practice. Int J Hyperthermia 2: 39–50

Emami B, Perez CA (1985) Interstitial thermoradiotherapy: An overview. Endocur/Hyperth Oncol 1: 35–40

Emami B, Perez CA, Leybovitch L, Straube W, Vongerichten D (1987) Interstitial thermoradiotherapy in the treatment of malignant tumours. Int J Hyperthermia 3: 107–118

Gautherie M, Cosset JM, Gerard JP, Horiot JC, Ardiet JM, Akoum HE, Alperovitch A (1988) Interstitial hyperthermia using implanted electrodes: A multicentric program of technical evaluation and clinical trials over 96 patients. In: Abstracts of the 5th International Symposium on Hyperthermic Oncology, 29 Aug–3 Sept 1988, Kyoto, Japan, p 126

Gerner EW, Oval JH, Manning MR, Sim DA, Bowden GT, Hevezi JM (1983) Dose-rate dependence of heat radiosensitization. Int J Radiat Oncol Biol Phys 9: 1401–1404

Goffinet DR, Prionas SD, Kapp DS, Samulski TV, Fessenden P, Hahn GM, Lohrbach AW, Mariscal JM, Bagshaw MA (1990) Interstitial ^{192}Ir flexible catheter radiofrequency hyperthermia treatments of head and neck and recurrent pelvic carcinomas. Int J Radiat Oncol Biol Phys 18: 199–210

Harisiadis L, Sung D, Kessaris N, Hall EJ (1978) Hyperthermia and low dose-rate irradiation. Radiology 129: 195–198

Hiraoka M, Jo S, Dodo Y, Ono K, Takahashi M, Nishida H, Abe M (1984) Clinical results of radiofrequency hyperthermia combined with radiation in the treatment of radioresistant cancers. Cancer 54: 2898–2904

Jones EL, Lyons BE, Douple EB, Dain BJ (1989) Thermal enhancement of low dose rate irradiation in a murine tumour system. Int J Hyperthermia 5: 509–523

Kabalin JN, Hodge KK, McNeal JE, Freiha FS, Stamey TA (1989) Identification of residual cancer in the prostate following radiation therapy: Role of transrectal ultrasound guided biopsy and prostate specific antigen. J Urol 142: 326–331

Kapp DS (1986) Site and disease selection for hyperthermia clinical trials. Int J Hyperthermia 2: 139–156

Kapp DS (1988) Areas of need for continued phase II testing in human patients. In: Paliwal BR, Hetzel FW, Dewhirst MW (eds) Biological, Physical and Clinical Aspects of Hyperthermia. Medical Physics Monograph No 16. American Institute of Physics, Inc., New York, pp 424–443

Kapp DS, Fessenden P, Samulski TV, Bagshaw MA, Cox RS, Lee ER, Lohrbach AW, Meyer JL, Prionas SD (1988) Stanford University institutional report: Phase I evaluation of equipment for hyperthermia treatment of cancer. Int J Hyperthermia 4: 75–115

Kapp DS, Petersen IA, Cox RS, Hahn GM, Fessenden P, Prionas SD, Lee ER, Meyer JL, Samulski TV, Bagshaw MA (1990) Two or six hyperthermia treatments as an adjunct to radiation therapy yield similar tumor responses: Results of a randomized trial. Int J Radiat Oncol Biol Phys 19: 1481–1495

Linares LA, Nori D, Brenner H, Shiu M, Ballon D, Anderson L, Alfieri A, Brennan M, Fuks Z, Hilaris B (1986) Interstitial hyperthermia and brachytherapy: A preliminary report. Endocur/Hyperth Oncol 2: S-39–S-44

Mechling JA, Strohbehn JW (1986) A theoretical comparison of the temperature distributions produced by three interstitial hyperthermia systems. Int J Radiat Oncol Biol Phys 12: 2137–2149

Moorthy CR, Hahn EW, Kim JH, Feingold SM, Alfieri AA, Hilaris BS (1984) Improved response of a murine fibrosarcoma (Meth-A) to interstitial radiation when combined with hyperthermia. Int J Radiat Oncol Biol Phys 10: 2145–2148

Moriyama E, Matsumi N, Shiraishi T, Tamiya T, Satoh T, Matsumoto K, Furuta T, Nishimoto A (1988) Hyperthermia for brain tumors: Improved delivery with a new cooling system. Neurosurgery 23: 189–195

Oleson JR, Sim DA, Manning MR (1984) Analysis of prognostic variables in hyperthermia in 163 patients. Int J Radiat Oncol Biol Phys 10: 2331–2339

Overgaard J (1980) Simultaneous and sequential hyperthermia and radiation treatment of an experimental tumor and its surrounding normal tissue in vivo. Int J Radiat Oncol Biol Phys 6: 1507–1517

Overgaard J, Overgaard M (1984) A clinical trial evaluating the effect of simultaneous or sequential radiation and hyperthermia in the treatment of malignant melanoma.

In: Overgaard J (ed) Hyperthermic Oncology, 1984, vol 1. Francis & Taylor, London, pp 383–386

Perez CA, Emami B (1989) Clinical trials with local (external and interstitial) irradiation and hyperthermia. Current and future perspectives. Radiol Clin N Am 27: 525–542

Petrovich Z, Langholz B, Gibbs FA, Sapozink MD, Kapp DS, Stewart RJ, Emami B, Oleson J, Senzer N, Slater J, Astrahan M (1989) Regional hyperthermia for advanced tumors. A clinical study of 353 patients. Int J Radiat Oncol Biol Phys 16: 601–607

Petrovich Z, Langholz B, Lam K, Luxton G, Cohen D, Jepson J, Astrahan M (1989) Interstitial microwave hyperthermia combined with iridium-192 radiotherapy for recurrent tumors. Am J Clin Oncol (CCT) 12: 264–268

Prionas SD, Fessenden P, Kapp DS, Goffinet DR, Hahn GM (1989) Interstitial electrodes allowing longitudinal control of SAR distributions. In: Sugahara T, Saito M (eds) Hyperthermic Oncology 1988, vol 2, Special Plenary Lectures, Plenary Lectures, and Symposium and Workshop Summaries. Taylor & Francis, London, pp 707–710

Puthawala AA, Syed AMN, Sheikh KMA, Rafie S, McNamara S (1985) Interstitial hyperthermia for recurrent malignancies. Endocur/Hyperth Oncol 1: 125–131

Rafla S, Parikh K, Tchelebi M, Youssef E, Selim H, Bishay S (1989) Recurrent tumors of the head and neck, pelvis, and chest wall: Treatment with hyperthermia and brachytherapy. Radiology 172: 845–850

Samulski TV, Fessenden P, Valdagni R, Kapp DS (1987) Correlations of thermal washout rate, steady state temperatures, and tissue type in deep-seated recurrent or metastatic tumors. Int J Radiat Oncol Biol Phys 13: 907–916

Shipley WU, Bagshaw MA, Prout GR (1987) The success of radiation therapy in controlling prostatic cancer within the treated field. In: Prostatic Cancer, Part B: Imaging Techniques, Radiotherapy, Chemotherapy, and Management Issues. Alan Liss, Inc, New York, pp 199–212

Stauffer PR (1989) Heat localization by interstitial hyperthermia. In: Sugahara T, Saito M (eds) Hyperthermic Oncology 1988, vol 2, Special Plenary Lectures, Plenary Lectures, and Symposium and Workshop Summaries. Taylor & Francis, London, pp 640–643

Strohbehn JW, Douple EB (1984) Hyperthermia and cancer therapy: A review of biomedical engineering contributions and challenges. IEEE Trans Biomed Eng BME-3: 779–787

Surwit EA, Manning MR, Aristizabal SA, Oleson JR, Cetas TC (1983) Interstitial thermoradiotherapy in recurrent gynecologic malignancies. Gynecol Oncol 15: 95–102

Takashima S, Fishman HM (eds) (1977) Electrical properties of biological polymers, water, and membranes. Ann NY Acad Sci 303: 1–446

Uzunoglu NK, Nikita KS (1988) Estimation of temperature distribution inside tissues heated by interstitial RF electrode hyperthermia systems. IEEE Trans Biomed Eng 35: 250–256

Valdagni R, Liu FF, Kapp DS (1988) Important prognostic factors influencing outcome of combined radiation and hyperthermia. Int J Radiat Oncol Biol Phys 15: 959–972

Visser AG, Deurloo IKK, Levendag PC, Ruifrok ACC, Cornet B, van Rhoon GC (1989) An interstitial hyperthermia system at 27 MHz. Int J Hyperthermia 5: 265–276

Vora N, Forell B, Joseph C, Lipsett JA, Archambeau JO (1982) Interstitial implant with interstitial hyperthermia. Cancer 50: 2518–2523

Vora NL, Luk KH, Forell B, Findley DO, Lipsett JA, Pezner RD, Desai KR, Wong JYC, Hill B (1988) Interstitial local current field hyperthermia for advanced cancers of the cervix. Endocur/Hyperth Oncol 4: 97–106

7

Clinical Experience with Different Interstitial Hyperthermia Techniques

C. Marchal[1], *M. Pernot*[2], *S. Hoffstetter*[2], *and P. Bey*[2]

[1] Radiotherapy Department,
[2] Brachytherapy Department, Centre Alexis-Vautrin, Vandoeuvre-Les-Nancy, France

Introduction

Modern brachytherapy procedures were designed and developed in France by PIERQUIN and CHASSAGNE (1966–1967) using iridium 192. The use of polyethylene tubes adapted for afterloading techniques has greatly simplified brachytherapy, allowing better implantations covering larger volumes, which explains its present success.

Brachytherapy alone or combined with external radiotherapy proved to be more efficient than external radiotherapy alone in a number of tumor sites such as cervix uteri (CHASSAGNE et al, 1966), oropharynx (PERNOT et al, 1980), base of the tongue (HOFFSTETTER et al, 1986), anal canal, vagina, ... In addition, a conservative treatment can often be carried out which is a considerable advantage over the damaging effects of surgery, especially as to head and neck tumors. Moreover, the local control rates obtained often exceed both those of surgery alone, and of surgery associated with external radiotherapy. In a variety of clinical conditions, brachytherapy is used after external irradiation of the tumor and nodal areas; it allows a higher dose to be applied to the residual tumor volume. Often, this residual tumor volume is so large that the question arises: what is the dose that should be delivered to obtain the best local control with acceptable toxicity, which is known to be proportional to the dose increase? For those patients, the aim is to increase the efficiency of brachytherapy without rising its toxicity by combining other therapeutic modalities. Hyperthermia could be one of these methods and its association with brachytherapy will be valuable only if it can be delivered routinely without disturbing conventional proved brachytherapy modalities.

Keeping this aim in mind, we have tried to apply and to develop various heating techniques which could be easily combined with conventional brachytherapy implantations.

Practical and clinical aspects of the main interstitial hyperthermia techniques currently used

Till now, four interstitial methods have remained under investigation: ferromagnetic seeds (FM), RF electrodes and coaxial microwave antennas (STROHBEHN, 1986) and hot water flow (HANDL-ZELLER, 1986).

The first technique uses Eddy currents induced by a magnetic field of a circular coil placed around the body inside intratumorally implanted metallic rods. The research is aiming chiefly at developing self-regulated seeds with Curie points around 50°C (BREZOVICH, 1981; LILLY, 1985; STAUFFER et al, 1984; CETAS et al, 1982). However the electromagnetic shielding of the treatment room and the perfect implantation of these seeds are required.

Usually, interstitial heating with RF electrodes is essentially conductive, produced by 0.5 to 1 MHz currents between electrically connected arrays of needles (ASTRAHAN et al, 1982). This technique was developed at Los Alamos by Doss et al (1976) and then renewed at Tucson by MANNING and CETAS (1982) and at the Institute Gustave Roussy by COSSET (1984, 1985). The geometry of implantation is critical because it is imperative that the wires are perfectly parallel and the distance between electrodes is equally satisfactory for hyperthermal homogeneity and for curietherapy dosimetry. This technique does not enable non-coplanar implantation of electrodes or loops. Moreover these rigid steel needles are directly matched to normal tissues and to the tumor, and local tolerance can be a problem. The future of this method should be the development of flexible electrodes of adapted length.

Interstitial hyperthermia by microwave antennas was developed by a number of groups (STROHBEHN, 1979, 1986; TAYLOR, 1978). One major advantage is that the catheter is a part of the antenna design (KING et al, 1983; TREMBLY, 1983). This technique is useful and applicable in various situations but, the natural resonant length is a constraint. The greatest problem is the control of the temperature distribution in the longitudinal direction and the control of the active length according to the geometry and the volume of the tumor (TREMBLY, 1985). In this way, work is in progress to modify the design of these antennas (LEE, 1986; STAUFFER et al, 1987; RYAN and STROHBEHN, 1987).

More recently hot water flow was proposed by BREZOVICH (1988) in USA and HANDL-ZELLER et al (1986–1988) in Austria as the most simple technique that could be easily combined with conventional brachytherapy techniques using plastic or metallic vectors.

Considering the clinical response, a short review of literature is reported in Table 1. It appears that the tumor response does not seem to be related to the interstitial hyperthermia technique used though the tolerance does. The techniques for which we are able to measure the maximum temperature will induce the lowest rate of toxic effect. Contrary to this, with the electromagnetic methods of heating which allow some coherent effects, the temperature increase depends not only on the blood flow but also on the dielectric properties of tissues. In this case we are not able to measure exactly the location and the level of the maximum temperature and therefore the tolerance is surely at its worst.

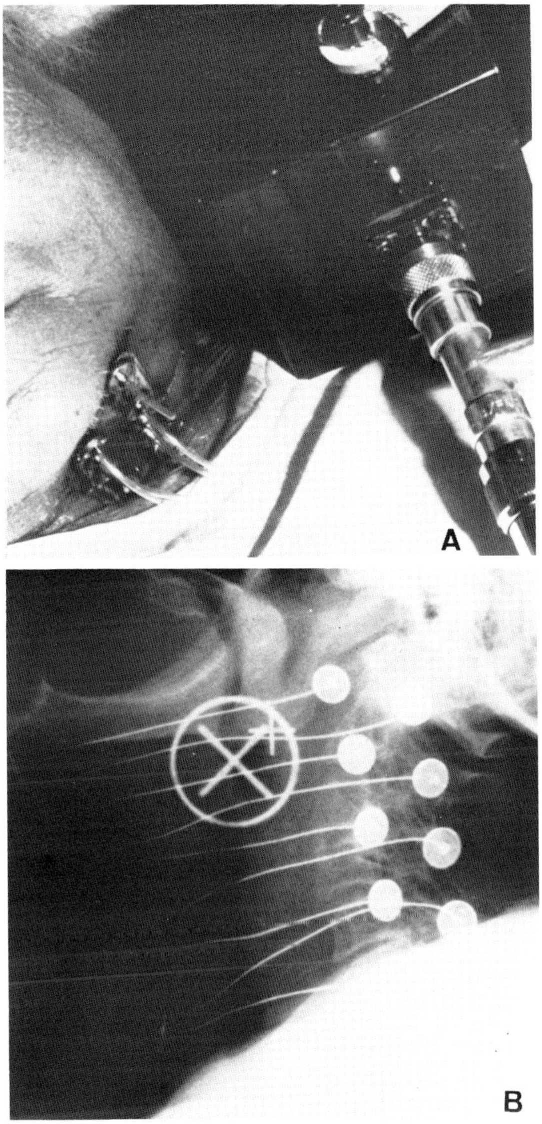

Fig. 1. Case of a large neck node recurrence after local irradiation treated by the combination of brachytherapy (60 Gy) and external microwave (434 MHz) hyperthermia using the implanted plastic tubes for thermometry. (**A**) During the hyperthermia session. (**B**) Lateral control radiograph

Clinical experience with different heating techniques

Drawing on the advantages and limits of these interstitial techniques and the practical experience gathered, we have developed therefore our own hyperthermia devices for use in combination with brachytherapy.

Brachytherapy implantation techniques used in our institution were described elsewhere (PERNOT et al, 1980–1988). Basically they apply the rules of the sytéme de Paris (PIERQUIN et al, 1967) with parallel implantations of multiple

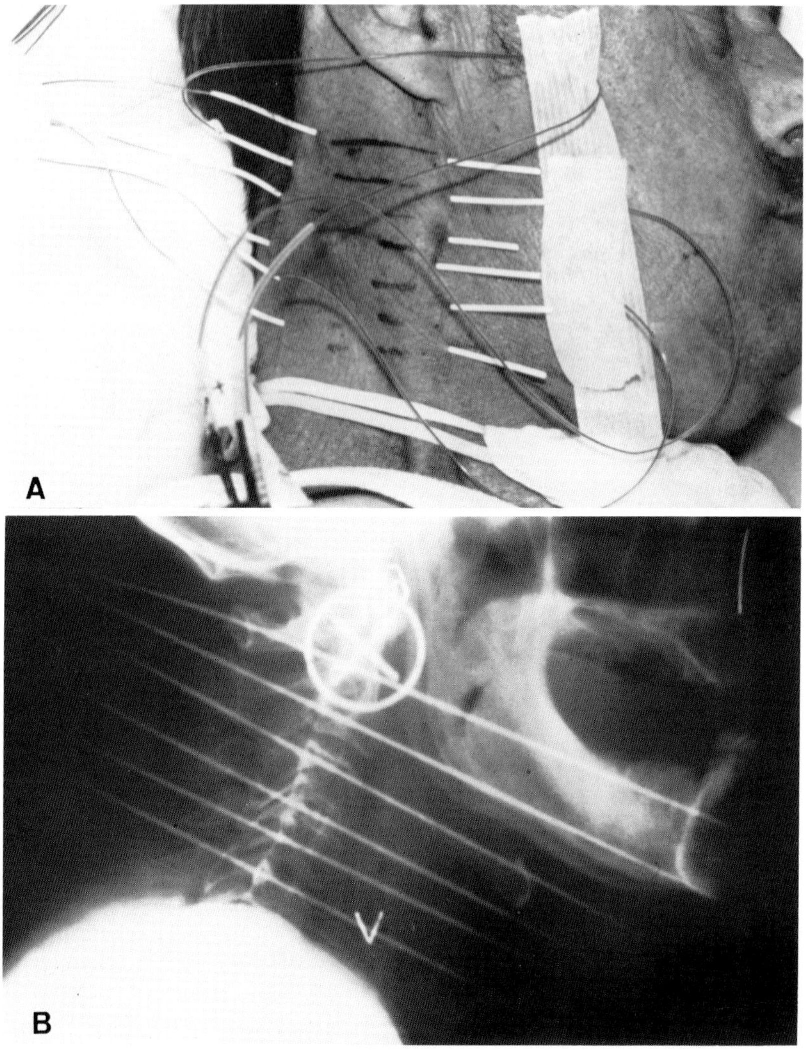

Fig. 2. Neck node recurrence of 3 cm in diameter in previously irradiated site. (**A**) View of the implantation with 6 parallel tubes during interstitial heating at 27 MHz. (**B**) Control radiograph

lines distant from 1.2 to 2 cm loaded by low dose rate Iridium 192 wires.

In 1982 for the first time we began to combine external hyperthermia induced by a rectangular waveguide operating at 434 MHz (MARCHAL et al, 1983) with brachytherapy using the plastic tubes for multiple thermometry. Fig. 1 shows the case of a neck node recurrence in site previously irradiated. The waveguide placed directly on the skin cannot induce enough homogeneous heating in the entire tumor volume, and temperature gradients of more than 5°C were measured in the axis of the nine plastic catheters implanted in two planes for brachytherapy. Tumors of the base of tongue and of floor of the mouth showed the same heterogeneities even when using water bolus and surface cooling pads.

Therefore in 1984 we developed our own interstitial method operating at 27.12 MHz (Marchal et al, 1985). It consists essentially in flexible conductor wires of which inserted length can be adjusted to the catheter implantation and to the tumor volume. We showed the feasibility of this type of interstitial method of heating (Marchal et al, 1989). The length of these flexible electrodes is not critical and can be designed according to the tumor site and volume. This method encompasses all the advantages of the other techniques while eliminating their main limits. The use of thin flexible electrodes, of which diameter can be selected, is possible. Each electrode can be fitted with a microsensor for temperature measurements. The co-planar fitting of the antennas is not essential and loops can be used. The length of each electrode can be adjusted to the tumor volume to be treated, and each electrode can be either inserted or not in plastic catheters making after-loading techniques possible. The catheter is then an integral part of the electrode design and eliminates the effects of high field concentrations at the edges of the inserted electrode. The energy is put in all along the catheter by a capacitive coupling throughout the tumor (Nadi et al, 1987). The radial S.A.R. distributions are quite similar to those obtained by microwave antennas (Van Rhoon, 1986) and a homogeneous heating along the length of the electrode, like for RF needles or ferromagnetic seeds, are observed. The heating homogeneity appears to be reasonably good with the advantage of a fairly uniform heating throughout the whole inserted length. Despite the real advantages of this heating technique, clinically, for patients non-premedicated, the feelings of pain in and outside the tumor volume are the main limiting factor. Different kind of tumors sites were treated, for example recurrences of neck node metastases in previously irradiated sites (Fig. 2), base of tongue tumors (Fig. 3) or primary tumors of the cheek (Fig. 4), with different brachytherapy techniques (coplanar or non co-planar implantations, loops or not). In all cases pain was induced during all hyperthermia treatments.

Other groups working with electromagnetic heating describe these phenomena that could be explained by undetected hot spots. That is to say we are not able, with electromagnetic heating, to control correctly the maximum temperature within the tumor volume which is related to toxicity.

Therefore more recently we preferred the more simple technique using hot water circulation in the plastic tubes implanted for brachytherapy (Handl-Zeller et al, 1988). Fig. 5 shows a treatment of a tumor of the base of tongue for which the thermal gradient found throughout the tumor was lower than 4°C, between 42.5 and 46°C. The main advantage of this method is that the level of the maximum temperature in the tumor volume is always lower than the temperature of the circulating water. With this method, the self-toxicity of hyperthermia can be controlled. The tolerance is excellent and the feelings of pain are rarely observed.

Discussion and conclusions

For most interstitial hyperthermia systems, using 434, 915, 2450 MHz microwaves, or 0.3, 0.5 MHz radiofrequencies or low frequencies at 27 MHz, implanting

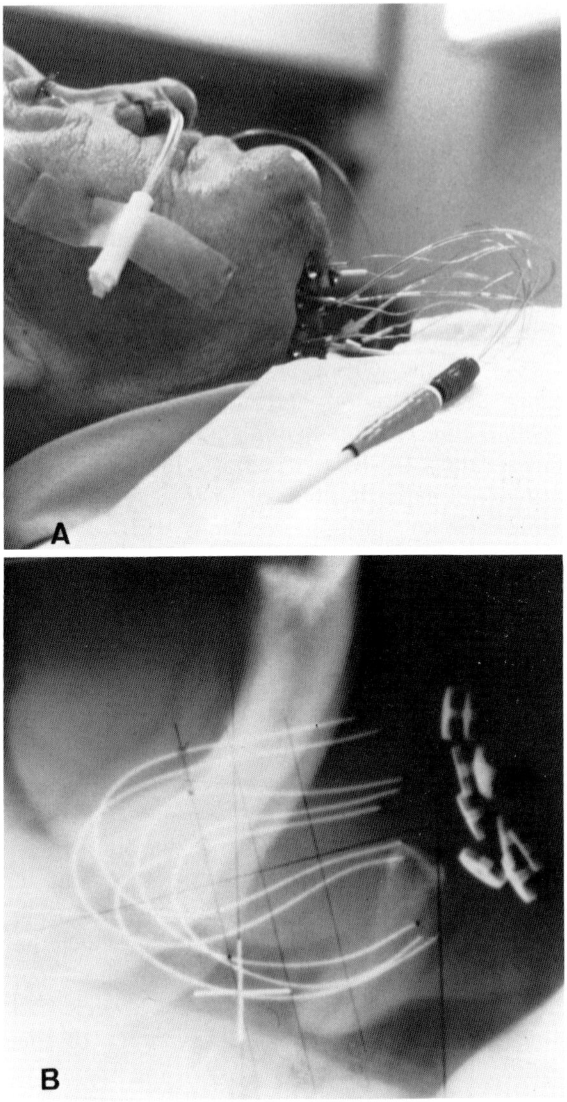

Fig. 3. Base of tongue tumor treated by external irradiation (50 Gy) and brachytherapy (30 Gy boost) followed by one session of interstitial hyperthermia. (**A**) View of the heating electrodes (27 MHz) inserted in the polyethylen tubes during the hyperthermia session. (**B**) Lateral control radiograph of the five implanted loops

of thermoseeds or thermal conduction through hot water circulation, an accurate geometrical implantation with parallel lines spaced about 1 cm apart is required. Those limits imposed by the laws of physics compel us to favour implantation for hyperthermia rather than optimal implantation for brachytherapy (PIERQUIN et al, 1987). These strict implantation conditions increase significantly the risk of hemorrhage for semi-deep regions such as base of tongue, cervical nodes and cannot be complied with in the case of tumors of oropharynx. These techniques are easily applicable to superficial skin tumors, to breast or pelvic tumors.

Considering heating techniques, micro-

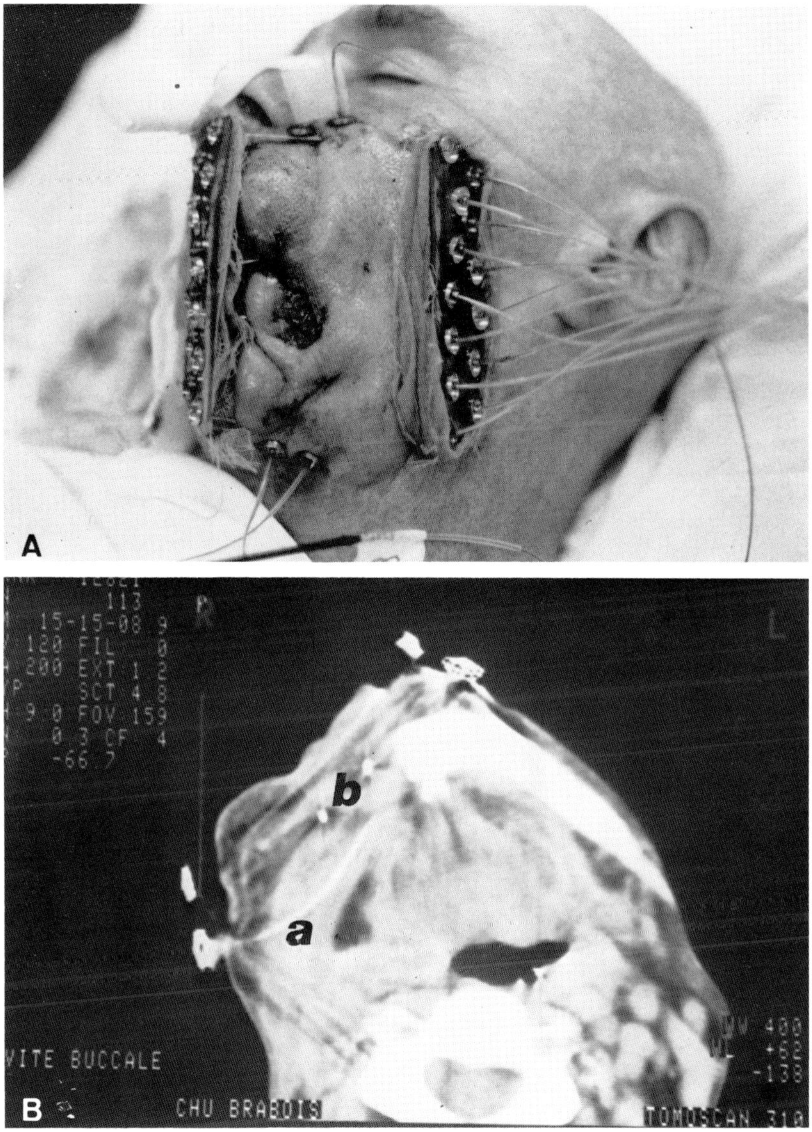

Fig. 4. Example of a squamous cell carcinoma of the cheek treated by 2 brachytherapy sessions combined with 27 MHz interstitial heating. (**A**) Implantation of thirteen parallel tubes for brachytherapy and the 2 catheters for axial thermometry (V). (**B**) CT scan view of the implantation, (a) brachytherapy lines, (b) thermometry lines

wave antennas do not induce a homogeneous distribution of temperature along each antenna (TREMBLY et al, 1985; MECHLING et al, 1986). Moreover, coaxial antennas have a resonant length for a given frequency and it is quite impossible to avoid it.

With asymmetric capacitive heating at

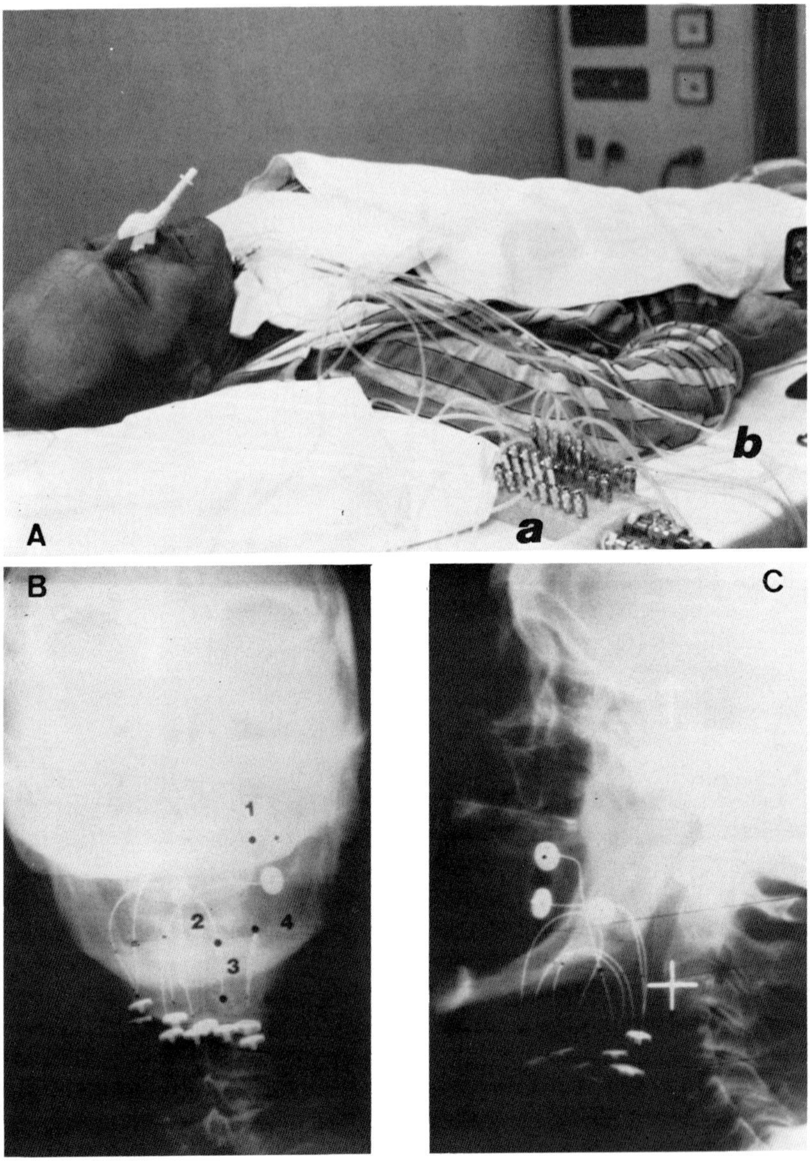

Fig. 5. Base of tongue tumor treated by brachytherapy loops and interstitial hyperthermia using hot water circulation. (**A**) View of the hyperthermia treatment with the manifold (a) and the silicon tubes (b). (**B**) Anterior radiograph of the implantation. (**C**) Lateral control radiograph

27.12 MHz there is no dependence on depth insertion and a good uniform heating is noticed along the total length of the inserted electrode. Since no coherent effects is possible at this frequency, an individual power regulation for each electrode is required.

Considering brachytherapy implanta-

Table 1. Short summary of literature on the tumor response and evaluated toxicity related to the technique used

Frequency	Authors	Nb tumors evaluable	Tumor response		Global response		Toxicity
			CR	PR	CR	PR	
915 MHz	• Emami et al (1987)	39	21	6	50%	15%	25%
	• Puthawala et al (1985)	43	32	11	74%	26%	21%
	• Petrovich et al (1988)	31	19	11	61%	35%	?
	• Inoue et al (1989)	10	1	7	10%	70%	?
	Total	123	73	35	59%	28%	≈23%
8 MHz	• Yabumoto et al (1989)	14	6	1	—	—	?
0.5 MHz	• Oleson et al (1984)	52	20	22	38%	42%	21%
	• Gautherie et al (1988)	96	59	13	61%	14%	26%
	• Vora et al (1989)	81	43	15	53%	18%	7%
	• Emami et al (1987)	9	5	1	55%	11%	?
	Total	238	127	51	52%	21%	≈18.5%
Hot water circulation	• Handl-Zeller et al (1989)	38	5	33	13%	87%	4%
	• Meredith et al (1989)	7	–	–	–	–	0%
	Total	45	–	–	–	–	≈ 2%
Ferromagnetic seeds	• Schimm et al (1989)	4	0	1	0%	25%	?

tions, in order to minimize the risks brought about for the patient by the combination with local hyperthermia, general anesthesia should not be prolonged. Moreover the treatments carried out under general anesthesia are time and labor-consuming (radiotherapists, anesthesists and nursing staff), and the local risk of burns is higher due to the loss of sensation. In all cases hyperthermia should not increase the local toxicity. That is to say the necrosis induced by thermobrachytherapy, burns or pains produced by thermotherapy, and hemorrhage by the use of an interstitial hyperthermia implantation is different from that used for conventional brachytherapy.

Physical, technical and clinical data have shown that the use of hot water circulation seems to be one of the best solutions allowing a complete control of the maximum temperature.

Acknowledgements: The authors are grateful to Mrs. J. Schaeffer for her technical assistance and to Miss D. Courtois for the care and time devoted to the typing of this manuscript. This work was supported by grants from the "Comité Départemental de Lutte Contre le Cancer de La Haute-Marne" and grants from F.N.C.L.C.C.

References

Aristizabal SA, Oleson JR (1984) Combined interstitial irradiation and localized current field hyperthermia: Results and conclusions from clinical studies. Cancer Res 44: 4757–4760

Astrahan MA, Norman A (1982) A localized current field hyperthermia system for use with Ir-192 interstitial implants. Med Phys 9: 419–424

Bicher HA, Wolfstein RW, Fingerhut AG, Frey HA, Lewinsky BS (1984) An effective fractionation regime for interstitial thermoradiotherapy: Preliminary clinical results. In: Overgaard J (ed) Hyperthermic Oncology, vol 1. Taylor & Francis, London, Philadelphia, pp 575–578

Brezovich IA, Atkinson WJ, Lilly MB (1984) Local hyperthermia with interstitial techniques. Cancer Res 44: 4652–4756

Brezovich IA, Young JH (1981) Hyperthermia with implanted electrodes. Med Phys 9: 79–84

Cetas TC, Hevezi JM, Manning MR, Ozimek EJ (1982) Dosimetry of interstitial thermoradiotherapy. Natl Cancer Inst Monogr 61: 505–507

Chan KW, Chou C, McDougal JA, Luk KH, Vora NL (1989) Changes in heating patterns of interstitial microwave antenna arrays at different insertion depths. Int J Hyperthermia 5(4): 499–507

Chassagne D, Pierquin B (1966) La plésiocuriethérapie des cancers du vagin par moulage plastique à l'iridium 192. J Radiol Electrol 46: 89–93

Cosset JM, Brule JM, Salama AM, Damia E, Dutreix J (1982) Low-frequency (0.5 MHz) contact and interstitial techniques for clinical hyperthermia. In: Biomedical Thermology. Alan R. Liss Inc., New York, pp 649–657

Cosset JM, Dutreix J, Gerbaulet A, Damia E (1985) L'association hyperthermie interstitielle-curiethérapie: Une technique de rattrapage des récidives en zones précédemment irradiées. In: Actualités Carcinologiques – Institut Gustave Roussy, Masson, Paris, pp 211–218

Cosset JM, Dutreix J, Gerbaulet A, Damia E (1984) Combined interstitial hyperthermia and brachyterapy: The Institut Gustave Roussy experience. In: Overgaard J (ed) Hyperthermic Oncology, vol 1. Taylor & Francis, London, Philadelphia, pp 587–590

Cosset JM, Dutreix J, Dufour J, Janoray P, Damia E, Haie C, Clarke D (1984) Combined interstitial hyperthermia and brachytherapy: Institut Gustave Roussy technique and preliminary results. Int J Radiat Oncol Biol Physics 10: 307–312

Cosset JM, Dutreix J, Haie C, Gerbaulet A, Janoray P, Dewar JA (1985) Interstitial thermoradiotherapy: A technical and clinical study of 29 implantations performed at the Institut Gustave Roussy. Int J Hyperthermia 1(1): 1, 3–13

Coughlin CT, Wong TZ, Strohbehn JW, Colacchio TA, Sutton JE, Belch RZ, Douple EB (1985) Intraoperative interstitial microwave-induced hyperthermia and brachytherapy. Int J Radiat Oncol Biol Phys 11: 1673–1678

Coughlin CT, Strohbehn JW, Ryan TP, Roberts DW, Colacchio TA, Douple EB (1989) Interstitial hyperthermia for deep seated malignancies. In: Proc 5th International Symposium on Hyperthermic Oncology, Kyoto, pp 596–597

Desmukh R, Damento M, Demer L, Forsyth K, de Young D, Dewhirst M, Cetas TC (1984) Ferromagnetic alloys with curie temperatures near 50°C for use in hyperthermic therapy. In: Overgaard J (ed) Hyperthermic Oncology, vol 1. Taylor & Francis, London, Philadelphia, pp 571–574

Doss JD (1975) Use of RF fields to produce hyperthermia in animal tumors. Proceedings of International Symposium on Cancer Therapy by Hyperthermia and Radiation. ARC, Washington DC, pp 226–227

Doss JD, McCabe A (1976) A technique for localized heating in tissue: An adjunct to tumor therapy. Medical Instrumentation 10: 16–20

Dutreix J, Cosset JM, Salama M, Brule JM, Damia E (1982) Experimental studies of various heating procedures for clinical application of localized hyperthermia. In: Biomedical Thermology. Alan R Liss Inc, New York, pp 585–596

Emami B, Marks J, Perez C, Nussbaum G, Leybovich L (1984) Treatment of human tumors with interstitial irradiation and hyperthermia. In: Overgaard J (ed) Hyperthermic Oncology, vol 1. Taylor & Francis, London, Philadelphia, pp 583–586

Emami B, Perez CA, Leybovich L, Straube W, Vongerichten D (1987) Interstitial thermoradiotherapy in treatment of malignant tumours. Int J Hyperthermia 3(2): 107–118

Emami B (1990) Applied techniques and clinical practice of local external and interstitial hyperthermia. Mallickrodt Institute of Radiology, Radiation Oncology Center, Washington University School of Medicine, St. Louis, Missouri, U.S.A.

Evans RG, Kimler BF, Morantz RA, Vats TS, Gemer LS, O'Kell V, Lowe N. A phase I-II study of the use fluosol-da 20% as an adjuvant radiation therapy in the treatment of primary high-grade brain tumors. Department of Radiation Oncology, University of Kansas Medical Center, Kansas City, KS, Brain Tumor Institute of Kansas City, MO, and Alpha Therapeutics Corporation, Los Angeles, CA, U.S.A.

Frazier OH, Corry PM (1984) Induction of hyperthermia using implanted electrodes. Cancer Res 44: 4854–4866

Gautherie M (1989) Interstitial hyperthermia: State of the art and prospects. Proc 5th International Symposium on Hyperthermic Oncology, Kyoto, pp 63–68

Gautherie M (1988) Clinical evaluation of the minerve hyperthermia system: Synthesis, T.V.P process

Handl-Zeller L (1989) Personnal communication

Handl-Zeller L, Schreier K, Kärcher KH, Budihna M, Lesnicar H. First clinical experience with the Viennese interstitial two-zone hyperthermia system. O. Handl Ges.m.b.h., Hetzendorferstr. 165A, A-1130 Wien, Austria; Inst. of Oncology, Zaloska 2, YU-61105 Ljubljana, Yugoslavia

Handl-Zeller L, Kärcher KH, Schreier K, Handl O (1987) Beitrag zur Optimierung interstitieller Hyperthermie-Systeme. Strahlentherapie 163: 460–467

Handl-Zeller L (1987) Entwicklung und Einführung neuer interstitieller Hyperthermie-Systeme. In: Hammer J, Kärcher KH (Hrsg) Forschritte in der interstitiellen und intrakavitären Strahlentherapie. Zuckschwerdt Verlag, Wien

Handl-Zeller L, Kärcher KH (1987) Hyperthermie als adjuvante Behandlung bei der Radiatio. In: Neugebauer H (Hrsg) Was gibt es Neues in der Medizin? Dr. Peter Müller Verlag, Wien

Handl-Zeller L, Kärcher KH, Lesnicar H, Budihna M, Schreier K (1987) Newly developed liquid heated interstitial hyperthermia system KHS-9/W18. Int J Hyperthermia 3: 567

Handl-Zeller L, Kärcher KH, Schreier K, Budihna M, Lesnicar H (1988) The interstitial Viennese system KHS-9/W18: Homogeneous hyperthermia with simultaneous radiation in deep seated tumors with integrated heat protection of normal tissue. In: Kärcher KH (ed) Progress in RadioOncology IV, Proc of the 4th Meeting on Progress in Radio-Oncology

Handl-Zeller L, Schreier K, Kärcher KH, Budihna M, Lesnicar H (1988) First clinical experience with the Viennese interstitial two-zone hyperthermia system. Proc 5th International Symposium on Hyperthermic Oncology, Kyoto, p 337

Hoffstetter S, Malissard L, Forçard JJ, Pernot M (1986) Carcinome épidermoïde de la base de langue (à propos de 108 cas traités au Centre Alexis Vautrin). J Eur Radiothérapie 7: 101–110

Inoue T, Masaki N, Ozeki S, Ikeda H, Nishiyama K, Matayoshi Y, Kozuka T (1989) Clinical experience of interstitial hyperthermia combined with external radiation using MA251 interstitial applicator. Proc 5th International Symposium on Hyperthermic Oncology, Kyoto, pp 598–599

Lee DJ, O'Neil MJ, Lam KS, Rostock R, Lam WC (1986) A new design of microwave interstitial applicators for hyperthermia with improved treatment volume. Int J Radiat Oncol Biol Phys 12: 2003

Lilly MB, Brezovich IA, Atkinson WJ (1985) Hyperthermia induction with thermally self-regulated ferromagnetic implants. Radiology 154: 243–244

Lin JC, Wang Y (1987) Interstitial microwave antennas for thermal therapy. Int J Hyperthermia 3: 37–47

Manning MR, Cetas TC, Miller RC, Oleson JR, Connor WG, Gerner EW (1982) Clinical hyperthermia: Results of a phase I trial employing hyperthermia alone or in combination with external beam or interstitial radiotherapy. Cancer 49: 205–216

Marchal C, Bey P, Escanye JM, Itty C, Hoffstetter S, Robert J (1983) 434 MHz microwave hyperthermia device applied in cancer therapy. J Eur Radiotherapy 4: 9–19

Marchal C, Hoffstetter S, Bey P, Pernot M, Gaulard ML (1985) Development of a new interstitial method of heating which can be used with conventional after-loading brachytherapy techniques using Ir 192. Strahlentherapie 161: 523–557

Marchal C, Bey P, Hoffstetter S, Roussey C, Nadi M, Gaulard ML (1986) Interstitial hyperthermia using 27.12 MHz string antennas. 8th European Meeting of E.S.H.O. Tiberias (Israel), 22nd–25th September

Marchal C, Nadi M, Hoffstetter S, Bey P, Pernot M, Prieur G (1989) Practical method of heating operating at 27.12 MHz. Int J Hyperthermia 5: 451–466

Mazeron JJ, Crook J, Benk V, Walop W, Pierquin B (1989) Iridium-192 implantation for T1 and T2 epidermoid carcinomas of the mobile tongue: The Creteil experience. Proc 31th ASTRO Meeting: 22

Mechling JA, Strohbehn JW (1986). A theoretical comparison of the temperature distributions produced by three interstitial hyperthermia systems. Int J Radiat Oncol Biol Phys 12: 2137–2149

Meredith RF, Brezovich I, Weppelmann B, Kim R, Salter M (1979) Interstitial thermoradiotherapy for head and neck cancer using brachytherapy catheters for perfusion heating. Proc 31th ASTRO Meeting: 22

Merrick HW, Milligan AJ, Woldenberg LS, Ahuja RK, Dobelbower RR (1987) Intraoperative interstitial hyperthermia in conjunction with intraoperative radiation therapy in a radiation-resistant carcinoma of the abdomen: Report on the feasibility of a new technique. J Surg Oncol 36: 48–51

Mitchell JB (1989) Radiobiology and Clinical Radiation Therapy: Mechanisms of Repair. Radiation Biology Section, Radiation Oncology Branch, National Cancer Institute, Bethesda

Nadi M, Marchal C, Tosser AJ, Roussey C, Gaulard ML (1988) New interstitial hyperthermia technique at 27 MHz. Innov Tech Biol Med 9: 105–115

Nadi M, Tosser AJ, Marchal C (1987) New interstitial hyperthermia using insulated wires at 27.12 MHz. In: Proceed IEEE/Ninth Annual Conf of the EMBS, Nov. 13–16, 1987, Boston, MA, U.S.A.

Oleson JR, Manning MR, Sim DA, Heuzinkueld RS, Aristizabal SA, Cetas TC, Hevez JM, Connor WG (1984) A review of the University of Arizona. Human clinical experience. In: Vaeth JM (ed) Frontiers of Radiation Therapy and Oncology, pp 136–143

Pernot M, Malissard L, Aletti P, Bey P, Hoffstetter S, Noel A (1980) Surdosage curiethérapique des tumeurs de la région veloamygdalienne. Technique par fils d'iridium sous tubes plastiques. J Eur Radiothér 1: 63–75

Pernot M, Malissard L, Hoffstetter S, Forçard JJ (1988) Association de radiothérapie externe et de curiethérapie pour le traitement des cancers épidermoïdes oropharyngés. J Français D'ORL 37: 243–249

Petrovich Z, Lam K, Astrahan M, Luxton G, Langholz B (1988) Interstitial radiotherapy combined with interstitial hyperthermia in the management of recurrent tumors. In: Recents in Cancer Research. Springer, Berlin, Heidelberg, New York, Tokyo, pp 136–140

Pierquin B, Dutreix A (1967) Towards a new system in curietherapy (endocurietherapy and plesiocurietherapy with non-radioactive preparation). Br J Radiol 40: 184–186

Pierquin B, Wilson JF, Chassagne D (1987) Modern Brachytherapy. Masson Publishing, New York

Puthawala AA, Nisar Syed AM, Sheikh Khalid MA, Rafie S, McNamara CS (1985) Interstitial hyperthermia for recurrent malignancies. Brachytherapy/Hyperthermia Oncology 1: 125–131

Ross D, Hugander A (1988) Design and test of microwave interstitial applicators with improved longitudinal heating pattern. Int J Hyperthermia 4(6): 609–615

Ryan TP, Strohbehn JW (1987) A comparison of power deposition for three microwave antennas used in hyperthermia cancer therapy. In: Proceed IEEE/Ninth Annual Conf of the EMBS, Nov. 13–16, 1987, Boston, MA, U.S.A.

Satoh T, Stauffer PR (1988) Implantable helical coil microwave antenna for interstitial hyperthermia. Int J Hyperthermia 4(5): 497–512

Schimm D, Cetas TC, Buechler D, Chen J, Dean S, Fletcher A, Haider S, Lutz W, Sinno R, Stauffer P, Cassady J (1989) Inductively heated, thermoregulating ferromagnetic seeds for interstitial thermoradiotherapy. Proc 5th International Symposium on Hyperthermic Oncology, Kyoto, pp 594–595

Schreier K, Budihna M, Lesnicar H, Handl-Zeller L, Hand JW, Prier MV, Clegg ST (1990) Preliminary studies of interstitial hyperthermia using hot water. Int J Hyperthermia 6: 431–444

Schwan HP (1957) Electrical properties of tissues and cells. Adv Biol Med Phys 5: 153–165

Stauffer PR, Satoh T, Suen SA, Fike JR (1987) Thermal dosimetry characterization of implantable helical coil microwave antennas. In: Proc IEEE/9th Annual Conf of the EMBS, Nov. 13–16, 1987, Boston, MA, U.S.A.

Stauffer PR, Cetas TC, Fletcher AM, de Young DW, Dewhirst MW, Oleson JR, Roemer RB (1984) Magnetic induction heating of ferromagnetic implants for inducing localized hyperthermia in deep-seated tumors. IEEE Trans Biomed Eng 31: 235–251

Stea B, Cetas TC, Lutz W, Lulu B, Shetter A, Rossman K, Obbens E, Guthkelch N, Iacono R, Schimm D, Cassady J (1989) Interstitial thermoradiotherapy of brain tumors: A phase I clinical trial. Proc 31st ASTRO Meeting: 116

Steeves RA (1989) The Radiologic Clinics of North America. Saunders, Philadelphia

Strohbehn JW, et al (1979) An invasive microwave antenna for locally induced hyperthermia for cancer therapy. J Microwave Power 14: 181–186

Strohbehn JW (1983) Temperature distributions from interstitial RF electrode hyperthermia systems: Theoretical predictions. Int J Radiat Oncol Biol Phys 9: 1655–1667

Strohbehn JW, Mechling JA (1986) Interstitial techniques for clinical hyperthermia. In: James RJ, Hand JW (eds) Physical Techniques in Clinical Hyperthermia. Research Studies Press, chapter 5, pp 210–287

Trembly BS (1985) The effects of driving frequency and antenna length on power deposition within a microwave antenna array used for hyperthermia. IEEE Trans Biomed Eng BME 32: 152–157

Visser AG, Van Rhoon GC, Hoogenboom J, de Ru V, Ledenvag PC (1986) (abstract) 27 MHz wire antennas for interstitial hyperthermia. 8th European Meeting of E.S.H.O., Tiberias (Israel), 22nd–25th September. Int J Hyperthermia 2: 413

Vora NL, Forell B, Luk KH, Pezner RD, Lipsett JA, Desai KR, Wong JYC, Chou CK, Chan KW (1989) Interstitial thermoradiotherapy (IT) in recurrent and advanced malignant tumors. Seven years of experience. Proc 5th International Symposium on Hyperthermic Oncology, Kyoto, pp 588–590

Waterman FM, Matthews J, Nerlinger RE (1987) Mapping temperature, specific absorption rate, and effective blood flow. In: Proc IEEE/Ninth Annual Conf of the

EMBS, November 13–16, 1987, Boston, MA, U.S.A.

Yabumoto E, Suyama S, Shou K, Yamazaki T (1989) A phase I clinical trial of radio-frequency interstitial hyperthermia combined with external radiotherapy. Proc 5th International Symposium on Hyperthermic Oncology, Kyoto, pp 591–593

8

Clinical Practice of Interstitial Microwave Hyperthermia Combined with Iridium-192 Brachytherapy

M. H. Seegenschmiedt[1,2], *R. Sauer*[1], *L. W. Brady*[2], and *U. L. Karlsson*[2]

[1] Strahlentherapeutische Klinik, Poliklinik der Universität Erlangen-Nürnberg, Erlangen, Federal Republic of Germany
[2] Department of Radiation Oncology and Nuclear Medicine, Hahnemann University, Philadelphia, Pennsylvania, U.S.A.

Introduction

Elevated temperatures in the range of 41 °C–45 °C in the whole body, in regional sections or localized areas of the human body in combination with radiotherapy have been used as a promising alternative to conventional treatment strategies, in particular for primary advanced tumors with a high probability for relapse and pretreated locally recurrent malignancies. Tumors of the head and neck, breast, brain as well as pelvic tumors may benefit from better local tumor control with impact on survival and quality of life (Kapp, 1986; Overgaard, 1989); improved local control may eventually result in a higher cure rate, better organ preservation and reduction of treatment morbidity. The clinical implementation of hyperthermia was stimulated by a better understanding of biological (Ben-Hur et al, 1974; Harisiadis et al, 1978; Miller et al, 1978; Gerner et al, 1983; Moorthy et al, 1984; Jones et al, 1989) and physiological effects (Dudar and Jain, 1984; Song, 1984; Reinhold and Endrich, 1986) on normal and tumor tissue as well as by newly developed heating techniques (Gautherie, 1989a; Hand, 1989), thermal modelling (Strohbehn et al, 1989) and improved invasive thermometry (Cetas, 1984). First promising clinical results (Kapp, 1989; Overgaard, 1989) have already been reported.

Compared to external hyperthermia techniques "interventional" heating techniques, microwave (MW), radiofrequency (RF) or hot-source (HS) interstitial hyperthermia (IHT) by means of ferromagnetic material (Brezovich et al, 1984; Neyzari and Cheung, 1985; Gautherie, 1989a) theoretically offer several advantages: (1) brachytherapy and IHT can be combined without major modification of each technique, (2) the confined treatment volume permits higher tumor doses and improved sparing of surrounding tissues, (3) where accessible deep-seated tumors can be treated, (4) sampling of invasive thermometry data and (5) improved treatment control by individual power steering.

Since 1986 at the Departments of Radiation Oncology of the University of Erlangen-Nürnberg (West Germany) and Hahnemann University Philadelphia (United States) a co-operative phase I/II clinical trial has been conducted to investigate the impact of interstitial thermo-radiotherapy (IHT/IRT) on initial and long-term local tumor response and related acute and late treatment toxicity. This report summarizes and updates the clinical practice using microwave (MW) IHT combined with Ir-192 brachytherapy and external radiotherapy (Phromratanapongse et al, 1990).

Clinical experience in head & neck and pelvic tumors

Patient and lesion characteristics

Since January 1986 a total of 56 malignant lesions of the head and neck, the pelvic region or other sites in 55 patients were treated with combined interstitial thermo-radiotherapy (IHT/IRT). In addition, three recurrent astrocytomas/glioblastoma multiforme of the brain have been treated with IRT/IHT, but are not included in this report due to special treatment conditions (Seegenschmiedt et al, 1987; Roberts et al, 1989) as well as three lesions in the head and neck, which have been recently treated with simultaneous radio-chemotherapy (RCT) combined with interstitial hyperthermia (IHT). All characteristic features of the patients and lesions (31 males, 24 females, age 6–81 years, mean: 61 years) are summarized in Table 1. The 56 lesions consisted of three groups: advanced primary (AP), local recurrent and local metastatic (LM) lesions. The AP lesions had not received prior radiotherapy and had undergone incomplete surgical resection prior to the beginning of the study, wheras all LR and LM lesions had been previously treated with a variety of treatment modalities: 30 (54%) had undergone prior external radiation therapy (ERT) with doses ranging from 40–72 Gy (mean: 56 Gy, SD ± 12) and 28 (50%) had received prior chemotherapy. 38 (68%) lesions were located in the head and neck, 13 (23%) in the pelvis and 5 (9%) in other body sites. The tumor dimensions were usually measured by using calipers in accessible sites or by careful evaluation of appropriate diagnostic imaging techniques (ultrasound, CT or NMR-imaging): 16 (29%) lesions were ≤ 25 ccm, 12 (21%) ≤ 50 ccm, 16 (29%) ≤ 100 ccm and 8 (14%) ≤ 150 ccm. Four tumor lesions (7%) had extensive volumes >225 ccm. One was a recurrent Ewing's sarcoma of the iliac crest, the others were large nodular metastases of breast carcinoma in the axilla or the neck respectively. The lesions ≤ 150 ccm averaged 4.5 × 4 × 3 ccm with volumes between 10–135 ccm (mean: 55 ccm, SD ± 33).

Thermo-radiotherapy treatment concept

The typical flow-chart of all treatment procedures is displayed on Table 2. Clinical staging, assessment of tumor dimensions and patho-histological confirmation preceded IRT and IHT, which were usually applied as the first step within the

Table 1. Characteristic features of patients and lesions

Patients: (N = 55)	Sex:	31 males, 24 females;
	Age:	6–81 years, mean: 63 years;
Lesions: (N = 56)	Type:	26 (46%) Advanced Primary (AP)
		22 (39%) Local Recurrent (LR)
		8 (14%) Local Metastases (LM)
Location:		38 (68%) Head & Neck Region
		13 (23%) Pelvic Region
		5 (9%) Other Body Sites
Tumors/H & N:		18 Base of Tongue/Tongue
		10 Floor of Mouth
		4 Tonsillar Fossa
		3 Pharynx
		3 Neck Nodes
/PEL:		5 Cervix
		3 Vagina
		2 Colo-rectal
		2 Urethra
		1 Anus
/OTH:		2 Chest Wall
		1 Abdominal Wall
		1 Iliac Crest
		1 Cheek
Histology:		45 (80%) Squamous Cell Carcinoma
		9 (16%) Adenocarcinoma
		2 (4%) Soft Tissue Sarcoma
Pretreatment (N = 56)		55 (98%) Incomplete Surgical Resection
		30 (54%) Adjuvant Radiation Therapy
		28 (50%) Adjuvant Chemotherapy

treatment schedule supplemented by ERT after a 1–2 week break. All patients entered the study with an anticipated life expectancy of at least 3 months; they had signed an informed consent form explaining the investigational nature of the study and the possible risks.

Interstitial Iridium-192 radiotherapy technique

The surgical implantation of afterloading probes was usually performed in the OR with the patient under general anaesthesia. Free hand implants were applied for the H & N lesions and well-established template techniques for pelvic lesions (Syed et al, 1978; Puthawala et al, 1982; Hilaris and Henschke, 1985; Perez et al, 1985; Goffinet et al, 1985; Mazeron et al, 1987): 19 gauge hollow stainless steel needles were distributed within the tumor volume and surrounding tissue about 1–1.5 cm apart according to the "Paris System" (Pierquin et al, 1978). The same distance separated individual planes of the implant. Afterwards thin leads of 16 gauge closed end plastic afterloading

Table 2. Treatment schedule and flow chart of procedures

Diagnostic Staging	Tumor Location, Tumor Volume, Tumor Type, Histology, Grading.
Surgical Procedure	Biopsy or Incomplete Surgery, Afterloading Probe Implantation.
Treatment Planning	IRT: Orthogonal X-rays, CT-scan, Isodose Distribution Planning. IHT: Antenna & Generator Set-Up and Thermometry Sensor Set-Up.
Interstitial Hyperthermia (IHT)	45–60 minutes at 41°C–44°C, 1 IHT before IRT/1 IHT after IRT.
Interstitial Radiotherapy (IRT)	Iridium-192, 20–30 Gy/50 cGy/h, total irradiation time 48–72 h.
	Afterloading Probe Explantation, 1–2 weeks break prior to ERT.
External Radiotherapy (ERT)	Depending upon prior radiation: up to 50 Gy photon/electron beam, 70–80 Gy total (IRT + ERT) dose, 110 Gy cumulative dose (LR lesions).
Follow-Up Examination	Clinical Evaluation: 6 and 12 weeks, 6, 12 and every 6 months ongoing.

tubes were threaded through the needles and the needles replaced by flexible Teflon tubes. These tubes were kept in place by a plastic template or plastic buttons on both sides of the implant. Fig. 1 displays a post-operative interstitial implant in the OR suite for a base of tongue carcinoma with the plastic afterloading tubes thread through the chin and floor of mouth. For brachytherapy low-dose Ir-192 seeds equidistantly inbedded in plastic tubes were inserted manually or by afterloading procedure.

LR and LM lesions, which had been previously irradiated with radiation doses between 40–70 Gy, received reduced doses ≤50 Gy for their relapse treatment course; between 20–40 Gy were applied locally by IRT, the rest by ERT; however, those lesions did not exceed a cumulative dose (previous RT plus current RT dose) of 110 Gy per site. In contrast, all AM lesions without prior RT received a total RT dose between 70–80 Gy consisting of 20–30 Gy local brachytherapy during one IRT session and 50–60 Gy local and regional conventional ERT (photons, electrons). Hence AP lesions had a therapeutic advantage receiving "high dose" RT compared to "low dose" RT of the LR/LM lesions. The applied IRT dose ranged from 17 to 48 Gy (mean 26.2 Gy, SD ± 8) and the specific dose rate from 25 to 70 cGy/h (mean 44 cGy/h,

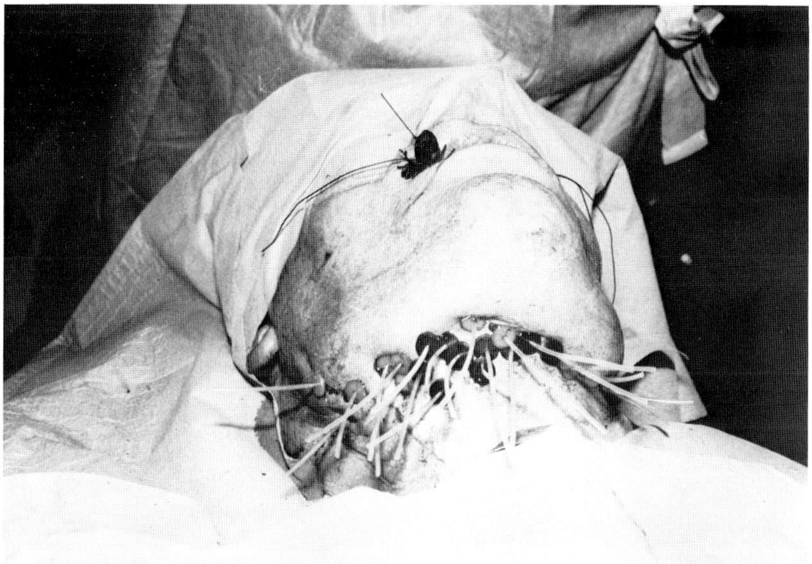

Fig. 1. Post-operative interstitial implant for a base of tongue carcinoma.

SD ± 12) resulting in an implantation period of 44–96 hours. The total applied dose (IRT + ERT dose) reached 31–82 Gy (mean 60 Gy, SD ± 18). 20 (36%) lesions received ≤ 50 Gy, 15 (27%) lesions between 51–70 Gy and 21 (38%) lesions >70 Gy.

Interstitial microwave hyperthermia technique

Two commercial heating systems (University of Erlangen-Nürnberg: Lund/Buchler System 4010, Lund Science AB, Sweden; Hahnemann University Philadelphia: Clini-Therm Mark VI/IX, Clini-Therm Corp., Dallas, Texas, U.S.A.) were employed. These systems provide an integrated interstitial 915 MHz MW treatment mode, which permits the output of the RF amplifier to by split into four variable attenuators, i.e. "channels", each controlling four interstitial MW antennae. Thus a total of 16 MW antennae can be simultaneously powered during one IHT session. Power balancing and individual steering capabilities of each "channel" as well as simultaneous survey of 32 independent thermometry sensors are controlled by a personal computer. At the end of each session an evaluation program analyzes the thermometry data and provides a summary printout.

The employed MW antennae are single node, semi-flexible coaxial dipole antennae, which provide a nearly ellipsoidal radiative heating pattern of about 6 cm longitudinal length (3 cm per lobe) and 1.5 cm axial length in the central plane when tested in an appropriate static muscle equivalent phantom (Chou et al, 1984). Many physical conditions, however, may change the typical heating pattern of the individual antenna and the heat distribution within the individual implant, e.g. coherent or incoherent mode of antennae activation, constructive and destructive interference, antenna insertion depth influencing the resonance status of the antennae, spacing and distribution among the individual antennae as well as specific anatomical conditions like muscle-bone interfaces (MECHLING and STROHBEHN, 1986; CHAN et al, 1989; JAMES et al, 1989; STAUFFER et al, 1989a). Head and neck tumors usually require an implantation length of 4–8 cm, but in pelvic tumors, this can range to between 10–15 cm.

The individual MW antennae distribution was primarily determined by established radiation dosimetry guidelines (PIERQUIN et al, 1978) and site-specific tumor conditions. Sometimes anatomical constraints, such as short insertion depth or vicinity to bony structures limited the use of some afterloading probes for heating purposes. Depending upon the specific treatment volume and catheter distribution 4–16 (mean 9, SD ± 4) antennae were used for lesions ≤150 ccm. However, large tumors >150 ccm could only be treated in a "sandwich mode" either with one part of the lesion being treated before and the other part after application of IRT, or separately within the same, but extended IHT session. Initially we intended to apply always two IHT sessions at 41 °C–44 °C for approximately one hour at therapeutic temperatures. 40 (71%) lesions were treated according to this concept, but 16 (29%) lesions received only one IHT session because of various problems, such as technical difficulties, patient's tolerance or management with co-operating clinics (probe implantation and explantation on working days).

At the beginning of each IHT treatment the specific power output of each attenuator was increased only gradually over a period of 10–15 minutes in order to avoid discomfort to the patient. Usually after 20 minutes "steady state conditions" with therapeutic tumor temperatures in the range of 41 °C–44 °C were reached and maintained for 60 minutes. During IHT several physical parameters, such as pulse rate, blood pressure and systemic body temperature, were carefully monitored. All but one patient were treated whilst awake with non-opiate analgesics and a mild sedative, which were applied intravenously as necessary throughout the treatment session. The only patient treated under general anaesthesia was a 6 year old child with a recurrent soft tissue sarcoma in the cheek.

Invasive thermometry technique

IHT provides the unique opportunity to obtain multiple "invasive" thermometry readings in close spatial and temporal distribution throughout the treatment. This allows in general a better control of the heating efficacy and an improved "targeting" of power steering. All invasive thermometry data were collected with the integrated thermometry devices of the employed hyperthermia systems, i.e. the fiberoptic technique of the Thermo Sentry 1200 System (Clini-Therm Mark VI/IX) and the non-perturbing thermistor technique of the Lund/Buchler Hyperthermia System 4010. Whereas fiberoptic thermometry analyzes the transmission change of infra-red light passing through Gallium Arsenide crystals, the thermistor thermometry technique measures the thermally induced change or resistivity in semiconductors (CETAS, 1985). Both techniques allow the use of single and multiple sensor probes with a 1.1 cm spacing.

A total of 8–40 (mean: 17, SD ± 7) thermometry sensors were used with 4–18 (mean: 8, SD ± 3) sensors within the tumor volume. At least one sensor array was placed close to the tumor center. At

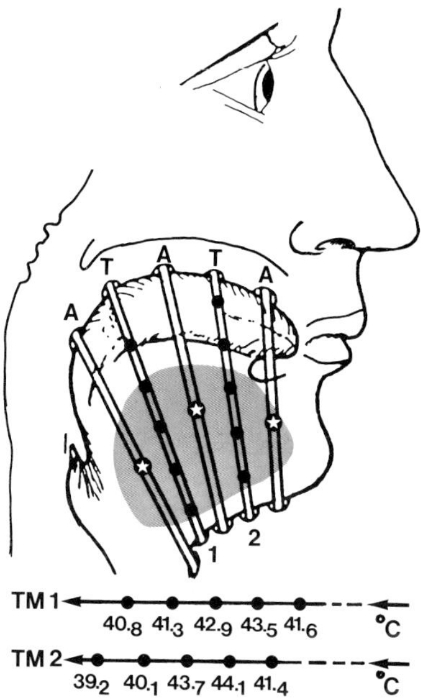

Fig. 2. Interstitial hyperthermia set-up in the base of tongue.

Agenda: Lateral view of an interstitial hyperthermia set-up in the central plane of a base of tongue carcinoma. The implant consists of antennae (A) and multi-sensor thermometry probes (T) in between. Thermal mapping is performed during IHT by "tracking" the central thermometry probes. Corresponding TM1 and TM2 profiles are displayed in the lower part of the figure with arrows indicating the direction of probe insertion.

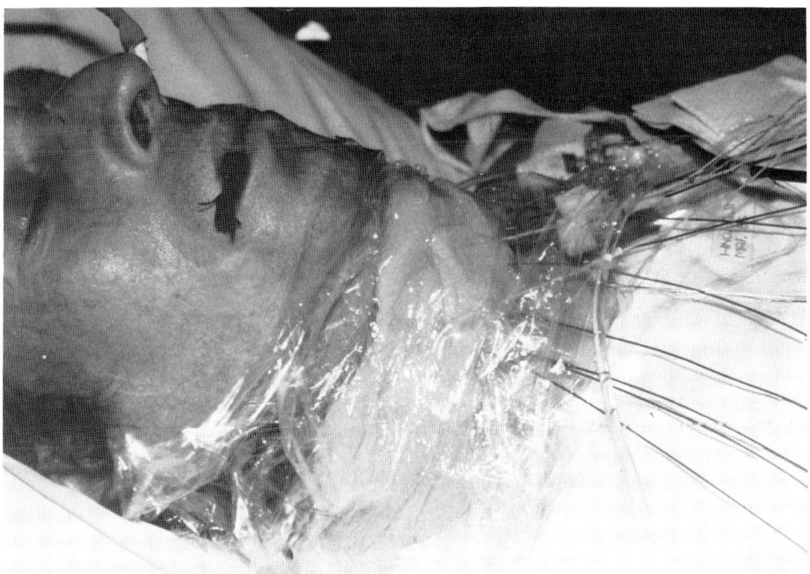

Fig. 3. Interstitial hyperthermia set-up for a base of tongue carcinoma.

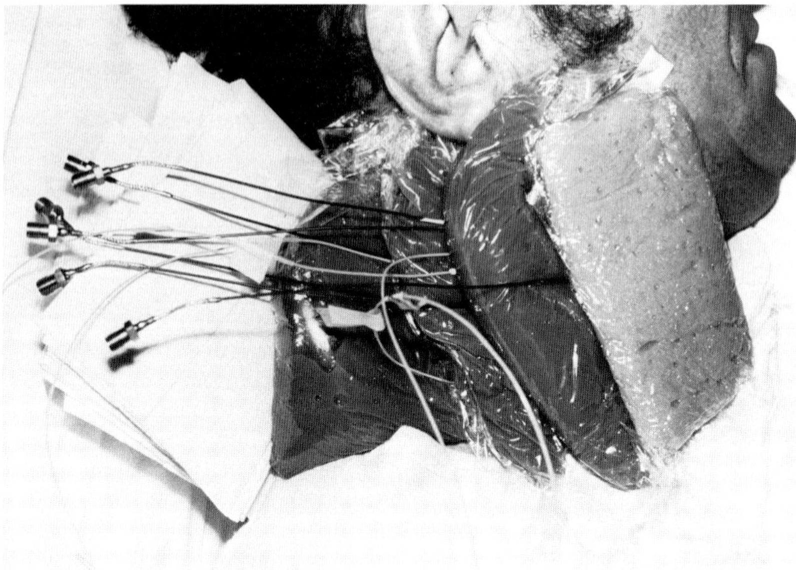

Fig. 4. Interstitial hyperthermia set-up for a large N3 neck node metastasis.

steady state conditions thermal mapping (TM) was performed in at least two perpendicular central planes, i.e. the probes were manually moved to record temperatures every 0.5 cm along the track. The documented temperature profile was compared to the established tumor dimensions. Fig. 2 demonstrates the lateral view of an interstitial implant of the base of tongue displaying the MW antenna and thermometry probe distribution with corresponding thermal mapping tracks and thermometry readings. Many aspects have to be considered in a treatment planning session prior to the commencement of IHT to assure appropriate quality assurance conditions and reliable evaluation of IHT treatment sessions (SEEGENSCHMIEDT et al, 1989).

The absolute and the mean tumor minimum (Tmin, Tmin/mean) and tumor maximum (Tmax, Tmax/mean) temperatures were recorded during each IHT session. The thermal quality (TQ) of each IHT session was calculated as the ratio of sensors in tumor tissue, which reached a mean thermometry level of ≥41 °C (TQ 41 °C), compared to all tumor sensors. If all tumor sensors exceeded 41 °C, the TQ 41 °C yielded 100% and the heating session was considered as "excellent"; similarly scoring for TQ 41 °C ≥ 75% was "good", for TQ 41 °C ≥ 50% "fair" and for TQ 41 °C < 50% "poor". A minimum of 4 tumor sensors was used, to avoid over-estimation of only one thermometry reading (CORRY et al, 1988). A typical complex treatment set-up for interstitial hyperthermia of a base of tongue tumor is demonstrated in Fig. 3 and in Fig. 4 for a large N3 neck node metastasis of an unknown primary tumor.

Criteria of tumor response and statistical methods

Due to the loco-regional character of the treatment approach the main intention

was to assess the local tumor response. Tumor size was measured before, during and after completion of IHT/IRT treatment and in further FU (every 3 months). The criteria of the WHO (World Health Organization, 1979) were applied to define the local tumor response: complete response (CR = total tumor disappearance), partial response (PR = >50% reduction in tumor size), no change (NC = ≤50% reduction and ≤25% increase of tumor size) and progressive disease (PD = >25% increase of tumor size). The evaluation was conducted on December 31, 1989, with a minimum FU ≥ 3 months; FU periods ranged from 3–45 months (mean: 18 months, SD ± 9). Initial response was defined at 3 months FU (56 lesions) and long-term response at 12 months FU for 40 (71%) lesions. 8 lesions had shorter FU periods due to the patient's death. Relapses after combined IRT/IHT were grouped as within (= local) or outside (= regional) of the treated volume.
(Acute) side-effects and/or (chronic) complications were evaluated as grade 0 for no side-effects or complications, grade 1 for minor complications, which did not require special care, i.e. blisters, mucositis, erythema, grade 2 for major complications, which depended on long-term medical care, i.e. deep burns and ulcerations, grade 3 for major complications, which required specific surgical intervention, i.e. fistulas and extensive tissue break-down, and grade 4 for fatal complications. Statistical values were determined by the established student-T and Fisher's exact tests (FISHER and YATES, 1963).

Clinical results

Initial tumor response

The initial local tumor response at 3 months FU revealed a total of 38/56 lesions (68%) with CR, 12/56 (21%) lesions with PR and 6/56 (11%) lesions with NC or PD. The total tumor response rate (CR + PR) yielded 50/56 (89%). 6/12 (50%) lesions with initial PR at 3 months subsequently developed local control (LC) at 12 months FU, whereas 4/12 lesions (33%) remained stable and 2/12 lesions (17%) suffered local-regional relapse or renewed progression of disease (Table 3).

Long-term tumor response

After 12 months FU, 8/55 patients (15%) had died. Three of them had reached CR as initial tumor response one dying from a carotid blow-out, the other two from pulmonary metastases. At death all lesions had local tumor control (LC) at the treatment site. One patient initially had PR and achieved CR at 6 months FU, but then died from a second primary tumor at 11 months. The other patients never responded to IRT/IHT and died at 4–9 months due to local and systemic progression. The analysis of long-term tumor response of 40 lesions with a minimum of 12 months FU revealed 35/40 (88%) lesions with LC and 5/40 (13%) with local relapse (REC). Including all 8 patients, who deceased prior to 12 months FU, (4 LC, 4 REC/PD), the total LC rate accounts for 39/48 (81%) and the local failure rate for 9/48 (19%) (Table 3). So far a total of 12/55 (22%)

Table 3. Initial and long-term tumor response at 3 and 12 months follow-up

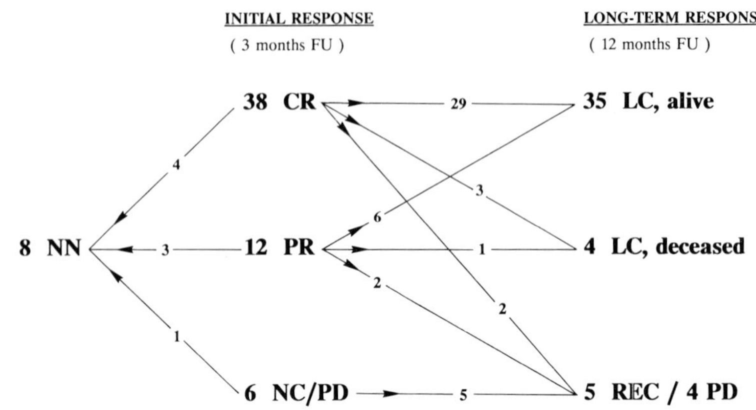

Agenda: Figures represent the number of lesions at follow-up (large) or changing response (small). NN = not reached follow-up 12 months; CR = complete remission, PR = partial remission, NC = no change, PD = progressive disease, REC = local recurrence, LC = local control

patients have developed distant metastases, but have still maintained local control within the treated volume.

Analysis of prognostic treatment factors

An analysis of various patient, tumor and treatment parameters was performed. No prognostic significance was found for age and sex of the patients, lesion site, tumor histology, tumor stage or grade, specific IRT isodose level and duration of the IRT treatment. Moreover lesions, which had two IHT sessions, had no advantage over those receiving only one IHT session. In contrast several other parameters were found to significantly correlate with tumor response, which are summarized in Table 4:

(1) SITE OF LESION: Response was independent of the location of the malignant lesions. Head and neck tumors yielded 26/38 (68%) CR compared to 9/13 (69%) CR for pelvic malignancies. 2/5 (40%) of the lesions at other locations achieved CR.

(2) TYPE OF LESION: AP lesions reached better response, 23/26 (88%) CR, compared to LR and LM lesions with a rate of 15/30 (50%) CR ($p \leq 0.005$).

(3) TUMOR VOLUME: "Small" lesions responded better than "large" lesions; an intrinsic "breakpoint" was found around 75 ccm, which may also reflect the mean number of 8 MW antennae per lesion with an estimated mean heating volume of about 10 ccm per antenna (i.e. the estimate of the 50% iso-SAR distribution in muscle equivalent tissue). The group of "small" lesions ≤75 ccm had a rate of 29/37 (78%) CR compared to "large" lesions >75 ccm with 9/19 (47%) CR ($p \leq 0.05$).

(4) RADIATION DOSE: The total radiation dose (IRT + ERT) influenced treatment outcome. Lesions

Table 4. Prognostic factors for interstitial thermo-radiotherapy

(N = 56)

			Clinical tumor response (at 3 months FU)			
			(CR)	(PR)	(NC)	p-value
Lesion type:						
	AP	+)	23(88%)	2(8%)	1(4%)	+) $p<0.01$
	LR/LM		15(50%)	10(33%)	5(17%)	
Tumor volume:						
	≤75 ccm	#)	29(78%)	7(19%)	1(3%)	#) $p<0.05$
	>75 cm		9(47%)	5(26%)	5(26%)	
Radiation dose:						
	≤50 Gy	§)	8(40%)	8(40%)	4(20%)	§) $p<0.005$
	>50 Gy		30(83%)	4(11%)	2(5%)	
Thermal dose:						
T min/mean	<41.0°C	$)	20(58%)	8(24%)	6(18%)	$) $p<0.25$
	≥41.0°C		18(82%)	4(18%)	—	nonsignificant
Thermal quality:						
TQ41°C	>75%	*)	26(87%)	4(13%)	—	*) $p<0.005$
	<75%		12(46%)	8(31%)	6(23%)	

treated with "low-dose" RT ≤ 50 Gy had 8/20 (40%) CR compared to lesions receiving "high-dose" RT > 50 Gy with 30/36 (83%) CR ($p \leq 0.005$). AP lesions received a higher mean radiation dose (70 Gy, SD ± 8) compared to LR/LM lesions (52 Gy, SD ± 17), and all lesions being treated with >70 Gy were AP lesions and achieved the best results with 19/21 (90%) CR.

(5) THERMAL PARAMETERS: Parameters linked to minimum tumor temperature influenced treatment outcome: lesions, which reached only a "low" mean minimum tumor temperature T min/mean <40°C responded worse, 6/13 (46%) CR, compared to lesions achieving "moderate" temperatures of 40°C–40.9°C, 14/21 (67%) CR, and "high" temperatures of ≥41°C, 18/22 (78%) CR, but these differences are not statistically significant ($p <0.25$). The impact of thermal quality (TQ), however, was significant: lesions with TQ 41°C ≥ 75%, i.e. "excellent or good heating" achieved 26/30 (87%) CR, compared to lesions with TQ 41°C < 75%, i.e. "moderate or poor heating", with 12/26 (46%) CR ($p < 0.005$). "Poor heating" with TQ 41°C

< 50% resulted in complete response only for 3/9 (33%) lesions (all with high RT dose) TM data revealed no significant difference probably due to the small number of thermometry points evaluated.

Toxicity evaluation

Acute side-effects, i.e. during or within 48 hours of IHT/IRT treatment, occurred in 16/55 (29%) patients. The following toxicity evaluations were observed: grade 1 (mucositis, blister) in 4/56 (7%) lesions, grade 2 (ulceration, fistula, deep burn) in 10 (18%) and grade 3 (soft tissue break-down) in two (4%) lesions. Fatal side-effects were not observed. The majority of patients 40/56 (71%) tolerated the treatment well without any toxicity. 12/55 (22%) patients or 12/16 (75%) lesions, who initially developed acute side-effects, subsequently experienced long-term complications: 9 (16%) lesions developed slowly healing ulcers or fistulas which cleared up with systemic or local antibiotics and antiseptic dressing over a period of 4–12 months (mean: 6 months, SD ± 3). Lesions in critical anatomical regions or with compromised perfusion, e.g. vesico-vaginal and recto-vaginal septum wall or scar tissues, were prone to ulcerations and fistulas. Three (5%) lesions needed surgery due to an extensive tissue break-down. One patient died from a carotid blow-out after initial CR at 9 months, which may be attributed to both IRT and IHT. Complications were more frequent in the pelvis (5/13 = 38%) compared to head and neck (9/38 = 24%). Maximum tumor temperatures ⩾ 45 °C seemed to induce thermal damage, i.e. for Tmax ⩾ 45 °C a total of 8/16 (50%) complications were noted compared to Tmax < 45 °C with only 8/40 (20%) complications, but this difference was not yet statistically significant.

Discussion of clinical results

The IRT/IHT treatment for AP, LR and LM lesions proved to be both effective and safe. High initial response (CR + PR = 89%), excellent local tumor control at 12 months FU (LC = 83%) and acceptable toxicity (complication = 22%) were noted. Besides objective tumor response considerable palliative effects were obtained in many patients, in particular prevention of bleeding and pain relief. Considering the aggressive pre-treatment of many lesions, the observed complication rate of 22% is quite tolerable and without significant difference between AP and LR lesions. IRT/IHT is still not a routine procedure even in our specialized clinic despite a dedicated team of surgeons, radiation oncologists, hyperthermia technologists and nurses, who are acquainted to patient care and technical procedures. Despite the expenses in time, personnel, material and the complex interdisciplinary cooperation, these encouraging results deserve further investigation by multicentric prospectively randomized phase III trials.

Our findings are supported by published data of other centers using microwave (MW) and/or radiofrequency (RF) IHT. The cumulative clinical experience of about 500 lesions offers promising results despite a variety of different treatment parameters, e.g. tumor size, location, timing and sequence of IRT/IHT and different technical equipment. The rate of complete tumor response (CR) ranges

Table 5a. Clinical results with interstitial microwave hyperthermia

Reference		Lesions	Clinical Response CR	PR	NC	uneval.	Toxicity	Follow-up (months)
BICHER et al,	1984	8	5(63%)	2(25%)	1(13%)	—	1(13%)	short
STROHBEHN et al,	1984	6	3(50%)	2(33%)	1(17%)	—	1(17%)	short
PUTHAWALA et al,	1985	43	32(74%)	11(26%)	—	—	9(21%)	>12
EMAMI et al,	1987	39	21(54%)	9(23%)	5(13%)	4	10(25%)	6–48
AOYAGI et al,	1989	10	2(20%)	4(40%)	4(40%)	—	2(20%)	—
INOUE et al,	1989	9	1(11%)	6(67%)	1(11%)	1	1(11%)	—
PETROVICH et al,	1989	44	28(64%)	15(34%)	1(2%)	—	9(20%)	3–36
Current Study	1990	56	38(68%)	12(21%)	6(11%)	—	12(21%)	6–45
Total Experience	MW-IHT	215	130(60%)	61(28%)	19(9%)	5	45(21%)	

Table 5b. Clinical results with interstitial radiofrequency hyperthermia

Reference		Lesions	Clinical Response CR	PR	NC	uneval.	Toxicity	Follow-up (months)
VORA et al,	1982	16	11(69%)	1(6%)	3(19%)	1	1(6%)	1–13
OLESON et al,	1984	52	20(38%)	22(42%)	10(19%)	—	11(21%)	3–18
COSSET et al,	1985	29	19(66%)	4(14%)	—	6	7(25%)	>2
LINARES et al,	1986	10	3(30%)	7(70%)	—	—	4(40%)	short
EMAMI et al,	1987	9	5(56%)	3(33%)	1(11%)	—	2(25%)	6–48
GAUTHERIE et al,	1989a	95	62(65%)	15(16%)	18(19%)	—	25(26%)	>2
YABUMOTO et al,	1989	13	7(54%)	2(15%)	4(31%)	—	4(31%)	3–13
VORA et al,	1989	75	42(56%)	11(15%)	21(28%)	1	13(17%)	6–74
Total Experience	RF-IHT	299	169(57%)	65(22%)	57(19%)	8	67(22%)	

between 11% – 74% and the total tumor response rate (CR + PR) between 60–100%. No significant difference between MW-IHT (130/215 lesions = 60% CR) (EMAMI et al, 1984; STROHBEHN et al, 1984; BICHER et al, 1985; PUTHAWALA et al, 1985; EMAMI et al, 1987; LAM et al, 1988; AOYAGI et al, 1989; INOUE et al, 1989; PETROVICH et al, 1989; PHROMRATANAPONGSE et al, 1990) and RF-IHT (169/299 lesions = 57% CR) (VORA et al, 1982; EMAMI et al, 1984; OLESON et al, 1984; COSSET et al, 1985; LINARES et al, 1986; GAUTHERIE et al, 1989; VORA et al, 1989; YABUMOTO et al, 1989). Even the rate of treatment toxicity was similar for MW-IHT (45/215 lesions = 21%) and RF-IHT (67/299 lesions = 22%) respectively. The majority of complications could be attributed to rapid tumor necrosis in critical anatomical areas. The currently available clinical data on MW- and RF-IHT are summarized on Table 5a/5b.

Several prognostic lesion and treatment parameters were idenified in our study predicting tumor response. A clear radiation dose-response relation was observed revealing increasing tumor response with higher radiation dose: in our study AP lesions had an intrinsic therapeutic advantage, as they received a higher mean dose (70 Gy, SD ± 8) compared to LR/LM lesions (52 Gy, SD ± 17). Similar observations have been reported by other investigators (Oleson et al, 1984; Cosset et al, 1985; Lam et al, 1988; Petrovich et al, 1989). The complex mechanisms of hyperthermic radiosensitization of ERT and IRT have not been investigated in a randomized study; so far it is not clear, to what extent IRT/IHT may improve tumor response compared to IRT alone or may allow for a reduced RT dose, in order to achieve equal or superior results. Recent results in murine tumors indicate a thermal enhancement ratio (TER) of 1.3–1.7 for interstitial IRT/IHT depending upon the sequence of both treatment modalities (Jones et al, 1989).

Whereas lesion site and tumor histology had neither in our nor in other studies any prognostic value, lesion type (Emami et al, 1984; Puthawala et al, 1985; Emami et al, 1987) and tumor volume (Emami et al, 1984; Dewhirst et al, 1986; Emami et al, 1987; Lam et al, 1988; Petrovich et al, 1989) influenced response significantly. In our experience the radiation dose advantage of AP lesions clearly influenced the better outcome for this group of patients compared to LR/LM as pointed out earlier. Another reasion for the worse results in LR lesions may be related to the socalled "tumor bed effect" (TBE), which positively correlates with the previously applied radiation dose, indicating a higher resistance to hyperthermia (thermotolerance) in pre-irradiated tumors (Urano and Tanaka, 1989). The impact of tumor volume on treatment outcome is due to several factors. As with superficial techniques, insufficient interstitial implantation coverage could result in poor heating due to insufficient power deposition characteristics and could lead to worse clinical results especially for extensive lesions. When analyzing the quality of the interstitial implant (QI) among our patient population by calculating the ratio between tumor volume (ccm) and the number of employed MW antennae (N), it became evident, that most lesions with a QI $\geq$ 10 ccm tumor volume per antenna indicating wide antennae spacing ("poor implant") did worse than lesions with a QI < 10 ccm tumor volume per antenna indicating narrow spacing ("good implant"). In the "poor implant" group only 6/16 (38%) lesions achieved CR compared to 32/40 (80%) CR for the "good implant" group ($p \leq 0.01$). Lesions with QI < 5 ccm tumor volume per antenna reached an even higher CR, 20/23 (87%); although our QI terms "good" and "poor implant" are somewhat semi-quantitative parameters and may depend on various specific technical and clinical conditions, it is obvious, that QI may influence both the characteristic IRT dose distribution as well as the "thermal dose" distribution of IHT throughout the target volume. Unfortunately all other published reports lack sufficient data on tumor volume and/or antenna distribution to assess a comparable QI index, Nevertheless the importance of quality assurance has been already emphasized by others (Nußbaum, 1984; Seegenschmiedt et al, 1989; Stauffer et al, 1989b).

A number of studies have revealed thermal parameters, which correlate with tumor and normal tissue response, either in animal studies (Dewhirst et al, 1984) and/or clinical studies (Dewhirst et al, 1984; Emami et al, 1984; Oleson et al, 1984; Dewhirst et al, 1986; Emami et al, 1987). Oleson et al examined 161 patients (52 lesions treated with IHT) and identified the minimum tumor temperature T min (mean) as the single most significant factor in predicting tumor response (Oleson et al, 1984). Dewhirst et al found that "thermal doses" (TD) of Tmin EQ 43°C < 1 did not achieve better results than in the RT control group, however, for Tmin Eq 43°C 1–5 the CR rate was doubled (Dewhirst et al, 1984; 1986). The extrapolation of this value according to the formula of Sapareto and Dewey (1984) translates into a mean minimum tumor temperature T min/mean = 41.3°C, which should inhibit repair of radiation induced sublethal damage. This figure seems to correspond nicely to our findings using the TQ 41°C value for assessment of heating quality throughout the tumor volume. Similarly Emami et al have emphasized the impact of "quality of heating" (Emami et al, 1987) on tumor response; they observed, that lesions with minimum temperatures ≤42°C did not achieve sufficient response compared to lesions with temperatures >42°C yielding 70% CR. No further details were provided for the number and specific locations of sensors applied.

In clinical practice, it is always difficult to monitor exactly the minimum tumor temperature throughout the tumor volume and the individual IHT session. The number and location of thermometry sensors, their physical performance pattern as well as the spatial and temporal resolution of TM procedures may influence the assessment of minimum temperature data. To avoid an overestimation of a small thermometry data base (Corry et al, 1988), in our approach we used as many thermometry sensors as possible within the tumor volume and in between antennae, i.e. at least 4 for small and 16 for large lesions. All tumor sensors (with a minimum of 4 sensors) were included for the analysis of the "thermal quality". Nevertheless we were unable to yield such high minimum tumor temperatures as reported by others (Emami et al, 1984; Oleson et al, 1984; Emami et al, 1987). We assume, that in our study more tumor sensors were used and included for analysis than in historic studies thereby increasing the likelihood to record lower minimum tumor temperatures. From a biological and clinical standpoint otherwise it is still not clear, if the whole tumor volume needs to be exposed to high cytotoxic temperatures. One effective IHT session around 41 °C might be sufficient to eradicate critical "radioresistant tumor cell pockets" and enhance the response in surrounding areas. Most interestingly we found no difference between one versus two IHT sessions among our patients.

The observed treatment toxicity (either acute side-effects and/or late complications) did neither correlate with the number of IHT sessions (one versus two) nor with any type of pre-treatment nor the lesion type (local recurrent versus advanced primary). Instead maximum temperatures, specifically temperatures ⩾45°C, ie Tmax/mean ⩾45°C, induced thermal toxicity. Clinical data from other institutions (Emami et al, 1984; Oleson et al, 1984; Dewhirst et al, 1984 and 1986; Emami et al, 1987; Lam et al, 1988; Petrovich et al, 1989) support our findings indicating thermal damage being induced by a single high thermal exposure beyond normal tissue tolerance. An objective evaluation of thermal toxicity, however, needs to differentiate between the intended tumorcidal effects, which can cause rapid tumor necrosis in infiltrated anatomical structures (e.g. recto-vaginal or recto-vesical wall), and undesired toxic effects on surrounding normal tissues.

From our clinical work we conclude that non-toxic but effective hyperthermia appears to be a "tricky walk on a small mountain ridge" lined by toxic and uneffective hazards: recommended minimum temperatures in tumor tissue should be uniformly above 41°C or even higher, whereas maxima in normal tissues should not exceed 44°C over long period of time.

Future perspectives

All phase I/II studies implementing IRT/IHT still need enforcement by prospectively randomized phase III trials to evaluate the various treatment factors responsible for the therapeutic impact of combined IRT/IHT. At present two trials have been initiated: one study conducted by the Radiation Therapy Oncology Group (RTOG), RTOG 84–19 (RTOG, 1987) and one study by the European Society of Hyperthermic Oncology (ESHO), 4–86 trial (Overgaard, 1987). These trials compare conventional IRT alone versus combined IRT/IHT for palliative or adjuvant tumor therapy respectively. The American study addresses a broad spectrum of recurrent or persistent lesions stratified by institution, histology, size of lesion, type of lesion, heating modality, prior and actual radiation dose. The European study only focusses on a small subset of tumors, primary T1–T3 base of the tongue lesions, eligible for treatment by ERT + IRT. Other tumor sites may deserve the adjuvant implementation of IRT/IHT (Kapp, 1986; Overgaard, 1989). New clinical approaches of "interventional hyperthermia" may arise from new types of clinical application (e.g. intraoperative IHT combined with IORT) and new applicators (e.g. intraluminal and intracavitary applicators, eye-plaque applicators). IRT/IHT and IHT alone in conjunction with chemotherapy (e.g. cisplatinum) also deserves intensive investigation.

In future IRT/IHT studies need improved heating and thermometry technology; technical research currently focusses on several details regarding heating devices (individual power steering and phase shifting of MW antennae, switching between coherent and in-coherent mode, multisegment or other antennae designs to vary the active heating length), thermometry devices (development of non-invasive thermometry techniques, automatic tracking of thermometry probes, implementation of thermal washout calculations) and computer software (fast screen or mouse controlled menues, implementation of various algorithms for thermometry data analysis). In addition, technical and clinical quality assurance programs have to be defined and implemented, to control and evaluate the variety of critical treatment parameters (Nußbaum, 1984; Corry et al, 1988; Seegenschmiedt et al, 1989; Stauffer et al, 1989b). Biological and physiological experiments are necessary to study the radiosensitizing effects of hyperthermia on low-dose radiation, the critical TER ratio, the tumor bed effect (TBE) or specific pharmaceutical methods to influence and take advantage of local tumor perfusion characteristics and intratumoral metabolic milieu. Ongoing prospective randomized studies should incorporate stratification by prognostic parameters, such as tumor volume, radiation dose and thermal factors. This approach will provide sufficient scientific credit to define the adjuvant and palliative therapeutic role and potential of thermo-radiotherapy.

Acknowledgements: The authors are extremely grateful to Mr. Richard Tobin and Mr. William Kempin, Radiation Therapy Service Engineers, Mr. Pramook Phromratanapongse, M.D., and Mrs. Patricia Guerieri, M.D., Postgraduate Research Fellows (all at Hahnemann University Philadelphia) as well as Mrs. Marianne Kettner and Mrs. Rosemarie Rössler, Radiation Therapy Technicians (all University Erlangen-Nürnberg) for their dedicated and skillful technical assistance, thorough data management and diligent patient care. This work was supported in part by the German Cancer Foundation (Dr. Mildred Scheel Stiftung).

Abbreviations

MW	microwave (hyperthermia)
RF	radiofrequency (hyperthermia)
HS	hot source (hyperthermia)
IHT	interstitial hyperthermia
IRT	interstitial radiotherapy
ERT	external radiotherapy
AP	advanced primary (lesions)
LR	local recurrent (lesions)
LM	local metastatic (lesions)
CR	complete response rate
PR	partial response rate
NC	no change (of tumor)
PC	progession of disease
LC	local (tumor) control
SAR	specific absorption rate
TER	thermal enhancement ratio
TBE	tumor bed effect (of heating)
TQ	thermal quality (of heating)
TM	thermal mapping (of temperatures)
QI	quality of (interstitial) implant

References

Aoyagi Y, Kanehira C, Kobori K, Hayakawa Y, Mochizuki S, Harada N (1989) Clinical experience with microwave interstitial hyperthermia. In: Sugahara T, Saito M (eds) Hyperthermic Oncology 1988, vol 1. Taylor & Francis, London, New York, Philadelphia, pp 601–603

Ben-Hur E, Elkind MM, Bronk BV (1974) Thermally enhanced radiosensitivity of cultered Chinese hamster cells; inhibition of repair of sublethal damage and enhancement of lethal damage. Radiat Res 58: 38–51

Bicher HI, Moore DW, Wolfstein RS (1985) A method for interstitial thermoradiotherapy. In: Overgaard J (ed) Hyperthermic Oncology 1984, vol 1. Taylor & Francis, London, Philadelphia, pp 575–578

Brezovich IA, Atkinson WJ, Lilly MB (1984) Local hyperthermia with interstitial techniques. Cancer Res (Suppl) 44: 4752–5756

Cetas TC (1985) Thermometry and thermal dosimetry. In: Overgaard J (ed) Hyperthermic Oncology 1984, vol 2. Taylor & Francis, London, Philadelphia, pp 9–41

Chan KW, Chou CK, McDougall JA, Luk KH, Vora NL, Forell BW (1989) Changes in heating patterns of interstitial microwave antenna arrays at different insertion depths. Int J Hyperthermia 5: 499–508

Chou CK, Chen GW, Guy AW, Luk KH (1984) Formulas for preparing phantom muscle tissue at various radiofrequencies. Bioelectromagnetics 5: 435–441

Corry PM, Jabboury K, Ong JS, Armour EP, McCraw FJ, LeDuc T (1988) Evaluation of equipment for hyperthermia treatment of cancer. Int J Hyperthermia 4: 53–74

Cosset JM, Dutreix J, Haie C, Gerbaulet A, Janoray P, Dewars JA (1985) Interstitial thermoradiotherapy: A technical and clinical study of 29 implantations performed at the Institute Gustave Roussy. Int J Hyperthermia 1: 3–13

Dewhirst MW, Sim DA, Sapareto S, Connor WG (1984) The importance of minimum tumour temperature in determining early and long-term reponse of spontaneous pet animal tumours to heat and radiation. Cancer Res (Suppl) 44: 43–50

Dewhirst MW, Sim DA (1986) Estimation of therapeutic gain in clinical trials involving hyperthermia and radiotherapy. Int J Hyperthermia 2: 165–178

Dudar TE, Jain RK (1984) Differential response of normal and tumor microcirculation to hyperthermia. Cancer Res 44: 605–612

Emami B, Marks JE, Perez CA, Nußbaum GH, Leybovich L, von Gerichten D (1984) Interstitial thermoradiotherapy in the treatment of recurrent residual malignant tumors. Am J Clin Oncol 6: 699–704

Emami B, Perez CA, Leybovich L, Straube W, von Gerichten D (1987) Interstitial thermoradiotherapy in treatment of malignant tumors. Int J Hyperthermia 3: 107–118

Fisher RA, Yates F (1963) Statistical Tables for Biological, Agricultural and Medical Research. Oliver and Boyd Ltd., Edinburgh, p 47

Gautherie M (1989a) Interstitial hyperthermia: State of the art and prospects. In: Sugahara T, Saito M (eds) Hyperthermic Oncology 1988, vol 2. Taylor & Francis, London, New York, Philadelphia, pp 63–68

Gautherie M, Cosset JM, Gerard JP, Horiot JC, Ardiet JM, El Akoum H, Alperovitch A (1989b) Radiofrequency interstitial hyperthermia: A multicentric program of quality assessment and clinical trials. In: Sugahara T, Saito M (eds) Hyperthermic Oncology 1988, vol 2. Taylor & Francis, London, New York, Philadelphia, pp 711–714

Gerner EW, Oval JH, Manning MR, Sim DA, Bowden GT, Hevezi J (1983) Dose rate dependence of heat radiosensitization. Int J Radiat Oncol Biol Phys 9: 1401–1404

Goffinet DR, Fee Jr WE, Wells J, Austin-Seymour M, Clarke D, Mariscal JM, Goode RL (1985) 192 Iridium pharyngoepiglottic fold interstitial implants. The key to successful treatment of base of tongue carcinoma by radiation treatment. Cancer 55: 941–948

Hand JW (1989) Heating techniques for clinical hyperthermia. In: Sugahara T, Saito M (eds) Hyperthermic Oncology 1988, vol 2. Taylor & Francis, London, New York, Philadelphia, pp 39–44

Harisiadis L, Sung D, Kessaris N, Hall EJ (1978) Hyperthermia and low dose rate irradiation. Radiology 129: 195–198

Hilaris BS, Henschke UK (1985) General principles and techniques of interstitial brachytherapy. In: Hilaris BS (ed) Handbook of Interstitial Brachtherapy. Publ. Sciences Group, Inc., Acton, MA, U.S.A., pp 61–86

Inoue T, Masaki N, Ozeki S, Ikeda H, Nishiyama K, Matayoshi Y, Kozuka T (1989) Clinical experience of interstitial hyperthermia combined with external radiation using MA-251 interstitial applicator. In: Sugahara T, Saito M (eds) Hyperthermic Oncology 1988, vol 1. Taylor & Francis, London, New York, Philadelphia, pp 598–600

James BJ, Strohbehn JW, Mechling JA, Trembly BS (1989) The effect of insertion depth on the theoretical SAR patterns of

915 MHz dipole antenna arrays for hyperthermia. Int J Hyperthermia 5: 733–747

Jones EL, Lyons BE, Douple EB, Dain BJ (1989) Thermal enhancement of low dose irradiation in a murine tumour system. Int J Hyperthermia 5: 509–524

Kapp DS (1986) Site and disease selection for hyperthermia clinical trials. Int J Hyperthermia 2: 139–156

Kapp DS (1989) Hyperthermia of superficial malignancies. In: Sugahara T, Saito M (eds) Hyperthermic Oncology 1988, Taylor & Francis, London, New York, Philadelphia, pp 51–56

Lam K, Astrahan M, Langholz B, Jepson J (1988) Interstitial thermoradiotherapy for recurrent or persistent tumours. Int J Hyperthermia 4: 259–266

Linares LA, Nort D, Brenner H, Shiu M, Ballon D, Anderson L, Alfieri A, Brennan M, Fuks Z, Hilaris B (1986) Interstitial hyperthermia and brachytherapy: A preliminary report. Endocurietherapy/Hyperthermia Oncol 2: 39–44

Mazeron JJ, Langlois D, Glaubiger D, Huart J, Martin M, Raznal M, Calitchi E, Ganem G, Faraldi M, Feuilhade F, Brun B, Marin L, Le Bourgeois JP, Baillet F, Pierquin B (1987) Salvage irradiation of oropharyngeal cancers using Iridium 192 wire implants: 5 year results of 70 cases. Int J Radiat Oncol Biol Phys 13: 957–962

Mechling JA, Strohbehn JW (1986) A theoretical comparison of the temperatures distributions produced by three interstitial hyperthermia systems. Int J Radiat Oncol Biol Phys 12: 2137–2148

Miller RC, Leith JT, Voemett RC, Gerner EW (1978) Effects of interstitial radiation therapy alone, or in combination with localized hyperthermia on a mouse mammary tumour. Radiat Res 19: 175–180

Moorthy CR, Hahn EW, Kim JH, Feingold BS, Alifieri AA, Hilaris BS (1984) Improved response of a murine fibrosarcoma (Meth-A) to interstitial radiation when combined with hyperthermia. Int J Radiat Oncol Biol Phys 10: 2145–2148

Neyzari A, Cheung AY (1985) A review of brachyhyperthermia approaches for the treatment of cancer. Endocurietherapy Hyperthermia Oncol 1: 257–264

Nußbaum GH (1984) Quality assessment and assurance in clinical hyperthermia: Requirements and procedures. Cancer Res (Suppl) 44: 4811–4817

Oleson JR, Manning MR, Sim DA, Heusinkveld M, Aristizibal SA, Cetas TC, Hevezi JC, Connor WG (1984) A review of the University of Arizona human clinical hyperthermia experience. Front Radiat Ther Oncol 18: 136–143

Overgaard J (1985) Rationale and problems in the design of clinical studies. In: Overgaard J (ed) Hyperthermic Oncology 1984, vol 2. Taylor & Francis, London, Philadelphia, New York, pp 325–338

Overgaard J (1987) Hyperthermia as an adjuvant to radiotherapy. Review of the randomized multicenter studies of the European Society of Hyperthermic Oncology. Strahlenther Onkol 163: 453–457

Overgaard J (1989) The current and potential role of hyperthermia in radiotherapy. Int J Radiat Oncol Biol Phys 16: 535–549

Perez CA, Kuske R, Glasgow GP (1985) Review of brachytherapy techniques for gynecologic tumors. Endocurietherapy/Hyperthermia Oncol 1: 153–175

Petrovich Z, Langholz B, Lam K, Luxton G, Cohen D, Jepson J, Astrahan M (1989) Interstitial microwave hyperthermia combined with Iridium-192 radiotherapy for recurrent tumours. Am J Clin Oncol 12: 264–268

Pierquin B, Dutreix A, Paine CH, Chassagne D, Marinello G, Ash D (1978) The Paris System in interstitial radiation therapy. Acta Radiol Oncol 17: 33–48

Phromratanapongse P, Seegenschmiedt MH, Karlsson UL, Brady LW, Sauer R, Herbst M, Fietkau R (1990) Initial results of phase I/II interstitial thermo-radiotherapy for primary advanced and local recurrent tumors. Am J Clin Oncol 13: 259–268

Puthawala AA, Syed AMN, Khalid MA, Rafie S, McNamara CS (1985) Interstitial hyperthermia for recurrent malignancies. Endocurietherapy/Hyperthermia Oncol 1: 125–131

Puthawala AA, Syed AMN, Flemming P, Disaia PJ (1982) Re-irradiation with interstitial implant for recurrent pelvic malignancies. Cancer 50: 2810–2814

Reinhold HS, Endrich B (1986) Tumour microcirculation as a target for hyperthermia. Int J Hyperthermia 2: 117–137

Roberts DW, Strohbehn JW, Coughlin CT, Ryan TP, Lyons BE, Douple EB, Fratkin JD (1989) Hyperthermia of brain tumor: The Dartmouth experience. In: Sugahara T, Saito M (eds) Hyperthermic Oncology 1988, vol 2. Taylor & Francis, London, New York, Philadelphia, pp 476–479

RTOG (1987) Radiation Therapy Oncology Group Reports. Philadelphia, PA, U.S.A., July 8–10, 1987, Vol. 1, pp 217–218

Sapareto SA, Dewey WC (1984) Thermal dose determination in cancer therapy. Int J Radiat Oncol Biol Phys 10: 787–800

Seegenschmiedt MH, Brady LW, Karlsson UL, Black P, McCormack T (1987) A critical review of interstitial thermoradiotherapy for recurrent malignant astrocytoma: Problems and promises. Int J Hyperthermia 3: 360–589

Seegenschmiedt MH, Sauer R, Herbst M, Thiel H-J, Fietkau R, Brady LW, Karlsson UL (1989) Interstitial hyperthermia for head and neck tumors: Treatment planning and quality assurance (QA). In: Sugahara T, Saito M (eds) Hyperthermic Oncology 1988, vol 2. Taylor & Francis, London, New York, Philadelphia, pp 524–527

Song CW (1984) Effect of local hyperthermia on bloodflow and microenvironment. Cancer Res (Suppl) 44: 4721–4730

Stauffer PR, Sneed PK, Suen SA, Satoh T, Matsumoto K, Fike JR, Phillips TL (1989a) Comparative thermal dosimetry of interstitial microwave and radiofrequency-LCF hyperthermia. Int J Hyperthermia 5: 307–318

Stauffer PR (1989b) Quality assurance requirements for interstitial hyperthermia. In: Sugahara T, Saito M (eds) Hyperthermic Oncology 1988, vol 2. Taylor & Francis, London, New York, Philadelphia, pp 577–578

Strohbehn JW, Douple EB, Coughlin CT (1984) Interstitial microwave antenna array systems for hyperthermia. Front Radiat Ther Oncol 18: 70–84

Strohbehn JW, Lynch K, Paulsen K, Yuan X (1989) Electromagnetic and thermal modelling for hyperthermic treatment planning. In: Sugahara T, Saito M (eds) Hyperthermic Oncology 1988, vol 2. Taylor & Francis, London, New York, Philadelphia, pp 45–50

Syed AMN, Feder FW, Neblett D (1978) Iridium-192 afterloaded implant in the retreatment of head and neck cancers. Brit J Radiol 51: 814–820

Urano M, Tanaka N (1989) The effect of preirradiated tumour bed on the response of a murine fibrosarcoma to elevated temperatures. Int J Hyperthermia 5: 617–624

Vora NL, Forell B, Joseph C, Lipsett JA, Archambeau J (1982) Interstitial implant with interstitial hyperthermia. Cancer 50: 2518–2523

Vora NL, Forell B, Luk KH, Pezner RD, Desai KR, Lipsett JA, Wong JYA (1989) Interstitial thermoradiotherapy in recurrent and advanced malignant tumors: Seven years experience. In: Sugahara T, Saito M (eds) Hyperthermic Oncology 1988, vol 1. Taylor & Francis, London, New York, Philadelphia, pp 588–590

World Health Organization (WHO) (1979) Handbook for Reporting Results of Cancer Treatment. Geneva, Switzerland: World Health Organization

Yabumoto E, Suyama S, Show K, Yamazaki T (1989) A phase I clinical trial of radiofrequency interstitial hyperthermia combined with external radiotherapy. In: Sugahara T, Saito M (eds) Hyperthermic Oncology, vol 1. Taylor & Francis, London, New York, Philadelphia, pp 591–593

9

Animal Experiments with Interstitial Water Hyperthermia

M. Budihna[1], *H. Lesnicar*[1], *L. Handl-Zeller*[2], and *K. Schreier*[2]

[1] Institute of Oncology, Ljubljana, Yugoslavia
[2] Clinic for Radiotherapy and Radiobiology, University of Vienna, Vienna, Austria

Introduction

Invasive hyperthermia methods have been developed as an alternative when noninvasive systems are inefficient or not adapted for producing therapeutic temperatures throughout the entire tumor volume, without overheating normal tissues. Another major interest is the synergistic effect of interstitial hyperthermia combined with irradiation (EMAMI et al, 1984; COSSET et al, 1985a). When interstitial irradiation is combined with external irradiation or is employed alone, the heating can be added using previously implanted catheters. Thus, the heating could be better localized and controlled than in noninvasive methods. This is particularly true for deep-seated tumors where hyperthermic levels cannot be always obtained by noninvasive methods (DUTREIX et al, 1982). The methods for interstitial hyperthermia mostly used at present are implantable microwave antennas, localized current fields, and ferromagnetic seeds (e.g. STROHBEHN and MECHLING, 1986; STAUFFER et al, 1989). The ferromagnetic seed technique differs from the other two in that the heating of tissue is completely dependent upon its thermal conduction and blood flow cooling. Thermal seeds are in this case "hot sources". Another hot source can be hot water circulating through an array of implanted tubes (HANDL-ZELLER et al, 1986) which are subsequently loaded with Ir-192 wires.

The aim of this chapter is to describe the animal experiments and results obtained by interstitial heating system using hot water. This hyperthermia system was developed at the University Clinic of Radiotherapy and Radiobiology, Vienna. The experiments were carried out at the Institute of Oncology, Ljubljana.

Material and methods

Hyperthermia unit and heating tubes

The interstitial hyperthermia unit (model KHS 9-W 18, Othmar Handl GmbH) consists of a water reservoir, a precision thermostat including heater and cooler, pressure and suction pumps, a proportional integral differential (PID) device

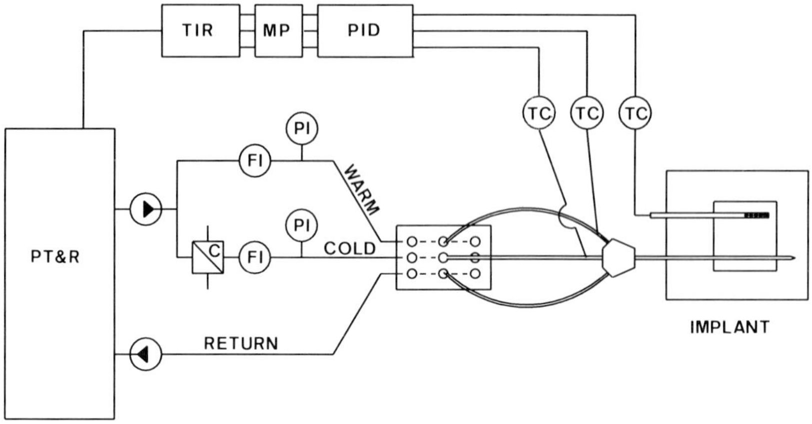

Fig. 1. Schematic presentation of the hyperthermia unit with the closed-ended counterflow needle and thermoprobe. MP = microprocessor, PID = controller, TIR = temperature indicator and registration, FI = flow indicator, PI = pressure indicator, TC = thermocouple, PT & R = precision thermostat and reservoir, C = cooler.

to control water temperature, a manually controlled device for pressure and flow rate, and the manifold to distribute water to the implant. The accuracy of the control system is ±0.1°C for temperature, ±0.1 bar for pressure and ±0.1 ml/s for flow (Fig. 1).

Two types of experiments were done: in one type the whole implant was heated, and in the second type only half of the implanted tissue was heated and the other half was cooled.

Metallic or plastic tubes 150 mm long with outer diameter (OD) 1.6 mm and inner diameter (ID) 1.4 mm allowing throughflow were used if the whole implant was heated. They were made from single material and in this respect differed from the plastic/metallic tubes used by Cosset et al (1985b) or Kapp et al (1988) for radiofrequency (RF) interstitial hyperthermia.

Closed-ended metal needles OD 1.8 mm, ID 1.6 mm with a sealed tip were used for the experiment in which one half of the implanted tissue was cooled and the other half heated. In this needle, hot water was brought to the tip through a smaller diameter metal tube inserted into the main needle through the entire length. Hot water from the tip flowed backwards in the main tube. Another, shorter tube, made of plastic material was also inserted into the main tube through which cold water flowed into the needle. The plastic tube can be easily moved and pushed into the metal tube as far as needed. In our experiment the tip of the cooling tube was fed into the middle of the thickness of the implanted tissue. Hot water returning from the end of the main needle met with cold water at the tip of the plastic tube and mixed with it. The mixture, several degrees cooler than hot water, flowed to the exit, rendering this part of the needle relatively cool. Thus, the "hot source" extended from the tip of the plastic tube to the end of the main tube (Fig. 2). The mixture of hot and cold water also caused a drop in the temperature of the heating water, flowing toward the tip of the main needle. Therefore, to achieve

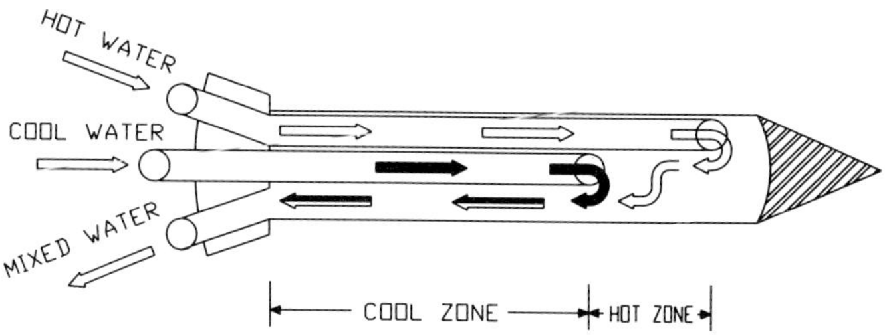

Fig. 2. Schematic presentation of the counterflow needle with cooling.

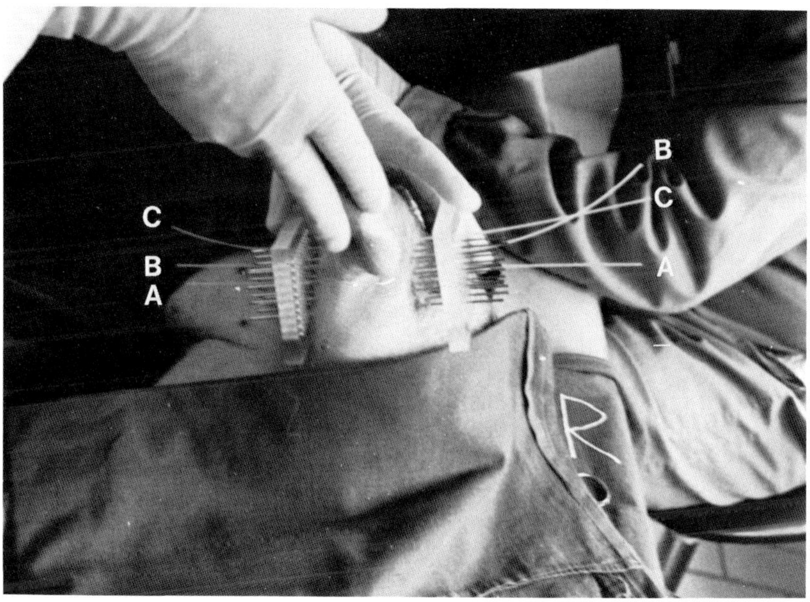

Fig. 3. The implanted pigs thigh plastic catheters for thermometry: A = center, B = halfway center to edge, C = 0.5 cm outside of the implant.

sufficient temperature of the "hot zone", the heating water had to be warmer than it was in experiments without cooling.

Experimental setup

Rabbits weighing 3.5 kg – 4 kg and pigs 15 kg – 20 kg were used in animal experiments. Rabbits were anesthesized with Thiopental injected intraperitoneally, and pigs by Halothane inhalation. Animals were covered to prevent their bodies cooling and to keep their body temperature as close to physiological level as possible. The room temperature was also kept constant (≅ 20°C) throughout the experiment. Sixteen (4 × 4) metallic or plastic tubes were implanted parallel to each other into the thighs of the animals with spacing of either 10 mm or 14 mm. Two plastic templates were used to obtain a good geometry of the implant (Fig. 3). The volume of the heated tissue ranged from 27 cc to 72 cc. Plastic catheters OD 1.6 mm, ID 1.4 mm were inserted parallel to the heating tubes in the

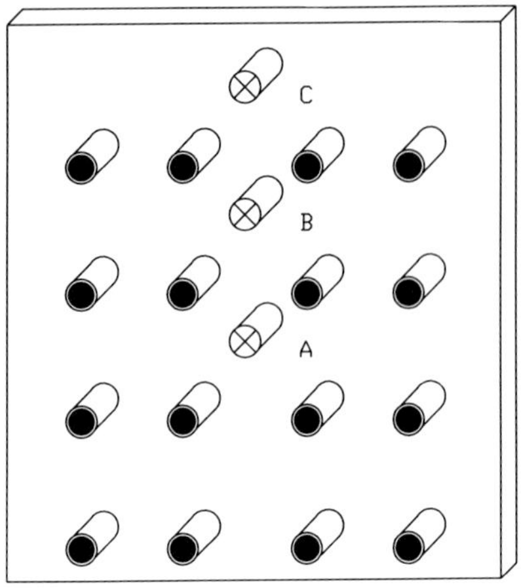

Fig. 4. The arrangement of the heating and temperature measurement tubes. A, B, C are temperature measurement tubes.

center (A), half way from the center to the edge of the implant (B) and 0.5 cm outside of the implant (C) (Fig. 4). Into these catheters a multijunction manganin/constantan thermocouple probe with 5 sensors placed at 5 mm intervals was inserted to monitor the temperature. The probe was moved in steps of 5–10 mm throughout the implanted region and temperatures were recorded for each step (this enabled up to 5 readings for each step). The temperature of the circulating water was measured in one of the heating tubes at both, the inflow and outflow.

To maintain the tissue temperature constant, water temperature had to be regulated manually. Starting from the initial 38°C it was then raised stepwise, 1°C per minute, to the final value of 45.5°C, 47°C or 48°C, (±0.3°C), as measured at the inflow point. It was considered that hyperthermia treatment started when the minimum tissue temperature of 42.5°C was obtained. The duration of heating was 45 to 60 minutes in order to simulate the situation in clinical hyperthermia treatment (Field and Morris, 1983). The flow rate of the heating water was between 1.5–2.5 ml/s per tube to minimize the difference between the inflow and outflow water temperature.

Results

Eight to 10 minutes were needed to raise the water temperature at the inflow point of the implant from 38°C to the required levels (45.5°C, 47°C or 48°C). It took approximately another 5 minutes for tissue temperature to reach the "steady

Table 1. Mean tissue temperature[a] in the implant with 10 mm spacing

	Rabbit	Rabbit	Pig
Water temperature	45.5	48	45.5
Line of measurement			
A	43.6 ± 0.5	47.2 ± 0.6	43.7 ± 0.6
B	43.5 ± 0.5	46.5 ± 0.7	43.7 ± 0.6
C	42.3 ± 0.6	44.5 ± 0.5	41.8 ± 0.5

[a] Mean values in °C ± standard deviation.

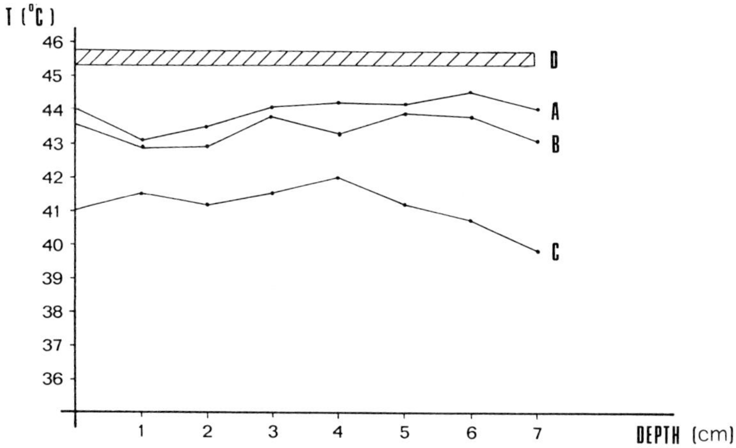

Fig. 5. The tissue temperature distribution in the throughflow metal needle implant along the measurement lines A, B and C, without cooling, D = the temperature of the heating water.

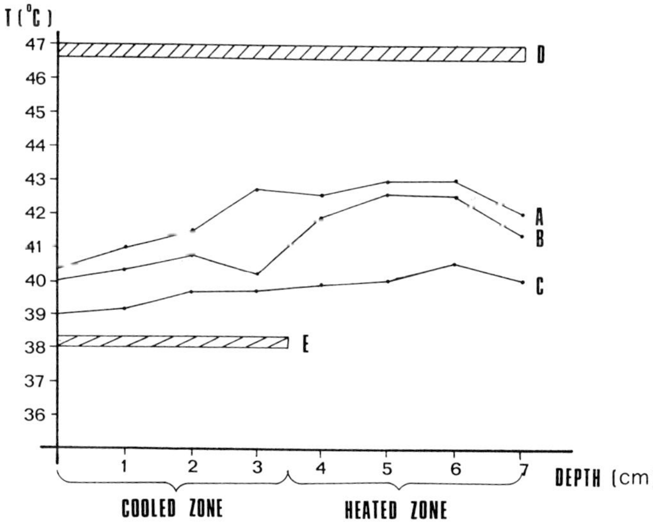

Fig. 6. The tissue temperature distribution in the counterflow metal needle implant along the measurement lines A, B and C, with cooling of the half of implant, D = the temperature of the heating water, E = the temperature of the cooling water.

state". Thus, 10 to 15 minutes were needed to reach treatment temperature levels in the tissue. Table 1 shows the temperature of the implanted tissue of rabbits' and pigs' thighs with 4 × 4 throughflow metal needles as measured in the lines A, B, C at the circulating water temperature 45.5°C and 48°C.

Table 2. Mean tissue temperature[a] in the implant with 14 mm spacing

	Pig	Pig
Water temperature	45.5	48
Line of measurement		
A	42.2 ± 0.4	42.7 ± 0.3
B	41.1 ± 0.3	42.5 ± 0.4
C	40.8 ± 0.2	41.7 ± 0.3

[a] Mean values in °C ± standard deviation.

In Fig. 5 the temperatures of the implanted tissue along the measurement lines A, B, C are shown in 4 × 4 metal needle implant with the spacing of 10 mm. The mean temperature of the heating water was 45.5°C.

Table 2 shows the temperature of the implanted tissue of the pigs' thighs using throughflow metal needles with 14 mm spacing as measured in lines A, B, C. The mean temperature of the heating water was 45.5°C and 48°C.

In the experiment with cooling, the tissue temperature of the cooled region was 2°C – 3°C lower than that of the heated part (Fig. 6).

When plastic tubes were used the temperature of heating water had to be about 2°C higher to achieve the same tissue temperature as with metal needles.

In our experiments the drop of the temperature from the inflow to the outflow point was less than 0.5°C if the flow rate per tube was more than 1.5 ml/sec.

Discussion

From the hot water tubes the heat is transferred only by thermal conduction. Thus, the interstitial hyperthermia with hot water is an example of "hot source" technique with sources having constant temperature. Ferromagnetic seeds or needles inserted in the tissue and heated by externally applied RF magnetic field (Brezovich et al, 1984; Partington et al, 1989), and implantable probes which are directly heated by simple resistive elements (Marchosky et al, 1988a,b) are also hot source techniques. The heating with ferromagnetic seeds or needles is rapid, stable and self-regulating (Partington et al, 1989) and that also applies to the heating with hot water. However, the heating with hot water, using our system, offers some advantages. First, the temperature of the hot source does not need to be preselected as it is in the case of ferromagnetic seeds, but can be easily varied according to demands of the individual situation. Second, the cooling system makes possible choosing optional length of each "hot source" which in turn means that the heating volume can be modified according to the tumor shape. The heating of the normal tissue to the cytotoxic levels can thus be avoided. This means that more selectivity in damaging the tumor tissue can be achieved. Third, the ferromagnetic seeds may change their temperature characteristic of the magnetic material in *in vivo* system where areas of sluggish blood flow may get higher temperatures than would be predicted from experiments *in vitro* (Partington et al, 1989), whereas heating with hot water is more predictable.

A general characteristic of heating with hot sources is that the spacing of the sources is more critical than it is in the case of microwave antennae (Strohbehn and MECHLING, 1986). Interstitial hyperthermia with microwave antennae, developed by a number of research teams (STROHBEHN et al, 1979; TAYLOR, 1980; COUGHLIN et al, 1983) is applicable in various situations, but the natural resonant length must be considered. The greatest problems concern temperature distribution control on the longitudinal axis, and the choice of active length according to the form and the volume of tumor (TREMBLY, 1985). In case of interstitial hyperthermia with hot water, in our experiments, there was no problem with longitudinal temperature distribution. In fact, in this respect the homogeneity of temperature distribution was better in hot water hyperthermia than that achieved with interstitial microwave antennas in experiments done by STAUFFER et al (1989). The volume of the implant seemed less important unless the flow rate of hot water was kept above 1.5 ml/s per tube: the temperature drop between the inflow and outflow measuring points was then bellow 0.5°C. So, the temperatures achieved in thighs of rabbits and pigs in our experiments were very similar although the implanted volumes differed considerably. If the spacing of needles was increased from 10 mm to 14 mm, the temperature of heating water had to be raised to 48°C in order to reach the tissue temperature above 42.5°C.

Low frequency electrodes produce conductive currents between electrically connected arrays of needles (DOSS and MCCABE, 1982; ASTRAHAN and NORMAN, 1982). This technique developed by MANING et al (1982) and by COSSET (1984a,b; 1985a) demands a perfect geometry of implantation: the needles must be parallel, of approximately equal length, and their spacing must be suitable for both, hyperthermal homogeneity and irradiation dosimetry. In the region of high blood flow the spacing should be approximately 10 mm, and for optimal power delivery and control either careful pretreatment selection of the connections to electrode pairs is required or a real time multiplexer is needed in which connections are chosen based on the information of temperature sensors (HAND et al, in press). In hot water technique it is very important to insert hot sources parallel. From our experiments with different spacings of the needles (10 mm and 14 mm), it could be inferred that any non-parallelism would cause cold or warm areas. However, hot areas cannot be warmer than the heating water. If the spacing was 10 mm, in the regions with high blood flow its cooling effect was easily counterbalanced by self-regulating heat transfer mechanisms associated with hot water technique: the actual values of the normalized power measured for this hyperthermia system, were in the range of 15 – 20 W/m/°K. If normal conductivity of muscle tissue is 0.5 W/m/°K, it can be calculated that there is 30 – 40 times power in reserve available (SCHREIER et al, 1990) before energy supply is exhausted at the constant circulating water temperature. This probably explains why in our experiments with the 10 mm spacing of needles and water temperature of 48°C the tissue temperature nearly reached the temperature of heating water (circulatory collapse?) (see Table 1). This differs from the prediction of HAND et al (in press) where in computer simulations a hot water temperature of 54°C is needed to heat the tissue to acceptable temperature in order to overcome the cooling effect of maximal blood flow. In this simulation the reserve power supply of hot water, when cooling of the tissue was increased, was probably not taken into account.

The temperature measurements in our experiments were easy to perform. There were no electromagnetic fields to interfere with the measurements. Since temperature distribution was relatively homogeneous (Fig. 5) the location of the controlling thermocouple within the heated volume was not very critical. A safety feature of interstitial hot water hyperthermia system is that the maximum temperature in the implanted tissue cannot exceed the temperature of the wall of heating tubes. According to the material used (plastic or metal) this temperature is about 1°C–2°C lower than the water temperature.

Conclusions

Our animal experiments show that rather homogeneous treatment temperatures can be achieved in a short time and are easily controlled throughout the treatment. The cooling system permits the modifying of the heated volume according to the tumor shape, and consequently, sparing much of the normal tissue from overheating. The relative homogeneity of temperature distribution and the lack of electromagnetic fields make the temperature measurement relatively easy. The interstitial hyperthermia with hot water seems to be a simple and safe method for heating, which can also be used in clinical practice.

Acknowledgement: The authors would like to thank to Dr. Miljenko Martinjak from Veterinary Service of Ihan-Emona pigs farm for his kind assistance at animal experiments.

References

Astrahan MA, Norman A (1982) A localized current field hyperthermia system for use with Ir-192 interstitial implants. Medical Phys 9: 419–424

Brezovich IA, Atkinson WJ (1984) Temperature distributions in tumor models heated by self-regulating nickel-copper alloy thermoseeds. Med Phys 11: 145–152

Cosset JM, Dutreix J, Gerbaulet A, Damia E (1984a) Combined interstitial hyperthermia and brachytherapy: The Institute Gustave Roussy experience. In: Overgaard J (ed) Hyperthermic Oncology, vol 1. Taylor and Francis, London, pp 587–590

Cosset JM, Dutreix J, Dufour J, Janoray P, Damia E, Haie C, Clarke D (1984b) Combined interstitial hyperthermia and brachytherapy: Institute Gustave Roussy technique and preliminary results. Int J Radiat Oncol Biol Phys 10: 307–312

Cosset JM, Dutreix J, Gerbaulet A, Damia E (1985a) L'association hyperthermie interstitielle-curietherapie: Une technique de ratrapage des recidives en zones precedemment irradiees. In: Institut Gustave Roussy (ed) Actualites Carcinologiques. Masson, Paris, pp 211–218

Cosset JM, Dutreix J, Haie C, Gerbaulet A, Janoray P, Dewar JA (1985b) Interstitial thermoradiotherapy: A technical and clinical study of 29 implantations performed at the Institut Gustave-Roussy. Int J Hyperthermia 1: 3–13

Coughlin CT, Douple EB, Strohbehn JW, Eaton WL, Trembly BS, Wong TZ (1983) Interstitial hyperthermia in combination with brachytherapy. Radiology 148: 285–288

Doss JD, McCabe A (1982) A technique for localized heating in tissue: An adjunct to tumor therapy. Medical Instrumentation 10: 16–20

Dutreix J, Cosset JM, Salama M, Brule JM, Damia E (1982) Experimental studies of various heating procedures for clinical application of localized hyperthermia. In: Biomedical Thermology. Alan R. Liss Inc., New York, pp 585–596

Emami B, Marks J, Perez C, Nussbaum G, Leybovich L (1984) Treatment of human tumors with interstitial irradiation and hyperthermia. In: Overgaard J (ed) Hyperthermic Oncology, vol 1. Taylor & Francis, London, pp 583–586

Field SB, Morris CC (1983) The relationship between heating time and temperature: Its relevance to clinical hyperthermia. Radiother Oncol 1: 179–186

Hand JW, Trembly BS, Prior MV (in press) Physics of interstitial hyperthermia. Radiofrequency and hot water tube technique. In: Urano M, Douple E (eds) Hyperthermia and Oncology, vol 3: Interstitial Hyperthermia. Zeist VSP Utrecht

Handl-Zeller L, Kärcher KH, Schreier K, Handl O (1986) Optimierung interstitieller Hyperthermie-Systeme. Strahlentherapie 163: 460–463

Kapp DS, Fessenden P, Samulski TV, Bagshaw MA, Cox RS, Lee ER, Lohrbach AW, Meyer JL, Prionas SD (1988) Stanford University institutional report. Phase I evaluation of equipment for hyperthermia treatment of cancer. Int J Hyperthermia 4: 75–115

Manning MR, Cetas TC, Miller RC, Oleson JR, Corner WG, Gerner EW (1982) Clinical hyperthermia: Results of a phase I trial employing hyperthermia alone or in combination with external beam or interstitial radiotherapy. Cancer 49: 205–216

Marchosky JA, Moran C, Fearnot N (1988a) A system for volumetric interstitial hyperthermia. Abstracts 36th annual meeting of Radiation Research Society. RRS, Philadelphia, Abstract Cc 8, p 32

Marchosky JA, Moran C, Fearnot N (1988b) Volumetric interstitial hyperthermia: Phase 1 clinical study. Abstracts 36th Annual Meeting of Radiation Research Society. RRS, Philadelphia, Abstract Ch-7, p 46

Partington BP, Steeves RA, Su SL, Paliwal BR, Dubielzig RR, Wilson JW, Brezovich IA (1989) Temperature distributions, microangiographic and histopathologic correlations in normal tissue heated by ferromagnetic needles. Int J Hyperthermia 5: 319–327

Schreier K, Budihna M, Lesnicar H, Handl-Zeller L, Hand JW, Prior MV, Clegg ST, Brezovich IA (1990) Preliminary studies of interstitial hyperthermia using hot water. Int J Hyperthermia 6: 431–444

Stauffer PR, Sneed PK, Suen SA, Satoh T, Matsumoto K, Fike JR, Phillips TL (1989) Comparative thermal dosimetry of interstitial microwave and radiofrequency-LCF hyperthermia. Int J Hyperthermia 5: 307–318

Strohbehn JW, Mechling JA (1986) Interstitial techniques for clinical hyperthermia. In: Hand JW, James RJ (eds) Physical Techniques in Clinical Hyperthermia. Research Studies Press, Letchworth, pp 210–287

Strohbehn JW, Bowers ED, Walsh JE, Douple EB (1979) An invasion microwave antenna for locally-induced hyperthermia for cancer therapy. J Microwave Power 14: 339–350

Taylor LS (1980) Implantable radiators for cancer therapy by microwave hyperthermia. Proc IEEE 68: 142–148

Trembly BS (1985) The effects of driving frequency and antenna length on power deposition within a microwave antenna array used for hyperthermia. IEEE Transactions BME 32: 152–157

10

Simultaneous Application of Combined Interstitial High- or Low-Dose Rate Irradiation with Hot Water Hyperthermia

L. Handl-Zeller[1] and *O. Handl*[2]

[1] Clinic for Radiotherapy and Radiobiology, University of Vienna, Austria
[2] Med-Research O. Handl Ges.m.b.H., Vienna, Austria

Introduction

A mild heat treatment which causes no measurable effect may enhance the response to ionizing radiation (RT) which is qualitatively similar to that following RT alone. This sensitizing effect is normally expressed in terms of thermal enhancement ratio (TER) defined at the ratio of doses of ionizing radiation to cause a given level of response in the presence or absence of hyperthermia (HT), respectively.

The HT strategy clinically used is a sequential treatment, which mainly utilizes the hyperthermic cytotoxicity against radioresistant cells. An interval between RT and HT however reduces the response of the combined treatment. Even a so called simultaneous treatment with only a small interval between heat and RT reduces the sensitizing heat effect (Overgaard, 1989). If up to half an hour is allowed between RT and HT the major effect of such treatment will be dominated by the hyperthermic cytotoxicity, although some radiosensitization may persist in both tumor and normal tissue. Simultaneous application of irradiation and heat results in equal sensitization of tumor and normal tissue (Field, 1990) and is hence, of no therapeutic gain (Overgaard, 1980). Although hyperthermic radiosensitization with simultaneous treatment is able to yield the highest thermal enhancement ratio (TER), the clinical applicability of this protocol was till now dubious due to technical problems.

We believe that a simultaneous thermoradiotherapy with radiofrequency (RF) and microwave (MW) due to reasons of the high technical problems inherent is difficult to achieve. The main space in the catheter is needed for the use for antennae and temperature sensors. Due to this reason it appears to us that the combination of HT and RT is not possible with standard size afterloading catheters. Also with constant heat sources as ferromagnetic seeds or hot-wire-technique the inner space of the catheter is occupied.

It was therefore our aim to enable a selective tumor heating while the normal tissue is being kept at body temperature.

Methods

The catheters used here are in each case those used as standard brachytherapy practise which are connected via a suitable coupling system to the HT device. In each case a heating and a cooling water tube are inserted into the center of the catheter (HANDL-ZELLER et al, 1987; HANDL-ZELLER et al, 1988; SCHREIER et al, 1990). In low dose rate (LDR) systems the cooling water tube at each time is also the carrier of the radioactive Ir 192 wire (HANDL-ZELLER, 1990) (Fig. 1).

In high dose rate (HDR) systems during the time the RT is being applied in the active catheter, the water supply which controls the temperature in that specific catheter is switched off by computer control. The water which has remained in the catheter is first removed by the vacuum pump then the radiation source is inserted through the same catheter into the correct position by computer control. There are two solenoids in the hot water radiation catheter system. The solenoid

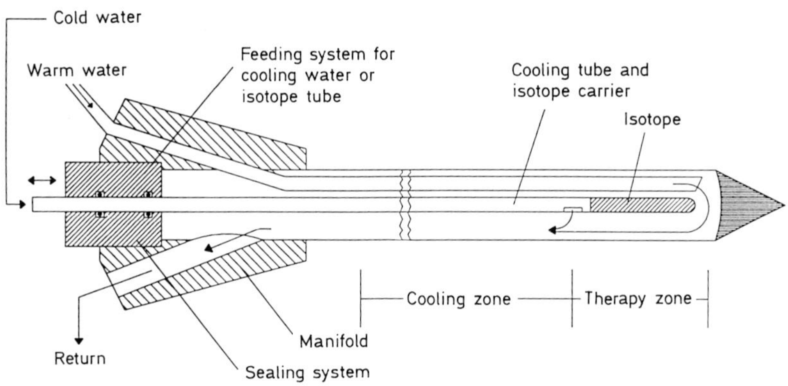

Fig. 1. Tube system for LDR-radiation.

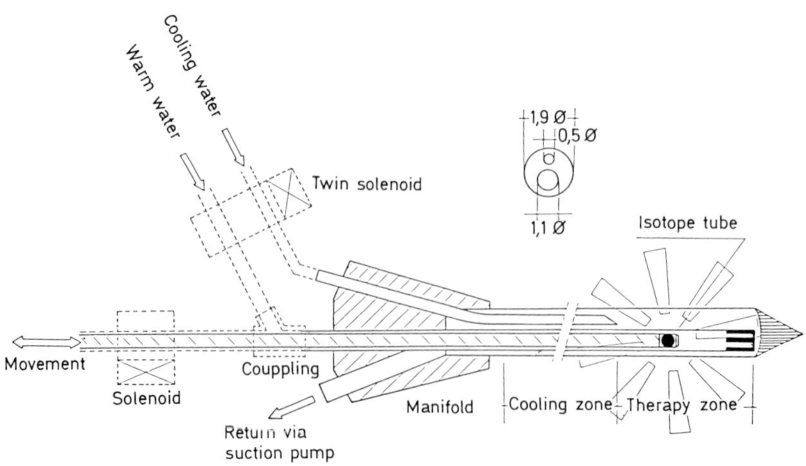

Fig. 2. Tube system for HDR-radiation.

for the RT remains closed when hot water is flowing. When the RT is to be applied the solenoid closes the hot water and the RT source enters the tube and supplies the active catheter (Fig. 2).
The reason for this control system is so that only the active catheter area looses the heat source during RT. All the other catheters continue to provide heat in a three-dimensional manner to the entire tumor volume. Data of localized HT in combination with LDR irradiation suggest that potentiation of LDR irradiation by a single heat treatment may be maximized if the HT is given either in the middle of, or simultaneously with the brachytherapy (JONES et al, 1989).

Timing of irradiation and heat administration for low and high dose rate irradiation

The sequencing of heat and radiation plays an important role in thermoradiosensitization and the interaction of the two types of damage. In general the TER is maximum when the two modalities are given simultaneously (SAPARETO et al, 1978; OVERGAARD, 1980).
DEWEY et al (1977) and SAPARETO et al (1979) have shown that when heat and irradiation are administered together to cells in vitro there is a greater cell kill then when heat is delivered more than 30 minutes before or after irradiation.

Timing of irradiation and heat administration for low dose rate irradiation

Data of JONES et al (1989) suggest that potentiation of low dose rate irradiation by a single heat treatment may be maximized if the hyperthermia treatment is given either in the middle of, or simultaneously with the brachytherapy.
Since our system is provided with a cooling system for normal tissue heat treatment can be confined to the tumor. Therefore therapeutic gain is not a critical limitation.

Timing of irradiation and heat administration for high dose rate irradiation

When high dose rate irradiation is administered at the beginning of the hyperthermia treatment then not only the supra-additivity between the hyperthermia and high dose rate irradiation is exploited, but also the potential for the hyperthermia to inhibit the repair of high dose rate irradiation induced potentially lethal damage is added (Personal communication, DOUPLE, 1990).

Results

The two zone catheter offers the possibility to conduct RT and HT simultaneously in order to confine this three-dimensionally with an accuracy of approximately ± 1 mm to the target volume. This functions because of the possibility to adjust the cooling water supply. That means that normal tissue can be cooled to body temperature (Fig. 4). For control temperatures are measured at inflow and outflow points directly at the catheter. Temperatures of tumor and normal tissue are mea-

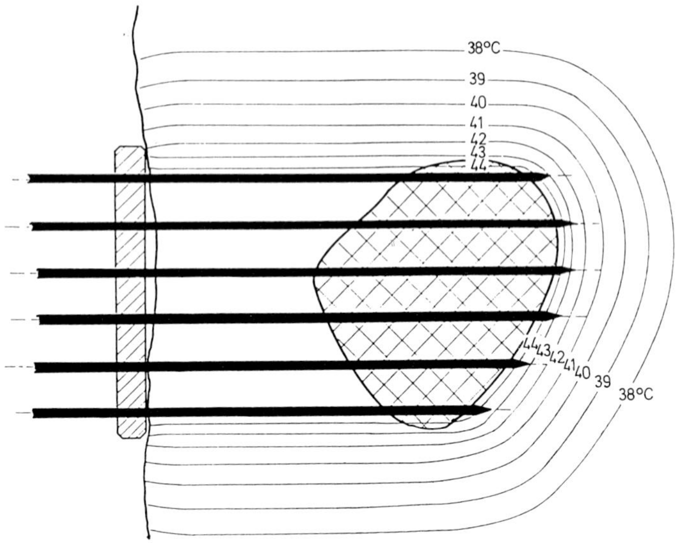

Fig. 3. Temperature course over the whole length of a catheter in healthy tissue.

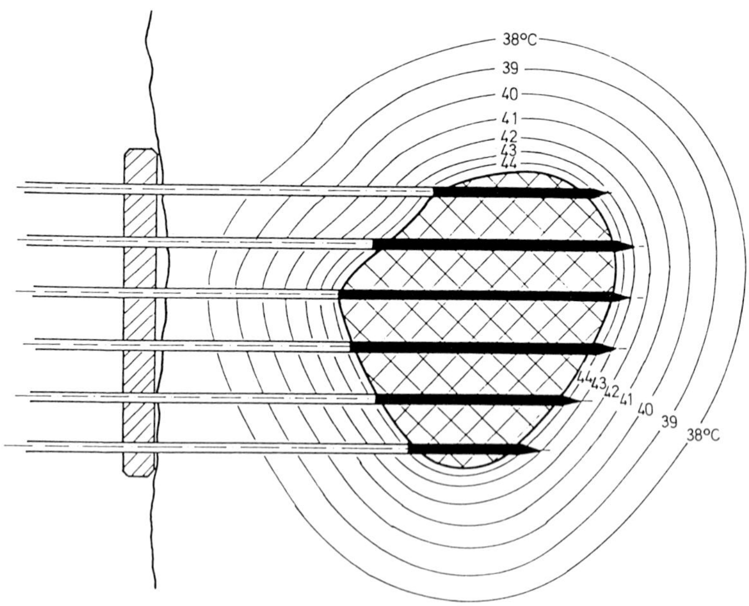

Fig. 4. Temperature course over the whole length of a catheter in tumor tissue.

sured in two axes with type T multipoint sensors which are moved in steps through the implanted region. Temperature measurements are carried out in all treatments.

A comparison between computer calculation and in vivo measurements with this system has been described elsewhere (SCHREIER et al, 1990). If localized HT treatment can be confined to the tumor, then therapeutic gain would not be a critical limitation. The measured temperatures confirm the values expected for the distribution of temperature both inside and outside of the tumor. Temperature measurements were carried out with a multipoint type T thermocouple measurement system. Readings from more than 100 completed treatments are available (Figs. 3, 4).

Discussion

Implants, as they are used for brachytherapy can also be used as interstitial sources of heat if hot water as energy carrier is used. The capability of bringing heat into muscle tissue is about 0.5 $Wm^{-1}{}^{\circ}C^{-1}$.

This means that water heated implants with the standard dimension of 1.6–2.0 mm diameter offer a high energy reserve and therefore can be seen as sources of heat at a constant temperature (BREZOVICH et al, 1984).

With heat sources of constant temperature one can expect a high homogeneity of distribution of temperature. Any increased cooling by blood flow can be successfully compensated for by the self-regulating heat transfer mechanism associated with the hot water tubes.

The actual values of the normalized power measured for this HT system were in the range of 15 to 20 $Wm^{-1}{}^{\circ}C^{-1}$. Assuming that the thermal conductivity of muscle tissue is 0.5 $Wm^{-1}{}^{\circ}C^{-1}$, it can be shown that a circulating water based HT system has 30 to 40 times the required power in reserve. In this respect hot water heated interstitial catheter systems can be considered to be a constant temperature system. Spacings for homogeneous isodose distribution (8–12 mm) are at the same time also the ideal spacings for HT with constant temperature sources. Due to the enormous power in reserve of our system it is not necessary to control the tubes individually as is demanded with radiofrequency and microwave systems.

It is also not necessary to insert catheters for temperature controlling. The catheters necessary for the RT are also used for the HT and are controlled collectively. This makes the system safe and simple to operate. Hot spots are excluded in the above described system since a higher temperature than that of the preselected system temperature cannot be reached. The maximum temperature in the system is approximately 3°C above treatment temperature. In interstitial RF and MW heating greater temperature differences longitudinally are one of the major problems.

Due to our system being heated at a constant temperature and a high flow rate and according to our counterflow system the temperature-gradient in the catheter is ± 0.2°C longitudinally.

The point of all our efforts was to be able to catch up on many years of demands by the biologists for simultaneous application in order to be able to achieve the maximum TER.

References

Brezovich IA, Atkinson WJ, Chakraborty DP (1984) Temperature distributions in tumor models heated by self-regulating nickel-copper alloy thermoseeds. Med Phys 11: 145–152

Dewey WC, Hopwood LE, Sapareto SA, et al (1977) Cellular responses to combinations of hyperthermia and radiation. Radiology 123: 464–474

Field SB (1990) In vivo aspects of hyperthermic oncology. In: Field SB, Hand JW (eds) An Introduction to the Practical Aspects of Clinical Hyperthermia. Taylor & Francis, London, New York, Philadelphia, pp 55–68

Handl-Zeller L (1990) Erhöhung der Thermal Enhancement Ratio durch simultane Applikation von Bestrahlung und Hyperthermie – Technische Möglichkeiten bei interstitieller Applikation. Strahlenther Onkol 166: 643–646

Handl-Zeller L, Kärcher KH, Schreier K, Handl O (1987) Beitrag zur Optimierung interstitieller Hyperthermiesysteme. Strahlenther Onkol 163: 406–463

Handl-Zeller L, Schreier K, Kärcher KH, Budihna M, Lesnicar H (1988) First clinical experience with the Viennese interstitial two zone hyperthermia system. In: Sugahara T, Saito M (eds) Hyperthermic Oncology. Proceedings of the 5th International Symposium on Hyperthermic Oncology, 1988, vol 1. Taylor & Francis, London, New York, Philadelphia, pp 814–816

Jones EL, Lyons BE, Douple EB, Darin BJ (1989) Thermal enhancement of low dose rate irradiation in a murine tumor system. Int J Hyperthermia 4: 509–523

Overgaard J (1980) Simultaneous and sequential hyperthermia and radiation treatment of an experimental tumor and its surrounding normal tissue in vivo. Int J Radiat Oncol Biol Phys 11: 1507–1517

Overgaard J (1989) The current and potential role of hyperthermia in radiotherapy. Int J Radiat Oncol Biol Phys 3: 535–549

Sapareto SA, Hopwood LE, Dewey WC (1978) Combined effects of x irradiation and hyperthermia on CHO cells for various temperatures and orders of application. Radiat Res 73: 221–233

Sapareto SA, Raaphorst GP, Dewey WC (1979) Cell killing and the sequencing of hyperthermia and radiation. Int J Radiat Oncol Biol Phys 5: 343–347

Schreier K, Budihna M, Lesnicar H, Handl-Zeller L, Hand JW, Prior MV, Clegg ST, Brezovich IA (1990) Preliminary studies of interstitial hyperthermia using hot water. Int J Hyperthermia 2: 431–444

11

Interstitial Warm-Water Hyperthermia Combined with Ir 192-HDR Implantation: Principle, Practical Application and First Clinical Experiences

K. S. Arian-Schad, H. Leitner, G. Stücklschweiger, L. Handl-Zeller, and *A. Hackl*

University Clinic of Radiology, Division of Radiotherapy, Graz, and University Clinic of Radiotherapy, Vienna, Austria

Introduction

The introduction of artificial radionuclides and the development of afterloading devices with computerized dosimetry calculation programs has led to a renewed interest in interstitial brachytherapy. To improve the therapeutic efficacy of interstitial radiotherapy combined effort has been directed to investigate the adjuvant use of hyperthermia. Whereas externally applied hyperthermia treatments cannot ensure uniform heat delivery, due in part to limitations in current technology, invasive techniques have proven themselves to be a reliable method of achieving relatively homogeneous thermal distributions within a defined volume with minimal damage to the neighbouring normal tissue.

So far, experiences in interstitial heat induction have been based on three principal methods, namely the use of microwave antennas, localized current fields or ferromagnetic seeds (Kapp et al, 1988; Shimm et al, 1988; Lam et al, 1988; Meredith et al, 1989).

Recently a new method of heating, utilizing hot water as an energy source circulating through either stainless needles or plastic catheters, has been introduced by Handl-Zeller and coworkers (1987, 1988, 1989) and Brezovich et al (1988). Preliminary results of studies in animal models and phantoms suggest that this method may represent not only a simple, but also a safe and efficient technique of inducing hyperthermia within the implanted volume (Schreier, 1990).

In collaboration with Handl-Zeller et al at the University of Vienna and the Institute of Oncology in Ljubljana (Lesnicar, 1988) this system has been investigated and adapted to the brachytherapy equipment at our institution. The clinical testing is still ongoing.

This chapter is to illustrate heat energy deposition profiles measured in phantoms using hot water flow with different needle implant spacings of 8 mm, 10 mm and 15 mm, and its practical application in combination with our Ir-192 HDR device and implantation technique. First clinical experiences in the conjunctive use of interstitial warm water flow for the treatment of primary anal carcinomas, vaginal recurrences and metastatic disease from malignant melanoma will be presented.

Interstitial brachytherapy

Set up

Interstitial radiation therapy is administered utilizing the MicroSelectron system (Nucletron International B.V.). This device consists of a treatment unit, in which a single high intensity Iridium 192 source with an activity of 370 GBq (10 Ci) stored within a shielded safe, is remotely afterloaded into a 18 channel indexing system. Optimum dose distribution can be achieved by gradual displacement of the source in steps of 0.25 cm or more at a maximum length of 12 cm with variable positioning and dwelling times of the source within each applicator. Either rigid hollow steel needles with an outer diameter of 1.9 mm (inner diameter 1.5 mm) or flexible plastic applicators are available for implantations.

The needle implant geometry for each volume to be treated is planned with a pre-implantation dose distribution calculation based upon the clinical and radiological findings.

After the insertion of the needles under general anesthesia a pair of orthogonal films are taken to assess the strictly parallel order of the implanted needles (Fig. 1a,b). If optimum geometry has been achieved the radiation can be delivered without delay. The duration of therapy lasts between 1.5 and 20 minutes depending on the source activity, the total dose applied, the geometry of needle placement and the treatment lengths of the needle.

With regard to the planned combination with interstitial hyperthermia a special custom-made template for needle volume implants for the treatment of anal and vaginal carcinomas has been designed (Fig. 2).

The lengths of the needles which are necessary for implantation of the tumor in each case are predetermined and marked with setscrews (A). To prevent the axial displacement of the needle after insertion these setscrews are wedged between two jigs made of plexiglas (B,C), which show identical patterns of bore with a centric fixed screw (D) at one end of a metal bolt (E).

To guarantee fixation of the template on the patient this metal bolt is connected to an hydraulic table fixature which is otherwise used for gynaecological applicators (Fig. 3), providing a much better fixation of the template than by sewing the same to the skin. The slit of the jig can be used to hold a supplementary vaginal applicator for anal implants, furthermore it provides a passage for an urethral metal catheter or permanent catheters used for implants of the vagina or urethra.

The drillings for the hollow needles are set at a distance of 8 mm, forming the corners of equilateral triangles placed side by side in a circle. In the center of gravity of each triangle a supplementary drilling allows in vivo measurements of temperature distribution (measurement lines P1, P2) during the hyperthermia treatment (Fig. 4b).

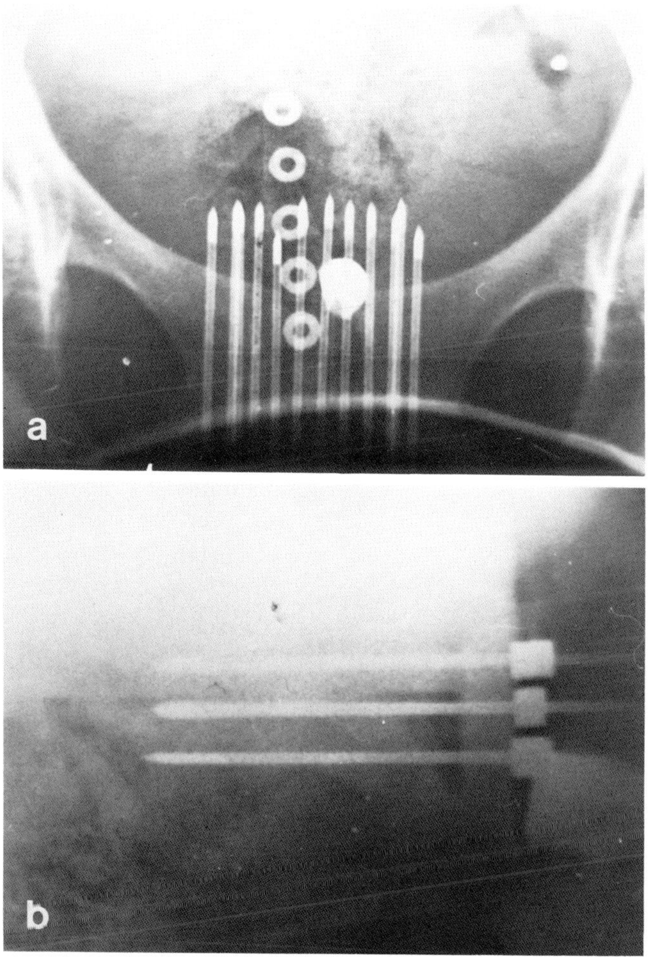

Fig. 1. Orthogonal films of a 12 needle volume implant for stage T3 anal carcinoma;
a anterior/posterior and
b lateral projections.

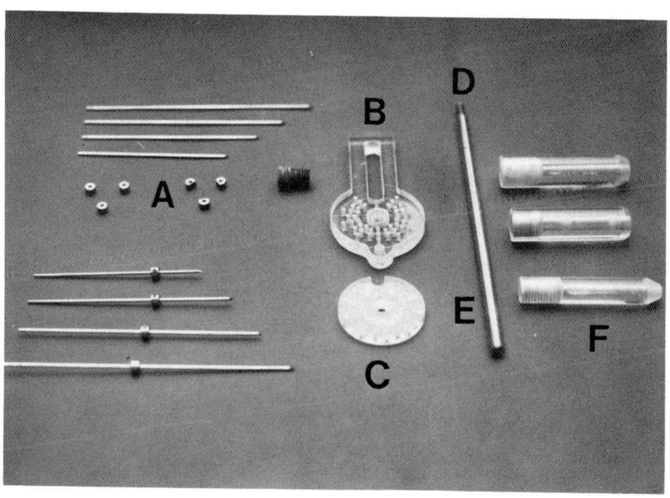

Fig. 2. Custom made template for anal and vaginal carcinoma with setscrews (A), two jigs with identical pattern of bore (B,C), metal bolt (E) with screw (D) for centric fixation. Various vaginal and rectal applicators (F).

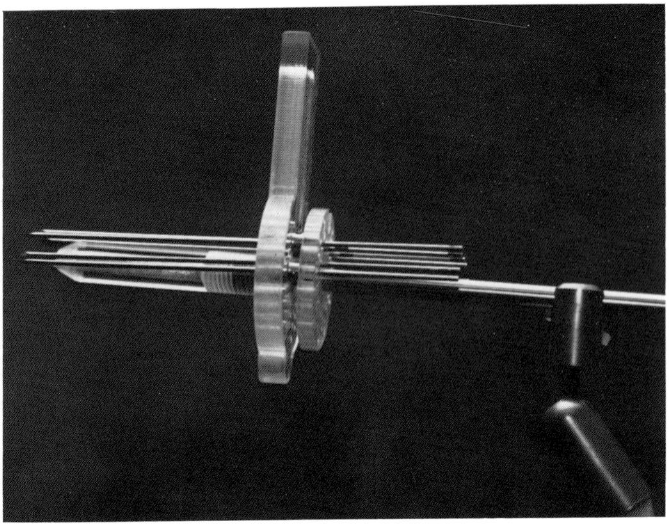

Fig. 3. Template with standard fixation.

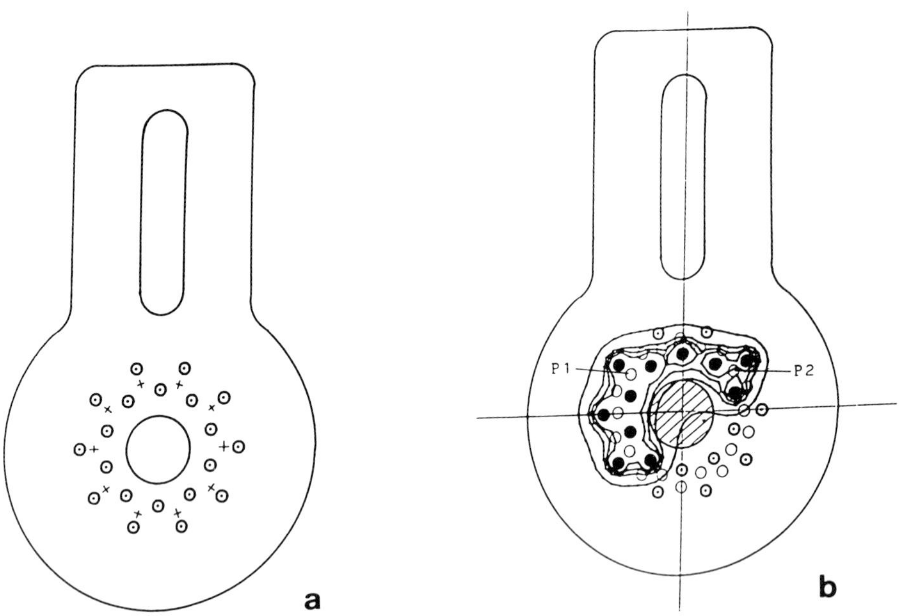

Fig. 4. Template with drillings for needle placement for radiation and thermometry.
a Reference point of dose (+).
b Loaded needles (.), calculated isodose (90%, 80%, 70%, 50%) measurement lines (P1, P2).

Dose calculation

A special program on an AT compatible computer for the calculation of the required treatment time has been developed at our institution. This program also enables one to calculate the 3-dimensional isodose distribution within the implanted volume and allows the visualization of the dose distribution in any orthogonal plane.

The theoretically possible coordinates of the pellet positions with each custom made template are stored in a data file and can be recalled for the jig currently in use.

After the geometrical pattern of placement and the active lengths of the needles have been determined, the treatment time for each source position is calculated. The calculation matrix is in maximum 40 cm to 40 cm with a pixel size of 1 mm to 10 mm. As reference point of dose the center of gravity of each equilateral triangle is used, from which the mean dose is calculated (Fig. 4a).

The treated volume is confined by the reference isodose surface which should enclose the planned target volume (Fig. 4b). A dose of 6–8 Gy per fraction is delivered to the target volume.

Interstitial hyperthermia

Subsequent to the radiation therapy the same hollow needles are used for the heating procedure.

We use the warm-water system KHS-9 developed by Otmar Handl GesmbH (Vienna), which has been described in detail previously (Handl-Zeller, 1987, 1988). This system is based on conductive heat transfer utilizing demineralized water with a preliminary temperature of approximately 46–48°C. The water is stored in a water reservoir in which the temperature is controlled by a precision thermostat. After the desired water temperature has been selected the fluid is distributed to the implanted needles via a manifold; a steady waterflow is ensured by a pressure and suction pump.

The synthetic connection system allows an axial flow through the needle as well as a coaxial contra-flow within the needle (1.5–2 ml/s/implant at 1–1.5 bar). Thus the implants may be used in stick-in (implants closed on one side) as well as in stick-through (implants open on both side) techniques. For thermometry measurements and temperature control multipoint mangan/constantin thermocouple probes are used.

To enable a continuous monitoring of tissue temperature two or more hollow needles are put into the prepared drillings for measurement purposes.

The temperature is taken in intervals of 5s as well by the autonomous measurement and control system inside the thermostat (water temperature: T_w), as by microelements next to the entrance/exit of the implant (entrance temperature: T_{in}, exit temperature: T_{out}) and a triplex analogue constructed thermoelement (T_A, T_B, T_C) placed at 5 mm intervals inside the tissue to be treated.

Phantom thermometry

Thermometry at the phantom has been done in order to test different mutual distances of needles set in equilateral triangles. The temperatures were taken

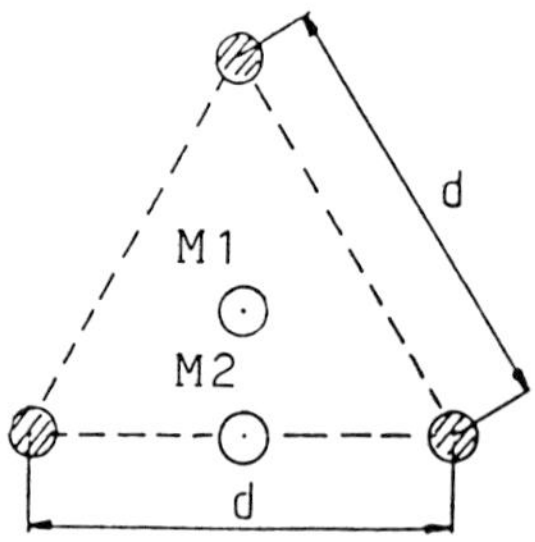

Fig. 5. Needle geometry for measurements in the phantom.

by thermocouple probes within hollow needles in the respective centers of gravity of the equilateral triangles (Fig. 5). The measured temperature sequel alongside the needle is projected for different basic distances of 8, 10 and 15 mm in the points of measurement M1 and M2 (Fig. 6).

To evaluate the longitudinal temperature distribution the thermoprobes were moved in steps of 5 mm through the implanted region.

The measurement values at a distance of at least 0.5 mm within the needle entrance and exit differed in the inquired cases less than ±0.5°C. Temperature measurements next to the exit/entrance of the implant (at the stick-through procedure ≤0.5 cm) showed a drop in temperature of max. 1°C due to the influence of room temperature.

For a manually preselected T_w of 47.5°C ± 0.5, the mean values of temperature calculated from point M1 showed to be 40.5°C for a basic needle distance of d = 15 mm (85.2% of the preselected T_w), 42.5°C for d = 10 mm (89.4%) and 44.7°C for d = 8 mm (94.2%).

As result of the reduction of the basic distance of 15 to 8 mm (at constant T_w) a rise in temperature of about 10% could be reached in point M1 in steady state. The mean deviation of temperature measured at point M2 (T_A, T_B, T_C) was less than 0.5°C as compared to the data obtained at point M1.

In vivo thermometry

Intratumoral temperature was recorded along the path of at least two tissue probes, dependent on the size of the treatment volume, with the measurement

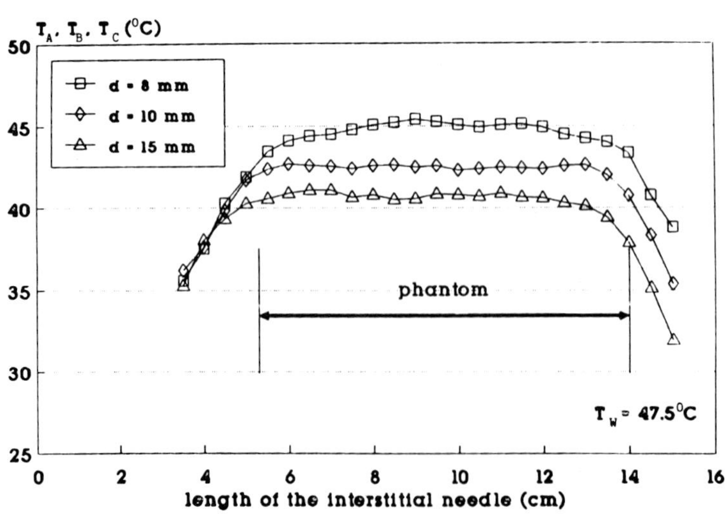

Fig. 6. Axial temperature distribution for different basic needle distances (d).

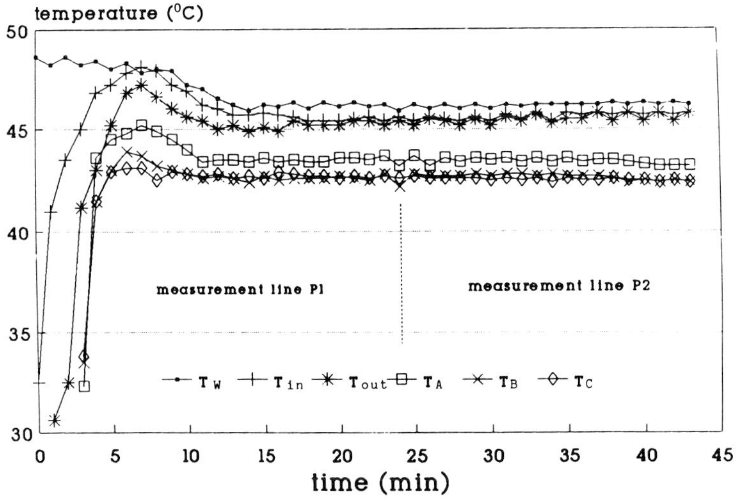

Fig. 7. In vivo thermometry of a vaginal implant. The thermocouple probe was placed from P1 to P2 after 20 minutes steady state temperature.

points A, B, C placed in the center of the lesion.

The therapeutic temperature was defined as 43.5°C. Treatment was started when any monitored intratumoral site reached 43.5°C and was then continued for additional 40 minutes. In all cases the water was preheated 30 minutes before the initiation of treatment.

The manually chosen T_w for the in vivo measurement illustrated in Fig. 7 was 48°C. The therapeutic temperature was reached as soon as 5 minutes after initiation of heating (T_A = 44.5°C, T_B = 43.3°C, T_C = 42.9°C). Since further measurements showed rise of temperature the T_w was manually lowered to 46.1°C. After the water had reached the prescribed value, measurements at the thermocouple over a time of 35 minutes showed a mean value of T_A = 43.3 ± 0.4°C, T_B = 42.6 ± 0.4°C, T_C = 42.6 ± 0.3°C (Fig. 7).

A change in position of the probe was undertaken 20 minutes after steady state had been reached. No difference in temperature was recorded.

During the course of all treatments the therapeutic temperature could be easily maintained by means of a preselected T_w of 46.1 to 48.5°C. The mean temperature difference between T_{in} and T_{out} in steady state never exceeded 0.2°C. In one patient the mean deviation of temperature inside the tumor was at maximum 1.5°C, whereas in the remainder the temperature difference never exceeded 1.1°C.

Patients' tumor and treatment characteristics

Between September 1988 and January 1990 seventeen treatments utilizing Ir-192 HDR radiation followed by interstitial warm water hyperthermia were performed in 9 patients (7 females, 2 males, aged 46 to 74 years) with a follow-up ranging from 1 to 17 months (mean 7; median 6 months).

Six patients had a diagnosis of primarily untreated anal canal carcinomas including 4 cases of squamous cell carcinoma and 2 tumors of cloacogenic origin. The stages comprised 4 stage T2 NO MO lesions (according to the UICC/TNM staging criteria 1987), one patient with stage T3 tumor and enlarged pelvic lymph nodes, who had declined surgery, and one case of stage T4 tumor with infiltration of the vagina and extensive perianal spread. In this case sufficient tumor shrinkage for a radical surgical approach of the primarily unresectable lesion was warranted, whereas in the remainder the aim was cure based on definitive external irradiation followed by two hyperthermia treatment in conjunction with Ir-192 high-dose-rate implantation. The implanted volume in this patient population ranged from 4 cm^3 to 130 cm^3 (median size 6 cm^3).

External radiation for patients with anal carcinomas was delivered using a split-course technique. In the first series a dose of 30 Gy (8 MeV photons) was applied through irregular shaped AP/PA fields encompassing the true pelvis and the inquinal lymph nodes with a daily fraction of 2 Gy, 5 times a week.

After a 2 week rest the interstitial Ir-192 high-dose-rate brachytherapy was performed, delivering a dose of 6–8 Gy per fraction to the target volume immediately followed by hyperthermia after the radioactive source had been removed. After a recovery period of 2 weeks external radiation treatment was continued to a total dose of 50 Gy. In the one patient, who had presented with enlarged pelvic nodes, an additional boost with 10 Gy was delivered to the pelvic and inquinal lymph node drainage.

As late as two months after completion of the external beam treatment a second implant in conjunction with hyperthermia was scheduled to allow optimum tumor shrinkage during this period of time.

Two patients were treated for vaginal lesions; one case was referred with recurrent disease from cervical cancer, the other was found to have a primary vaginal cancer stage T2 after having been successfully treated for endometrial carcinoma 10 years before. Since both patients had a history of prior full dose external radiation, the treatment was limited to interstitial thermoradiother-

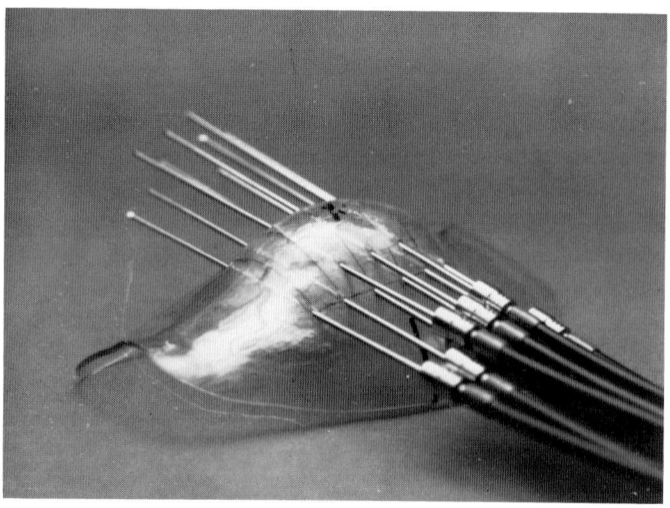

Fig. 8. Individually shaped implant aid with drillings for the treatment of a subcutaneous metastasis from malignant melanoma.

apy, which up until now has been applied twice, with an interval of 2–3 weeks.
Both implants encompassed two thirds of the vaginal wall and the entire length of the vagina with inclusion of the urethra into the treatment volume. The tumor volume at the beginning of therapy was 38 cm^3 and 50 cm^3, respectively.
One lady with metastatic lesions from malignant melanoma, who had failed to respond to large single fraction external beam therapy, was treated for palliation only. In this case a large subcutaneous metastasis infiltrating the entire right lower cervical, supra- and infraclavicular region with fixation to the upper chest wall was irradiated and heated using a special mould made of a 3 mm layer of Simona PVC GEOS. This material, otherwise used as positioning aid for the treatment of head/neck and brain tumors was designed to fit the lesion perfectly. Predetermined drilled holes provided a strictly parallel placement of the needles in this particularly large and irregular shaped subcutaneous lesion (tumor volume 240 cm^3). The second metastasis (80 cm^3) treated in the same patient was located at the dorsum of the left foot and was implanted using the same implant aid (Fig. 8).

Clinical response and side-effects

Of the patients treated for anal carcinomas in 4 of 6 cases a complete histopathological response was obtained. No interference with sphincter function was observed at a follow-up time ranging from 4 to 16 months (median 6.5, mean 8.5 months).
In the patient with stage T3 disease, in whom a complete clinical tumor regression had been assessed, a deep biopsy 4 months after the second implant revealed microscopic foci of squamous cell carcinoma within areas of pronounced scarring. This patient, who had first declined operation and chemotherapy subsequently underwent radical surgery. In the histologic specimen, however, no residual tumor was found at the previous tumor site. The pelvic nodes, which had been enlarged in this patient before initiation of external beam therapy were found to be free of tumor, while microscopic involvement of one lymph node beyond the pelvis was diagnosed.
In the case of stage T4 anal carcinoma only minor response of the marked perianal infiltration was achieved. This patient finally suffered recurrence at the perineum despite of radical surgery.
Partial response was obtained in both cases of vaginal tumors as soon as 14 days after the first implant. Since the time elapsed after the second treatment is of insufficient length the final response cannot as yet be evaluated.
A remarkable result was obtained in the patient with metastatic melanoma. There was a rapid reduction in the size of the mass at the right supra/infraclavicular region 2 weeks after treatment with continuous regression stated at further follow-up examinations over a period of 6 months (Fig. 9a,b,c). Although only one implant was performed in that particular case, pronounced teleangiectasis and loss of skin pigmentation as soon as 4 weeks after the treatment was noted. At the second treatment site on the dorsum of the foot only moderate reduction in size was observed over a 6

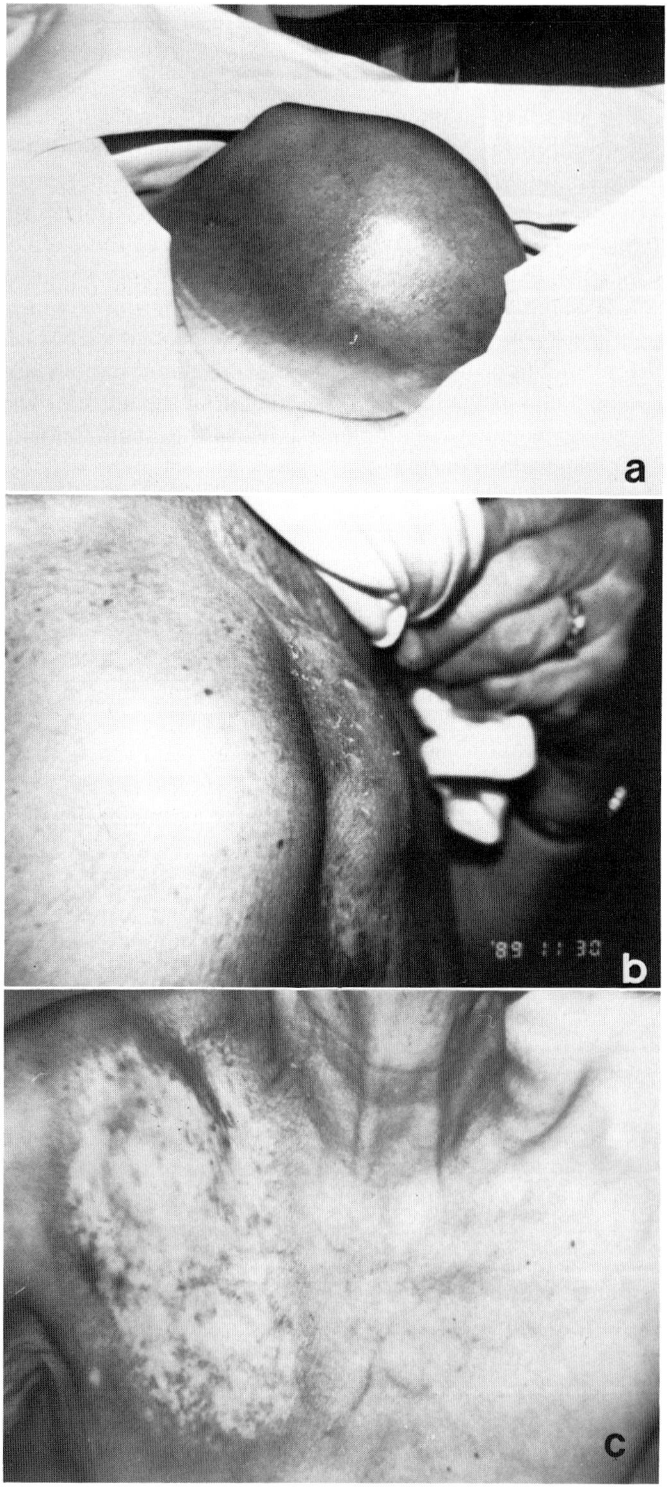

Fig. 9. Huge metastasis from malignant melanoma at the right supra/infraclavicular region.
a Lesion before initiation of thermoradiotherapy.
b 4 weeks and **c** 6 months after treatment.

months period with sudden necrosis and ulceration of the tumor without signs of marginal regrowth.

Interstitial thermoradiotherapy was well tolerated. None of the patients experienced any pain which might have been connected with the treatment. Acute reactions such as erythema, desquamation or blisters did not occur. Intravaginal bleeding after removal of the implant in one case required local compression over a few hour period.

All patients could be discharged from their hospital stay after a 24-hour observation period.

The only visible reaction observed was skin atrophy associated with depigmentation and teleangiectasis delineating the former extent of the lesion in the case of metastatic melanoma. The ulceration of the second lesion in the same patient might have been due to radiation overdosage based on the relatively large volume implant for the size of the lesion in conjunction with the thermotoxic effect of the heating procedure.

Conclusion

The axial temperature distribution for different basic needle distances of 15, 10 and 8 mm was evaluated using a tissue equivalent phantom. For that task a needle placement geometry in use for high-dose-rate therapy at our institution was chosen. The needles for the heating procedure were implanted forming the corners of an equilateral triangle; at the center of gravity of each triangle a thermocouple probe was placed parallel to the implanted needles and temperatures were recorded in steps of 5 mm through the treatment volume.

As a result of monitoring, an increase of 10% in temperature was obtained by reducing the basic needle distance to 8 mm. The mean deviation of temperature was recorded as being less than 0.5°C.

Analysing the temperature data of in vivo measurements the maximum deviation of temperature was (in one particular case), found to be 1.5°C whereas in the remainder, the temperature deviation was not found to exceed 1.1°C.

At a needle spacing of 8 mm, the temperature required for clinical application could be maintained in all heat treatments with a predetermined water temperature of 48°C, even at locations with high blood flow.

An essential advantage of the warm-water device exists due to the fact, that by preselection of temperature, the maximum temperature in the implanted volume cannot exceed the temperature at the wall of the implanted needle. Thus hot spots are avoided at any point of the treated tissue. Furthermore, no special isolation or shielding of the treatment room, as warranted for microwave advices, or adjacent facilities for power supply or monitoring are necessary. Thermometry can be performed during the treatment course without constraints with regard to heating artefacts associated with other modalities.

Taking these points into account the warm-water system represents a practical and safe technique for clinical application, which can also be easily adjusted to current brachytherapy systems in use.

The thermometry results obtained compare favorably to the experimental data reported by Brezovich et al (1988), Schreier et al (1990) and suggest good homogeneity of thermal distribution at therapeutic levels. Based on the fact, that so far adjunctive heating has been applied at our institution in a small number of patients and cases, in which interstitial radiation alone might have been sufficient to achieve local control, the clinical results have to be interpreted with caution. The local remissions in patients with recurrent or advanced lesions, however, appear promising and were remarkable in the case of malignant melanoma. Further work is to be carried out to support the efficacy of this device in clinical use.

References

Brezovich I, Meredith R, Henderson R, Brawner W, Weppelmann B, Salter M (1988) Hyperthermia with water perfused catheters. In: Sugahara T, Saito M (eds) Hyperthermic Oncology 1988, Proceedings of the 5th International Symposium on Hyperthermic Oncology, August 29–September 3, 1988, vol. 1. Taylor & Francis, London, New York, Philadelphia

Handl-Zeller L (1987) Entwicklung und Einführung neuer interstitieller Hyperthermiesysteme. In: Hammer J, Kärcher KH (Hrsg) Fortschritte in der interstitiellen und intracavitären Strahlentherapie. Zuckerschwerdt, Wien, pp 10–14

Handl-Zeller L, Kärcher KH, Lesnicar H, Budihna M, Schreier K (1987) Newly developed liquid heated interstitial hyperthermia system KHS-9/W 18. Int J Hyperthermia 6: 567

Handl-Zeller L, Kärcher KH, Schreier K, Handl O (1987) Beitrag zur Optimierung interstitieller Hyperthermiesysteme. Strahlenther Onkol 163: 406–463

Handl-Zeller L, Kärcher KH, Schreier K, Budihna M, Lesnicar H (1988) The interstitial Viennese system KHS-9/W 18. Homogeneous hyperthermia with simultaneous radiation in deep seated tumors with integrated heat protection of normal tissue. In: Kärcher KH (ed) Proceedings of the Fourth Meeting on Progress in Radio-Oncology, Vienna, 1988, ICRO, pp 267–269

Kapp DS, Fessenden P, Samulski TV, Bagshaw MA, Cox RS, Lee ER, Lohrbach AW, Meyer JL, Prionas SD (1988) Stanford University institutional report. Phase I evaluation of equipment for hyperthermic treatment of cancer. Int J Hyperthermia 4: 75–115

Lam K, Astrahan M, Langholz B, Jepson J, Cohen D, Luxton G, Petrovich Z (1988) Interstitial thermoradiotherapy for recurrent or persistent tumors. Int J Hyperthermia 4: 259–266

Lesnicar H, Budhina M, Handl-Zeller L, Schreier K (1988) Interstitial hyperthermia with circulating water-results of animal experiments. In: Kärcher KH (ed) Proceedings of the Fourth Meeting on Progress in Radio-Oncology, Vienna, 1988, ICRO, pp 263–266

Meredith RF, Brezovich IA, Weppelmann B, Henderson RA, Brawner WR, Kwapien RP, Bartolucci AA, Salter M (1989) Ferromagnetic thermoseeds: Suitable for an afterloading interstitial implant. Int J Radiat Oncol Biol Phys 17: 1341–1346

Schreier K, Budhina M, Lesnicar L, Handl-Zeller L, Hand JW, Prior MV, Clegg ST, Brezovich IA (1990) Preliminary studies of interstitial hyperthermia using hot water. Int J Hyperthermia 6: 231–444

Shimm DS, Cetas TC, Oleson JR, Cassady JR, Sim DA (1988) Clinical Evaluation of Hyperthermia Equipment: The University of Arizona Institutional Report for the NCI Hyperthermia Equipment Evaluation Contract, vol 4, pp 39–52

12

Interstitial Hyperthermia with Ferromagnetic Seed Implants: Preliminary Results of a Phase I Clinical Trial

B. Stea, D. Shimm, J. Kittelson, and *T. Cetas*

Department of Radiation Oncology, University of Arizona Health Sciences Center, Tucson, Arizona, U.S.A.

Introduction

Although the first use of hyperthermia in the treatment of cancer was reported in the 19th century, the use of hyperthermia as a treatment modality has been developing rapidly only over the last ten to fifteen years. Response rates have varied, depending on the size and location of the tumor, but hyperthermia combined with irradiation consistently appears to improve the complete response rate over that seen with irradiation alone by a factor of two, and to increase the response duration as well (OVERGAARD, 1987, 1989).

Interstitial techniques represent a promising approach to heating tumors which are poorly addressed by externally applied hyperthermia, and offer the following advantages. First, these techniques allow more efficient and uniform deposition of power directly into the tumor compared with externally-applied hyperthermia, without transit through overlying normal tissue. Second, because the implant is confined to the target volume, there is less heating of normal tissue. Third, because implantation is invasive, it is usually performed under general anesthesia, and therefore allows more extensive temperature measurements than other hyperthermia techniques. Fourth, because of the relatively homogeneous heating, and the possibility of extensive thermometry, implants are well suited for thermal modeling. On the other hand, interstitial hyperthermia does have drawbacks, as well. Implantation does require general anesthesia in most instances, and because of its invasive nature, it is not suitable in patients with bleeding disorders or altered mental status.

Inductively heated, thermally regulating ferromagnetic seed implantation is one of the more recent techniques to be introduced into the clinic (CETAS et al, 1989; HAIDER et al, 1987). The principal advantage of ferromagnetic implants is that power deposition depends only on the implant materials and the array configuration. The technique is readily compatible with interstitial brachytherapy, requiring that only minimal additional consideration be given to the hyperthermic aspects of the implantation, over and above that required for radiation dosimetry. The implantation procedure is

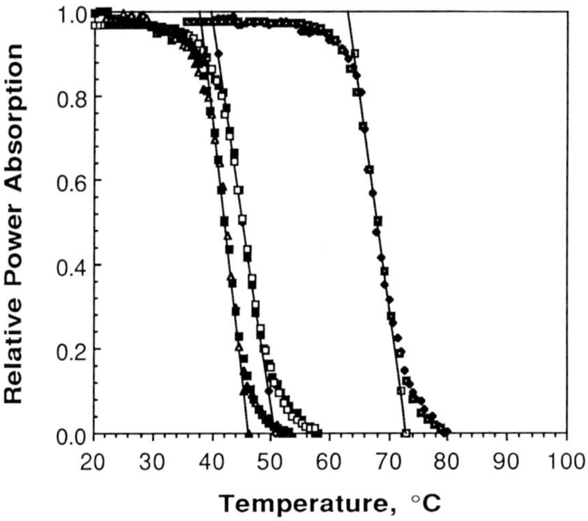

Fig. 1. Relative power absorption as a function of temperature for thermally regulating ferromagnetic seeds with three different Curie points. The Curie point of each seed, the temperature at which the magnetic permeability decreases to that of free space, is obtained by extrapolating the linear portion of the curve down to a relative power absorption of zero, and are approximately 46°, 50°, and 73 °C, respectively, for the three seeds graphed

performed in the operating room, independent of the hyperthermia treatment. Little danger exists of excessive local temperatures since the seeds are the hottest elements and their temperature is self-limited by intrinsic design, as specified by the Curie point, defined as the temperature at which the magnetic permeability decreases to that of free space (Fig. 1). The major difficulties with ferromagnetic implant heating are that a relatively dense array is required, since heating relies upon thermal conduction alone, and, second, that the treatment must be planned in advance with little possibility for altering the heating pattern apart from exchanging the seeds for some with a different Curie point. Here, we review our initial experience with interstitial thermoradiotherapy using thermally regulating ferromagnetic seeds in primary and recurrent intracranial gliomas, and in extracranial malignancies.

Methods

System description

Ferromagnetic seed heating has been the subject of several preliminary reports (Au et al, 1989; Shimm et al, 1989a,b; Stea et al, 1989; Deshmukh et al, 1984). Briefly, implantation of extracranial sites was performed using commercially-available 14-gauge afterloading catheters, with the aid of a template for gynecologic applications, or freehand, either percutaneously or following operative exposure, for other extracranial sites. For intracranial implants, catheters were placed stereotactically using a modified Brown-Roberts-Wells frame and a 3-dimensional treatment planning program, as described earlier (Lulu et al, 1989). Ferromagnetic seeds were fabricated of nickel-silicon alloy to have Curie points between 55°C and 80°C (Chen et al, 1988). Seeds are 1 mm in diameter and 10–12 mm in length, and are strung together 2–3 mm apart in heatshrunk Teflon tubing. Recently, we have used

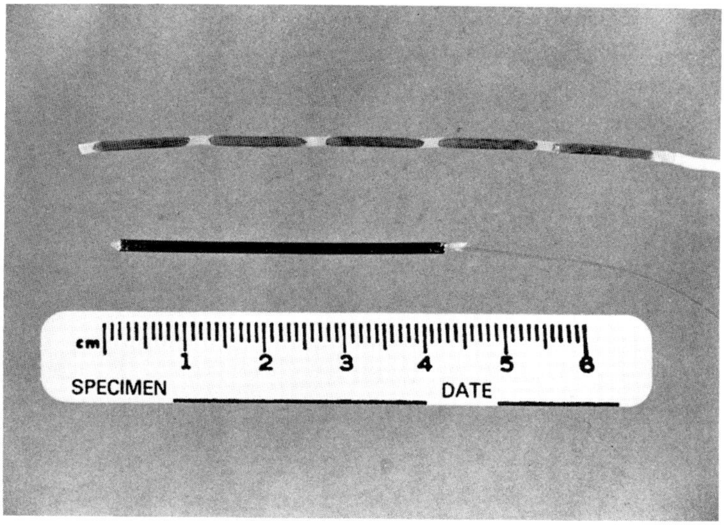

Fig. 2. Arrangement of ferromagnetic seeds or wires.
A discontinuous array of five ferromagnetic seeds, contained in a heat shrinkable Teflon catheter, is shown above; each seed measures 1 mm in diameter and 10–12 mm in length. A ferromagnetic stranded wire is shown below; six individual wires each measuring 0.45 mm in diameter are stranded together and cut to any desired length

ferromagnetic materials in the form of continuous wires (each 0.45 mm in diameter); six of these wires are stranded together to form ribbons measuring 1.4 mm in diameter which are cut to a length adequate to cover the thickness of the tumor (Fig. 2). Heating was achieved using an axially applied external magnetic induction field (1500–2400 A/m) operating at a frequency of 85–95 kHz, at power of 3–6 kW. The seeds or wires were aligned as close to parallel with the magnetic field as possible; however, the system is relatively tolerant of deviations from parallel of up to 20°. Copper-constantan thermocouple probes or fluoroptic thermometers with multiple sensors at 1 cm intervals along their length were used for temperature measurement. There were insignificant temperature perturbations using these probes within the magnetic field. Temperatures were monitored every 2–5 seconds using a computerized data acquisition system, and were stored automatically for later analysis. In these patients, orthogonal films were taken and a seed-finding program was used to locate seeds and thermometers in any plane in the treated volume (SIDDON and CHIN, 1985).

Patient population and tumor characteristics

Since June 1987 a total of 29 patients have been treated with ferromagnetic seed implants on a phase I clinical trial combining interstitial hyperthermia with brachytherapy. Fourteen patients had intracranial tumors, [anaplastic astrocytoma (AA) or glioblastoma multiforme (GBM)] and 15 patients were treated for a variety of extracranial tumors (see below). To be eligible for the brain tumor study, patients had to be older than 21 years of age, had to have a life expectancy of at least three months and a performance status of at least 50. Patients were excluded from the study if the target volume exceeded 100 cm^3, although 2 patients with implant volumes of 112 and 119 cm^3 were treated early in the study (see below). Furthermore, tumors located in the posterior fossa or the brainstem and multicentric tumors were also excluded from this trial. Our patient population included 10 females and 4 males with a median age of 51 years (range: 21–69 yrs) and a median performance status of 90 (range: 50–95). Three patients had a diagnosis of AA while 11 had GBM. Five of these 11 patients had recurrent GBM and had been heavily pretreated with external beam radiotherapy and/or chemotherapy. The implant volumes in these patients included the area of contrast enhancement on CT scan with an additional 1–2 cm margin depending on the area of surrounding edema on CT scans or on T_2-weighted MRI scans. The implant volumes ranged from 9 to 119 cm^3 (median: 61.5 cm^3). The median number of treatment catheters per patient was 19 (range: 7–27) and the median number of thermometry probes was 4 (range: 2–5). Patients with previously untreated tumors first received a course of external beam radiotherapy (40–41.4 Gy) at 1.8–2.0 Gy per fraction daily over 4–5 weeks. Two to four weeks later, the patients underwent an interstitial implant with Iridium-192 which delivered a dose of 32–40.2 Gy (median: 39.8 Gy) at a dose rate of 40–70 cGy per hour. Patients who presented to our department with recurrent GBM received only an interstitial implant which delivered a median dose of 40 Gy (range: 13.9–50 Gy) depending on the amount of prior radiation. The hyperthermia treatment was given immediately before loading the radioactive sources; 5 patients received a second heat treatment after completion of irradiation.

In addition, we have treated 17 advanced or recurrent extracranial tumors in 15 patients since 1987. Seven patients had head and neck tumors recurrent after irradiation, 3 patients had previously untreated advanced head and neck tumors which had achieved a complete regression after external beam radiotherapy, and 5 patients were treated for pelvic tumors: 2 for advanced cervical cancer, 2 for recurrent rectal cancer and 1 patient for pelvic sarcoma. Fourteen tumors were squamous cell carcinoma, 2 were adenocarcinoma and 1 was liposarcoma. The median tumor volume implanted was 12 cm^3, ranging up to 212 cm^3. The total radiation doses delivered with either implant alone or a combination of external radiation and brachytherapy ranged from 22.4 to 95.0 Gy, with a median dose of 59.6 Gy. In this patient population, hyperthermia was administered only once, before radiation. Five tumors were heated using non-thermally-regulating stainless steel seeds, and the remainder with thermally-regulating ferromagnetic seeds. Informed consent was obtained from all the patients before the procedure.

Results

Thermal dosimetry

Of 14 patients with high-grade gliomas, 12 were able to complete at least one heat treatment, and 5 received a second hyperthermia treatment after the radioactive sources were removed. Two pa-

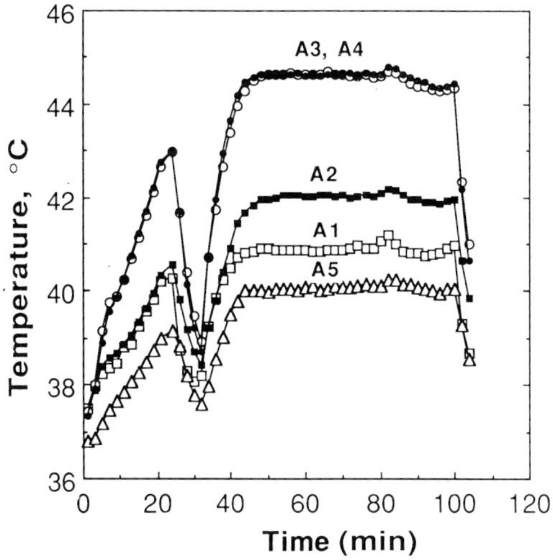

Fig. 3. Temperature versus time curves for a brain tumor treatment.
Continuous temperatures were monitored for five sensors spaced 1 cm apart along the same catheter. Sensor A_1 is located in the deepest part of the implant and A_5 is the most superficial. After 22 minutes of treatment, power was temporarily turned off in this patient so that some of the ferromagnetic seeds could be changed with others of a higher Curie point

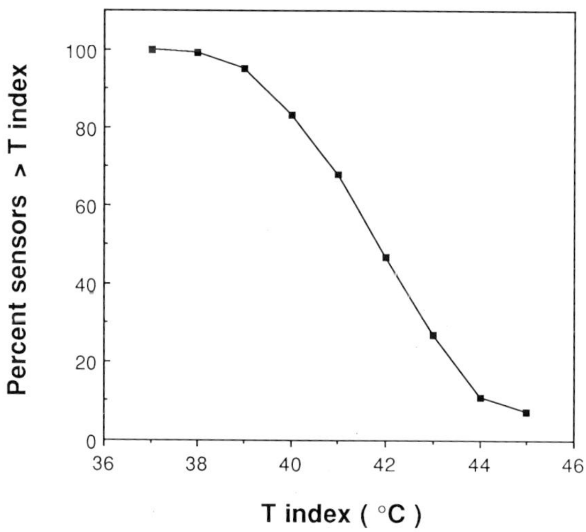

Fig. 4. Temperature distribution in twelve brain tumors.
A total of 175 intratumoral points were continuously measured in 12 patients with high grade gliomas (mean: 15 sensors per patient). Time-averaged mean temperatures were calculated over the entire duration of treatment (60 min.) and the proportion of sensors exceeding a given index temperature was plotted as a function of the index temperature

tients were unable to complete treatment due to poor tolerance (see below). In those patients who received two heat treatments, the second treatment usually yielded higher temperatures than the first (data not shown). Only the better of the two treatments was used to compute temperature distributions. In all patients, temperatures were continuosly monitored during the course of treatment, and a typical temperature vs time curve is shown in Fig. 3. A total of 175 points were monitored in the 12 patients who received a full heat treatment. Time-averaged mean temperature achieved during the 60 minute hyperthermia treatment were calculated for each of the sensors, and their distribution is shown in Fig. 4. Forty seven percent of all the sensors achieved and maintained a mean intratumoral temperature greater than 42°C. We have also calculated the fre-

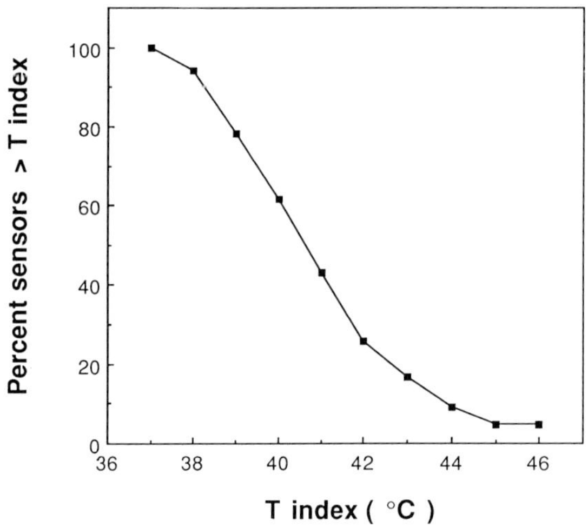

Fig. 5. Temperature distribution in 17 extracranial tumors.
A total of 206 temperature points were continuously monitored in 15 patients harboring 17 malignant tumors (mean: 12 sensors per tumor). Some of the sensors were in adjacent normal tissue and no attempt was made to separate these sensors from those located within the tumor. The proportion of sensors exceeding a given index temperature was plotted as a function of the index temperature

quency of temperature distributions as a function of the sensors' location within the target volume. We have found that 89% (25 of 28) of the sensors located in the center of the tumor achieved temperatures greater than 42°C, whereas 39% (58 of 147) of the sensors located in the periphery of the tumor (outermost 1 cm shell of the implant volume) achieved a similar temperature; this difference is statistically significant ($p < 0.001$, Chi-square).

Seventeen advanced or recurrent extracranial tumors in fifteen patients were heated with ferromagnetic implants. Thermometry data is available for 16 of these tumors; a mean of 12 sensors were monitored for each of these tumors. Time-averaged mean temperatures were calculated for each of these treatments and their distribution is plotted in Fig. 5. No attempt was made in these patients to discriminate between sensors located in tumor and sensors located in adjacent normal tissue. As shown in Fig. 5, only 25.7% of the sensors achieved a time-averaged mean temperature >42°C. The reason for somewhat lower mean temperatures in the extracranial sites when compared to the brain tumors is not clearly apparent. One possible explanation may be that the brain tumor implants were performed with the aid of a template (Lulu et al, 1989), thus permitting adherence to strict geometric guidelines for both the heating catheters' and the thermometers' location. This probably led to a more uniform distribution of heat sources, hence better heating, and to better temperature sampling, than in the extracranial tumor implants. The majority of the latter implants were performed by freehand technique. The second possible explanation is that the extracranial implants were performed with the first seed configuration which has only about half the efficiency of power absorption of the stranded wire configuration (Haider, 1988). That is, more power is absorbed by the stranded wire configuration thus providing more heat to replace that removed by thermal conduction and blood flow.

The influence of the geometry of the implant (intercatheter spacing) on the efficiency of heating was studied theoretically (Haider et al, 1987), and experimentally in the brain tumor implants

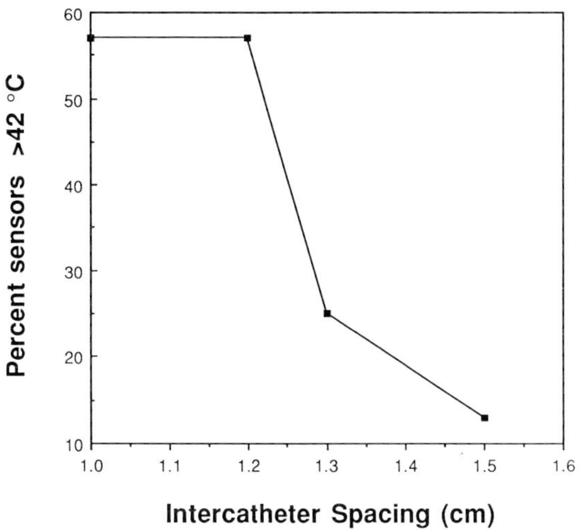

Fig. 6. Influence of intercatheter spacing on heating efficiency in brain tumor implants.
A total of 175 intratumoral points were monitored in 12 brain tumours implanted with different templates having an intercatheter spacing between 1.0 and 1.5 cm. The proportion of sensors with a time-averaged mean temperature >42 °C was plotted as function of the intercatheter spacing

(Fig. 6). A spacing of 1.0 to 1.2 cm appears to yield better temperatures than an implant with a wider spacing ($p < 0.001$, Chi-square).

Clinical response

Of the 14 patients with high-grade gliomas treated with ferromagnetic implants, 5 were treated for recurrent disease, while 9 had an implant as part of the initial treatment. Although all patients are routinely followed with serial neurological examinations and CT or MRI scans, it is often difficult to assess response to treatment in brain tumor patients. Therefore, survival remains the best indicator of the effectiveness of treatment in this patient population. Of the 9 patients who presented with previously untreated brain tumors, 6 are still alive 7 to 19 months after diagnosis, while 3 have died at 2, 6 and 9 months, respectively, from the diagnosis. One of these patients died as a result of complications from the treatment (see below). Among the 5 patients who were treated for recurrent brain tumors, 4 have already died, with a median survival time of 16 weeks from the time of treatment with hyperthermia.

Among the 17 extracranial tumors treated in 15 patients there have been 9 complete responses (CR) (53%), and 1 partial response (PR), for a total response rate of 59%. When analyzed by site, 6 of the 12 head and neck tumors achieved a CR, as did 3 of the 5 pelvic tumors. Analysis by histology reveals that 7 of the 14 squamous cell tumors achieved a CR, compared with 2 of the 3 other tumors. Finally, when responses were analyzed as a function of size, we found that of 12 tumors with evaluable measurements, 4 of 5 tumors with a volume of $< 11\ \text{cm}^3$ achieved a CR compared to only 2 of 6 tumors with a volume $> 11\ \text{cm}^3$. The median duration of response for the 17 extracranial tumors was 7 months, with the latest failure occurring at 10 months.

Patient tolerance and complications

Two of the 14 patients with brain implants were unable to complete their heat treatment due to poor tolerance. One patient developed a focal seizure, while the other one lost consciousness. Both of these episodes occurred in the initial ten minutes of the heat treatment, and both patients recovered completely without long-term sequelae. A third patient developed focal seizure activity which responded to diazepam, and was able to complete the heat treatment. The remaining 11 patients tolerated their treatment well without discomfort. However, there have been 3 serious complications associated with the procedure in these 14 patients. One patient developed transient brain edema which resolved with conservative medical management. Another patient developed hydrocephalus after implantation of the catheters but before the heat treatment, and required a ventriculostomy. The most serious complication was encountered in a patient who presented with a tumor volume of 119 cm^3 which required the implantation of 33 treatment catheters. This patient developed progressive brain edema following the implant, which worsened after hyperthermia, and culminated in herniation and eventually death. In retrospect this patient was a poor candidate for interstitial thermoradiotherapy due to the large size of her tumor and the presence of a mass effect with hemispheric shift prior to the implant.

Among the patients with extracranial tumors, only 1 patient suffered a complication (bone exposure) after the implant of a tumor that involved the floor of mouth and mandibular aveolar mucosa. This patient, however, later developed a local recurrence and it is unclear whether the bone exposure resulted from the treatment or rather was associated with the recurrence.

Discussion

Hyperthermia as an adjuvant to radiation therapy has been shown to increase the probability of achieving a complete response both in historical series (see Overgaard, 1989 for review) as well as in controlled (Scott et al, 1984) and phase III clinical trials (Arcangeli et al, 1985; Corry et al, 1982; Hiraoka et al, 1984; Marmor and Hahn, 1982; Valdagni et al, 1988.) However, our ability to control deep seated tumors has been limited by the availability of equipment that allows heating of deep seated structures (Shimm et al, 1988a & b). Interstitial thermoradiotherapy offers the advantage of allowing accurate delivery of hyperthermia and radiation to the tumor, while sparing normal tissues, with thc potential of improving the therapeutic ratio. This consideration is especially important for those tumors located in or near critical structures with limited tolerance to radiation (e.g. brain). Between 1977 and 1986 at the University of Arizona we have treated patients with deep-seated tumors with interstitial radiofrequency currents and interstitial microwaves (Shimm et al, 1990); since 1987 we have been using interstitial ferromagnetic implants. This technique offers several advantages: first, power deposition is a function of the implant geometry and of the ferromagnetic properties of the seeds; second, seeds are thermally self-regulating and their power absorption is a function of the temperature achieved (Fig. 1); third, this type of implant is compatible with currently performed brachytherapy techniques; fourth, treatment catheters can be differentially loaded with seeds of different

Curie points to optimize temperature distributions (Fig. 3).

Our limited experience with 17 extracranial tumors has been encouraging so far. Heating has generally been well-tolerated and there has been only one complication. The response rate of 59% for extracranial tumors is superior to that achieved with interstitial radiofrequency currents or interstitial microwaves at our institution (SHIMM et al, 1990) and is comparable to the results from other institutions published in the literature.

Interstitial hyperthermia of brain tumors has been attempted with several techniques including single-thermal probes (SUTTON et al, 1971), interstitial microwave antennae (ROBERTS et al, 1986; SALCMAN et al, 1981; SAMARAS et al, 1982; WINTER et al, 1985), RF electrodes (TANAKA et al, 1984), and more recently with inductively heated ferromagnetic implants (KIDA et al, 1989; STEA et al, 1989). Our experience with 14 brain tumors has shown that these tumors can be effectively heated, since 47% of all the sensors achieved a time-averaged mean temperature >42°C. Although we are more successful in heating the central (often necrotic) portion of the tumor, where 89% of the sensors were above 42°C, there is still room for improvement at the highly perfused periphery of the tumor, where only 39% of the sensors achieved the same temperature.

Although this is a phase I clinical trial and follow-up is limited, preliminary analysis of the data shows that 6 of 9 previously untreated brain tumor patients are still alive with a follow-up of 7–19 months. However, treatment of recurrent brain tumor has been unrewarding, as 4 of the 5 patients have died with a median survival of only 16 weeks. Despite the induction of seizures in two patients and loss of consciousness in another, hyperthermia of brain tumors by ferromagnetic induction appears to be well tolerated, and we believe it can safely be performed when the implant volume is kept below $100\,cm^3$.

Since the results reported here are from a phase I study, analysis of response has to be interpreted with caution. Many of the patients entered on the study had a very poor prognosis and only a small chance of responding to standard therapy. Furthermore, the implant technique and seed technology have evolved during the course of the study so that higher temperatures and better temperature distributions can be achieved now compared to the initial phase of the study. In conclusion, we believe that hyperthermia with thermally regulating, inductively heated ferromagnetic seeds, although still experimental, offers a promising and new approach to the delivery of heat to deep seated tumors. More clinical work however is needed to establish both the safety and efficacy in this technique in the treatment of human tumors.

Acknowledgement: This work was supported by the American Cancer Society Grant PDT310, NCI grants CA29653 and CA39468; Cancer Center Core Grant CA23074 and Hyperthermia Program Project Grant 17343. Dr. Stea and Dr. Shimm are recipients of American Cancer Society Clinical Oncology Career Development Awards.

References

Arcangeli G, Benassi M, Cividalli A, Lovisolo G, Mauro F (1987) Radiotherapy and hyperthermia: Analysis of clinical results and identification of prognostic variables. Cancer 60: 950–956

Au K, Cetas T, Shimm D, Chen J, Sinno R, Haider S, Buechler D, Lutz W, Cassady J (1989) Interstitial ferromagnetic hyperthermia and brachytherapy; preliminary results of a phase I clinical trial. Endocurietherapy/Hyperthermia Oncology 5: 127–136

Cetas T, Buechler D, Chen J, Sinno R, Haider S, Chen Z, Stauffer P, Lutz W, Lulu B, Poirier D, Demer L (1989) Physical aspects of ferromagnetic implants. In: Sugahara T, Saito M (eds) Hyperthermic Oncology 1988 – Proceedings of the 5th International Symposium on Hyperthermic Oncology, vol 1. Taylor & Francis, London, pp 863–864

Chen J-S, Poirier DR, Damento MA, Demer LJ, Biancaniello F, Cetas TC (1988) Development of Ni-4 wt.% Si thermoseeds for hyperthermia cancer treatment. J Biomed Materials Res 22: 303–319

Corry P, Spanos W, Tilchen E, Barlogie B, Barkley H, Armour E (1982) Combined ultrasound and radiation therapy treatment of human superficial tumors. Radiology 145: 165–169

Deshmukh R, Damento M, Demer L, Forsyth K, DeYoung D, Dewhirst M, Cetas TC (1984) Ferromagnetic alloys with Curie temperatures near 50°C for use in hyperthermic therapy. In: Overgaard J (ed) Hyperthermic Oncology. Taylor & Francis, London, Philadelphia, pp 571–574

Haider SA (1988) Ferromagnetic Implants in Hyperthermia: An Analytical, Numerical and Experimental Study. M.S. Thesis, Dept. of Electrical and Computer Engineering, University of Arizona, 1988

Haider SA, Chen Z-P, Cetas TC, Roemer RB (1987) Interstitial ferromagnetic implant heating: Practical guidelines for use. In: Proceedings of the Ninth Annual Conference of the IEEE Engineering in Medicine and Biology Society 3: 1626–1628

Hiraoka M, Jo S, Dodo Y, Ono K, Takahashi M, Nishida H, Abe N (1984) Clinical results of radiofrequency hyperthermia combined with radiation in the treatment of radioresistant cancers. Cancer 54: 2898–2904

Kida Y, Kobayashi T, Tanaka T (1989) Local hyperthermia of brain tumor by implant heating system: Preliminary clinical report. In: Sugahara T, Saito M (eds) Hyperthermic Oncology 1988 – Proceedings of the 5th International Symposium on Hyperthermic Oncology, vol 1. Taylor & Francis, London, New York, Philadelphia, pp 393–394

Lulu B, Lutz W, Cetas T (1989) CT based treatment planning of template guided stereotactic brain implants with ferromagnetic seeds. In: Sugahara T, Saido M (eds) Hyperthermic Oncology 1988 – Proceedings of the 5th International Symposium on Hyperthermic Oncology, vol 1. Taylor & Francis, London, New York, Philadelphia, pp 859–860

Marmor J, Hahn G (1980) Combined radiation and hyperthermia in superficial human tumors. Cancer 46: 1986–1991

Overgaard (1987) The design of clinical trials in hyperthermic oncology. In: Field S, Franconi C (eds) The Physics and Technology of Hyperthermia. Martinus-Nijhoff, Dordrecht, pp 598–622

Overgaard J (1989) The current and potential role of hyperthermia in radiotherapy. Int J Radiat Oncol Biol Phys 16: 535–549

Roberts D, Coughlin C, Wong T, Fratkin J, Douple E, Strohbehn J (1986) Interstitial hyperthermia and iridium brachytherapy in treatment of malignant glioma: A phase I clinical trial. J Neurosurg 64: 581–587

Salcman M, Samaras GM (1981) Hyperthermia for brain tumors: Biophysical rationale. Neurosurg 9: 327–335

Samaras G, Salcman M, Cheung A, Abdo H, Schepp R (1982) Microwave-induced hyperthermia: An experimental adjunct for brain tumor therapy. Natl Cancer Inst Monogr 61: 477–482

Scott R, Johnson R, Story L, Clay L (1984) Local hyperthermia in combination with definitive radiotherapy: Increased tumor clearance, reduced recurrence rate in extended follow-up. Int J Radiat Oncol Biol Phys 10: 2119–2123

Shimm D, Cetas T, Buechler D, Chen J, Dean S, Fletcher A, Haider S, Lutz W, Sinno R, Stauffer P, Cassady J (1989) Inductively heated, thermoregulating ferromagnetic seeds for interstitial thermoradiotherapy. In: Sugahara T, Saito M (eds) Hyperthermic Oncology 1988 – Proceedings of the 5th International Symposium on Hyperthermic Oncology, vol 1. Taylor & Francis, London, New York, Philadelphia, pp. 594–595

Shimm D, Stea B, Cetas T, Buechler D, Carter LP, Chen J, Dean S, Fletcher A, Guthkelch AN, Haider S, Hodak J, Iacono R, Lutz W, Obbens E, Rossman K, Sinno R, Spetzler R, Cassady JR (1989) Clinical results of interstitial hyperthermia using thermally regulating ferromagnetic seeds. In: Sugahara T, Saito M (eds) Hyperthermic Oncology 1988 – Proceedings of the 5th International Symposium on Hyperthermic Oncology, vol 1. Taylor & Francis, London, New York, Philadelphia, pp 536–539

Shimm D, Kittelson JM, Oleson JR, Aristizabal SA, Barlow LC, Cetas TC (1990) Interstitial thermoradiotherapy: Thermal dosimetry and clinical results. Int J Radiat Oncol Biol Phys 18: 383–387

Shimm D, Cetas T, Oleson J, Cassady J, Sim D (1988) Clinical evaluation of hyperthermia equipment. The University of Arizona institutional report for the NCI hyperthermia equipment evaluation contract. Int J Hyperthermia 4: 39–51

Shimm D, Cetas T, Oleson J, Gross E, Buechler D, Fletcher A, Dean S (1988) Regional hyperthermia for deep seated malignancies using the BSD annular array. Int J Hyperthermia 4: 159–170

Siddon R, Chin L (1985) Two film brachytherapy reconstruction algorithm. Med Phys 12: 77–83

Stea B, Cetas T, Lutz W, Lulu B, Shimm D, Cassady JR, Chen JS, Sinno R, Fletcher A, Dean A, Guthkelch N, Iacono R, Rossman K, Shetter A, Hodak J, Haider SA, Obbens E (1989) Interstitial hyperthermia of brain tumors with ferromagnetic seed implants. In: Sugahara T, Saito M (eds) Hyperthermic Oncology 1988, vol 1. Taylor & Francis, London, New York, Philadelphia, pp 391–392

Sutton CH (1971) Tumor hyperthermia in the treatment of malignant gliomas of the brain. Trans Am Neurol Assoc 96: 195–199

Tanaka R, Yamada N, Kim CH, Saito Y (1984) RF hyperthermia of human malignant brain tumor. In: Overgaard J (ed) Hyperthermic Oncology. Taylor & Francis, London, New York, Philadelphia, pp 747–750

Valdagni R, Amichetti M, Pani G (1988) Radical radiation alone versus radical radiation plus microwave hyperthermia for N_3 (TNM-UICC) neck nodes: A prospective randomized clinical trial. Int J Radiat Oncol Biol Phys 15: 13–24

Winter A, Laing J, Paglione R, Sterzer F (1985) Microwave hyperthermia for brain tumors. Neurosurg 17: 387–399